Fast Oscillations in Cortical Circuits

Computational Neuroscience
Terrence J. Sejnowski and Tomaso A. Poggio, editors

Fast Oscillations in Cortical Circuits

Roger D. Traub, John G. R. Jefferys, and Miles A. Whittington

A Bradford Book
The MIT Press
Cambridge, Massachusetts
London, England

This book was set in Palatino by DeskTopPro$_{/UX}$® and was printed and bound in the United States of America.

Library of Congress Cataloging-in-Publication Data

Traub, Roger D.
Fast oscillations in cortical circuits / Roger D. Traub, John G.R. Jefferys, and Miles A. Whittington.
p. cm.—(Computational neuroscience)
"Bradford book."
Includes bibliographical references and index.
ISBN 0-262-20118-6 (alk. paper)
1. Neural circuitry. 2. Oscillations. 3. Cerebral cortex.
4. Hippocampus (Brain) I. Jefferys, John G. R. II. Whittington, Miles A. III. Title. IV. Series.
QP363.3.T73 1999
612.8'25—dc21   98-34707
                                                                           CIP

It must be confessed, moreover, that perception *and that which depends on it* are inexplicable by mechanical causes, *that is, by figures and motions. And, supposing that there were a machine so constructed as to think, feel and have perception, we could conceive of it as enlarged and yet preserving the same proportions, so that we might enter it as into a mill. And this granted, we should only find on visiting it, pieces which push one against another, but never anything by which to explain a perception. This must be sought for, therefore, in the simple substance and not in the composite or in the machine. Furthermore, nothing but this (namely, perceptions and their changes) can be found in the simple substance. It is also in this alone that all the* internal activities *of simple substances can consist.*

—Leibniz, *The Monadology,* translated by George Martin Duncan

Contents

Series Foreword

Computational neuroscience is an approach to understanding the information content of neural signals by modeling the nervous system at many different structural scales, including the biophysical, the circuit, and the systems levels. Computer simulations of neurons and neural networks are complementary to traditional techniques in neuroscience. This book series welcomes contributions that link theoretical studies with experimental approaches to understanding information processing in the nervous system. Areas and topics of particular interest include biophysical mechanisms for computation in neurons, computer simulations of neural circuits, models of learning, representation of sensory information in neural networks, systems models of sensory-motor integration, and computational analysis of problems in biological sensing, motor control, and perception.

Terrence J. Sejnowski
Tomaso A. Poggio

Preface

The present book is a continuation of an earlier monograph, *Neuronal Networks of the Hippocampus* (Traub and Miles 1991). The theme of the earlier work concerned the interaction between intrinsic cellular properties, synaptic organization, and network properties in the hippocampus. Our thinking was influenced by research analyzing invertebrate central pattern generating circuits (Marder and Calabrese 1996), but the approach in mammalian brain was of necessity modified, owing to the large number of neurons in mammals and to the absence therein of neurons with specific identities. In consequence, the connectivity in large networks of mammalian neurons can only be described in statistical terms rather than by specifying which particular neurons connects to which particular other neuron.

The scientific questions considered in the earlier monograph had to do with in vitro models of epilepsy, for epileptiform events represented the type of network phenomenon most readily induced experimentally in brain slices. The epilepsy model studied in most detail was the model obtained by blockade—either complete or partial—of $GABA_A$ receptor-mediated inhibition, with resultant "epileptic" events that consisted of one or more synchronized bursts. A burst is a series of three or more action potentials, usually riding on a depolarizing wave.

The approach in the previous monograph—as in the present one—was to analyze the behavior of large networks of neurons,

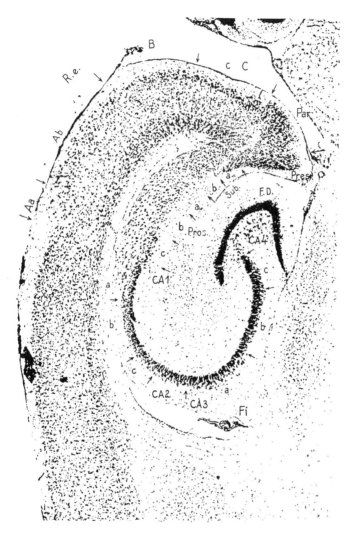

Figure P.1
Hippocampus and related structures: horizontal section of mouse brain. The tissue
was prepared with Nissl stain, which reveals neuronal somata. CA1, CA2, CA3, and
CA4 (hilus) are portions of the hippocampus. Other symbols are *F.D.*., fascia dentata
(dentate gyrus); *R.e.*, regio entorhinalis (entorhinal cortex); *Par.*, parasubiculum;
Sub., subiculum; *Pres.*, presubiculum; *Pros.*, prosubiculum; *Fi*, fimbria. (From Lorente de Nó, 1934.)

using a combination of electrophysiological and computer modeling techniques. In order to understand synchronization of bursting, it was necessary to analyze:

1. How excitation spreads through recurrently connected networks of intrinsically bursting neurons. Intrinsically bursting implies that the neuron possesses such a repertoire of membrane conductances that allow it to burst in response to a brief current pulse alone without a requirement for sustained synaptic excitation. Intrinsic bursting is characteristic of CA3 pyramidal cells when the membrane potential is in an appropriate range.

2. How the extent of synchrony (on a time scale of tens of ms) is regulated by synaptic inhibition.

3. How partial blockade of inhibition leads to interesting population phenomena, such as oscillation of the population as a whole but without oscillation of individual cells, and in which the cellular composition of individual population waves is random.

The mathematical concepts that influenced our thinking came in part from percolation theory (Fisher 1961), although the language used to express our ideas was mostly biological. We showed that a small number of principles on intrinsic bursting and on the ability of bursting in one neuron to induce bursting in another could explain interictal spikes but not sustained epileptic afterdischarges. An interictal spike is a brief—tens of ms—EEG event, which at the cellular level consists of synchronized bursting among a population of neurons. Our results raised the question that an inaccurate model of individual cells might be one reason why the network model could not replicate afterdischarges, another reason perhaps being the failure to include excitatory synaptic actions lasting tens of ms or more.

Several advances in the past seven years have motivated the writing of a new monograph. Below is a list of some of these advances, omitting for now details and citations to the literature:

1. Patch clamp techniques, applied both to acutely isolated neurons and to neurons in slices, have led to a more accurate kinetic description of membrane voltage-dependent currents, including calcium currents. Patch clamp techniques applied to dendrites have also extended earlier observations based on dendritic recordings with sharp electrodes and have allowed better definition of the spatial distribution of ionic conductances over the cell membrane.

2. These data in turn allow one to model single pyramidal cells more accurately. Once a model had been developed in which repetitive dendritic calcium spikes could be generated, as in real pyramidal cells, it became possible to understand in vitro afterdischarges produced by blockade of synaptic inhibition. Subsequently, progress has been made in understanding certain other experimental epilepsies as well and in understanding some of the underlying principles common to the epilepsies.

3. It was demonstrated that pharmacologically isolated networks of interneurons could produce synchronized bursts, resembling in form interictal spikes. These data suggested that interneuron networks might also generate interesting population phenomena under more physiological conditions.

4. It was shown that pharmacologically isolated interneuron networks could produce gamma-frequency (> 30 Hz but often simply called 40 Hz) oscillations in vitro, and this behavior could be explained using physical ideas of Wang and Rinzel and of Destexhe and Babloyantz. The discovery of gamma oscillations in slices implied that in vitro methods could be useful in elucidating cellular mechanisms of a phenomenon that many (including these authors) believe is important for perception and cognition.

5. It next became possible to induce 40 Hz oscillations in slices by tetanic stimulation so that both pyramidal cells, as well as interneurons, fired. Furthermore, such oscillations could synchronize over distances of several mm. Such in vitro oscillations not only share a

number of phenomenological features with in vivo oscillations, such as long latency to onset, but in slices, it was possible to analyze cellular mechanisms with electrophysiological and computer modeling techniques. In this way, one could account for long-range synchrony, even if inhibitory synaptic connectivity is localized and axon conduction is slow; the fast and reliable synaptic communication between pyramidal cells and interneurons plays a crucial role in this long-range synchrony.

6. Finally, it has been shown that 40 Hz oscillations themselves can induce synaptic plasticity, and the resultant plastic changes in turn influence the oscillations, as well as leading to a different sort of oscillation: beta (10–25 Hz). If 40 Hz oscillations are indeed relevant to perception, then these data suggest a connection between perception and memory.

The above-listed advances, their background and ramifications, and the in vivo context into which they fit, all make up the content of the present monograph. There is, of course, great interest in gamma oscillations among in vivo neurophysiologists because the manner in which such oscillations are induced by sensory stimulation—including global features of the stimulus—suggests some connection of the phenomenon with perception or cognition. Furthermore, it seems likely that gamma oscillations are produced by the brain for some fundamental, if still elusive, reasons. Oscillations are found in phylogenetically old parts of the brain (the olfactory system) and in the visual cortex of ancient types of vertebrates, for instance, reptiles (Prechtl 1994). Oscillations are also found in the olfactory systems of invertebrates (Laurent and Davidowitz 1994). One particular set of ramifications to be considered includes the mechanism of action of general anesthetics and the means by which opiates induce cognitive dysfunction.

Why include epileptic events and gamma oscillations as part of the same story, apart from the authors' having worked on both phe-

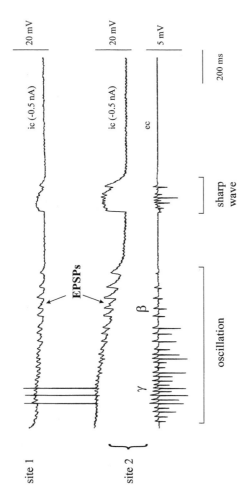

Figure P.2
Population phenomena which can be induced in the hippocampal slice by repetitive electrical stimulation. Recordings were made at two sites in the CA1 region, intracellular at site 1 and both intracellular (above) and extracellular (below) at site 2. Both neurons were hyperpolarized by passage of current through the electrodes. Repetitive electrical stimulation (20 pulses at 100 Hz) was delivered to both sites (this portion of the recording truncated). Following the stimulus, after a variable time interval, there is a population oscillation—visible in the extracellular recording—at about 45 Hz (gamma frequency, > 30 Hz), followed by an oscillation at about 11 Hz (beta frequency, 10–25 Hz), a pause, and then a synchronized burst (sharp wave). EPSPs are apparent in both cells during the beta oscillation and large EPSPs occur during the synchronized burst, this latter being considered epileptiform. These phenomena are discussed in detail in later chapters, especially chapters 9 and 10. (M. A. Whittington, unpublished data.)

nomena? After all, the relevant frequencies are not the same: synchronized bursts during afterdischarges usually occur at frequencies of 15 Hz or less and interictal spikes occur at frequencies less than 1 Hz. Furthermore, $GABA_A$ receptors play contrasting roles in the two phenomena. Hyperpolarizing $GABA_A$ actions are an absolute requirement for gamma oscillations to occur, and blockade of such receptors leads first to loss of long-range synchronization and then to abolition of the oscillations. In contrast, loss of hyperpolarizing $GABA_A$ synaptic actions or development of prolonged depolarizing $GABA_A$ effects both promote the occurrence of epileptiform discharges.

We offer several reasons for considering epilepsy and gamma oscillations together. First, from a conceptual viewpoint, it is interesting to contrast the different mechanisms of synchronization, primarily excitation between pyramidal cells in the one case (epilepsy) and primarily shared inhibition among pyramidal cells in the other case (gamma). Second, from a biological viewpoint, gamma oscillations and epilepsy may form part of a continuum of neuronal network behaviors. Tetanic stimulation evokes gamma oscillations, but if the stimulus becomes more intense, the gamma waves are followed by a beta oscillation (about 10–25 Hz), which depends on recurrent excitation between pyramidal cells. If the stimulus becomes even more intense, either interictal bursts or an afterdischarge can follow the gamma waves, both of these phenomena also depending critically upon recurrent excitation between pyramidal cells. Thus, the enhancement of recurrent excitation that gamma oscillations produce could predispose the neuronal network to epileptogenesis. Finally, gamma oscillations, at least in vitro, depend critically on metabotropic receptor activation, and metabotropic receptors may be important in prolonging afterdischarges (Taylor, Merlin, and Wong 1995; Merlin and Wong 1997).

We state now one theme that will keep recurring, as a leitmotiv of this book. The principles involved in globally synchronized oscillations, or of oscillations synchronized between two distant sites, build on the principles governing synchrony of local oscillations. In general, however, global/distant synchrony is more delicate than local synchrony. That is to say, global synchrony will prove more sensitive to parameter changes than local synchrony. If, in addition, global synchrony is required for higher brain functions, we can understand, in principle, specific means by which cognition can be disrupted, without necessarily losing the ability to generate gamma oscillations locally.

Acknowledgments

This book is dedicated to the memory of Dr. Robert Traub (1916–1996). The authors are indebted to their wives and children for their understanding. We owe a special debt to Rodolfo Llinás for encouragement and moral support, extending over twenty years. Our research was funded by IBM, the Wellcome Trust, the Human Frontier Science Program, and the Medical Research Council (U.K.). RDT is a Wellcome Principal Research Fellow. Erling Pytte provided much appreciated moral support at IBM. For their kindness and help with figures, we thank Eberhard Buhl, Mircea Steriade, Robert K. S. Wong, Charles M. Gray, Nelson Spruston, Nace Golding, David McCormick, Hillary Michelson, Dan Johnston, Mogens Andreasen, J. D. C. Lambert, György Buzsáki, Brian MacVicar, Alex M. Thomson, Arthur Konnerth, Peter Jonas, X-J Wang, Donald Barth, and Lisa Merlin. For important discussions we thank Diego Contreras, György Buzsáki, Robert K. S. Wong, Hillary Michelson, Richard Miles, Nancy Kopell, Bard Ermentrout, Charles M. Gray, Eberhard Buhl, Hannah Monyer, Mircea Steriade, Ivan Soltesz, Nelson Spruston, Arthur Konnerth, Andrea Bibbig, and Rodolfo Llinás. Andrea Bibbig critically read through the text at an early stage. The work was assisted by students and Research Fellows, including Simon B. Colling, I. M. Stanford, Cornelius Borck, Howard Faulkner, Helen C. Doheny, and John Fox. For invaluable help with computing issues, we thank Robert Walkup, Joefon Jann, Nick Hall, Will Weir, and Peter Mayes.

Fast Oscillations in
Cortical Circuits

1   Oscillations: What They Are, What They Might Be Good For

In mathematical physics, oscillations can be given a precise definition, for example, as a periodic solution of a set of differential equations. Oscillations of this sort arise in a number of contexts, including propagating electromagnetic and other kinds of waves. An example of a wave equation with periodic oscillations would be:

$$\nabla^2 E - \varepsilon\mu\partial^2 E/\partial t^2 - g\mu\partial E/\partial t = 0,$$

where the vector E is the electric field, ε is permittivity, μ is permeability, and g a constant relating current density to the electric field (Reitz and Milford 1960). In modeling biological oscillators, Kopell (1988) describes the properties of dynamical systems that can be used to represent the biological oscillator: the system should have a periodic orbit that is a limit cycle, that is, where certain stability criteria of the orbit are met. These criteria can, however, be defined precisely (Hirsch and Smale 1974).

How is one to define a biological oscillation itself, as distinct from the equations used to model the oscillation, especially given that phenomena in physiology that are called oscillatory are not precisely periodic? This issue is of practical importance in in vivo recordings, which tend to be noisy (see also below). Most investigators use an operational approach something like this: the recorded signal is fit with some standard function with free parameters, for example a Gabor function, a Gaussian-damped sinusoid:

$$G(x) = c_1 + c_2 \exp\left(-\, c_3\, x^2 \,/\, 2\right) \cos\left(c_4 x + c_5\right),$$

the c_i being constants to be fit to the data. The investigator determines, according to precise statistical criteria, whether the $G(x)$ so determined is distinguishable from a constant or from some randomly generated function. Different investigators may use different functions for fitting the data and different criteria for assessing the statistical significance of the fit.

One desires an approach where one concentrates on the underlying mathematical system that represents the neuronal network generating a signal, but unfortunately, such mathematical systems are in general not available. In most cases (and in the approach which we have used), the neuronal network is represented by a simulated network, which—from a mathematical point of view, if not from a conceptual one—is itself rather complicated. Until the function of neuronal network oscillations is better defined, it is not clear how to formulate a precise definition that captures what is biologically relevant. We shall simply present the data and let the reader judge whether the signals should be called oscillations.

Some examples where oscillatory phenomena arise in the real world include these:

1. Where a large task must be broken into a series of smaller identical tasks that are serially repeated—walking a long distance, swimming, sawing a log, chewing, birds flying, and so forth. Not all of these activities are rhythmic: one could saw a log with intervals of five seconds alternating with intervals of one hour, for example, although it would be inefficient to do so. The laws of aerodynamics prevent such a strategy from working with flying, of course, unless gliding is possible.

2. Where spatially separated parts of a machine must work together in an organized way. This process happens with logic gates in a computer, where a clock determines when information is to be transmitted between gates. The issue here is that the logic gates perform synchronously. Thus in principle, the clock need not be rhythmic, although making the clock rhythmic will increase efficiency by allowing more operations to be performed per second. Another "machine" with separate parts is a string quartet, for when the members of the quartet play asynchronously, it distresses the listener. In this case, rhythmicity of the playing can be important because past time intervals can be used by the musicians to anticipate future intervals, allowing them to keep in time with each other. In other words, oscillations can be used for prediction.

3. Where an organism may possess an oscillator in order to couple its activities to an oscillation presented to it by the external world, for example, circadian rhythms.

4. Where a population of N neurons may oscillate as a way of increasing the probability that k of the N neurons fire within a small time window. Thus, if the firing rates of the neurons are fixed, but the oscillation allows the neurons only to fire during certain small time intervals, then the probability of coincident firing will be increased. Such an effect can be important in at least two ways: (a) if downstream neurons act as threshold devices, only firing if at least k of their inputs fire within the given time window, so-called coincidence detection, or (b) for plasticity of synapses within the population, if such plasticity is Hebbian, i.e., requires nearly simultaneous firing of pre-and postsynaptic neurons.

Neuronal population oscillations are to be found throughout neurobiology and clinical neurology. To list but a few examples, there are central pattern generating circuits for gastrointestinal function, locomotion, swimming, and breathing (Marder and Calabrese 1996; Sigvardt et al. 1985; Smith et al. 1991); gamma and epileptic rhythms, as we have mentioned; the EEG alpha rhythm, 8–13 Hz in adult humans; sleep spindles (about 14 Hz in adult humans, see also Contreras and Steriade 1996); physiological tremor; and the slow sleep rhythm (Amzica and Steriade 1995). Some of these activities, including epilepsy (Bragin et al. 1997), involve oscillations on multiple time scales. Of the oscillations in the above list, gamma rhythms and seizures are distinguished in that they can be elicited readily in cortical circuits in vitro.

Classification of Types of in Vivo Gamma Oscillations

Gamma oscillations are found in many parts of the brain, including cortex, hippocampus, diencephalon, and cerebellum; similar appearing oscillations are present in invertebrate nervous sytems, including insect olfactory systems. Writing about gamma oscillations in mammalian brain, Galambos (1992) proposed the following useful classification: a) *spontaneous;* b) *induced,* not time-locked to the stimulus, hence disappearing in averages over repeated stimulations; c) *evoked,* time-locked to the stimulus; d) *emitted,* a type of oscillation that we shall not consider that follows an omitted stimulus in a train. To these types we might add e) *epileptic,* occurring during or after a seizure (Leung 1987; Jensen and Yaari 1997). An example of spontaneous gamma would be the waves recorded in rat hippocampus simultaneously with theta waves during ketamine/xylazine anesthesia (Soltesz and Deschênes 1993; Sik et al. 1995). Examples of induced gamma include after visual stimulation in neocortex (Eckhorn et al. 1988; Gray and Singer 1989), after a 1,000 Hz tone burst in human supratemporal auditory cortex (Pantev et al. 1991), after a physiological sharp wave in the hippocampus (Traub, Whittington, et al. 1996), and after stimulation of the pedunculopontine tegmental (PPT) nucleus (Steriade and Amzica 1996). Finally, an example of evoked gamma would be in the auditory cortex after a click (Galambos et al. 1981).

This monograph will concern, in large part, in vitro oscillations that capture some of the phenomenology of spontaneous and induced gamma. In vitro data suggest a set of working hypotheses: a) spontaneous gamma arises from persistent activation of muscarinic receptors in interneurons and possibly pyramidal cells; b) induced gamma results from transient delayed activation of metabotropic glutamate receptors in pyramidal cells and interneurons (with some contribution from muscarinic receptors); and c) immediate evoked gamma corresponds to the oscillation evoked by a single shock after a conditioning tetanic stimulation. These hypotheses will provide the reader with a conceptual framework for relating the in vitro observations to in vivo ones.

There are two fundamental sorts of mechanism which contribute to oscillations of single cells or populations of cells and/or to the synchrony of firing: *intrinsic cell properties* and *synaptic interactions*. Individual neurons, when the membrane potential is in an appropriate range, may develop—alone or in combination—subthreshold voltage oscillations, repeating single action potentials or repeating bursts of action potentials. When populations of neurons receive common synaptic inputs, including oscillatory inputs, the neurons will tend to oscillate in phase with each other, and this tendency can be enhanced if the neurons are synaptically coupled. It is all simple enough if the common oscillatory input is generated somewhere else, but not so simple if the common synaptic inputs emerge from the population itself! This caveat is especially relevant if axon conduction delays are present so that coupling between distant neurons would—one imagines at first—tend to be desynchronizing. Analysis of some of these emergent oscillations forms a major part of this monograph.

The oscillations that we shall be considering involve populations of neurons. Observation of such population oscillations with only one or two electrodes requires, of course, that the activities of the constituent neurons be synchronized. As was pointed out before

(Traub and Miles 1991), synchrony can only be defined in terms of some relevant time scale. In the present case, the time scale for synchrony should be significantly smaller than the period of the oscillation. For example, the period of epileptic synchronized bursts may be several seconds; therefore, when cells begin to burst within 10 ms of each other, they are considered to be synchronized. But during a gamma oscillation, with period about 25 ms, synchrony to within 1 or 2 ms is more appropriate to consider.

Importance of Technical Considerations in Recording Gamma Oscillations

There has been controversy over whether high-frequency cortical oscillations even exist (Horikawa et al. 1994; Young et al. 1992). The EEG recorded from the pial surface of the cortex or with depth electrodes in the hippocampus can show a broad spectrum across high frequencies (e.g., Bragin et al. 1995), and even have a $1/f$ character (Barrie et al. 1996). Problems can arise from the nonstationary frequency of the neuronal activity, from either averaging the activities of multiple neuronal populations or averaging over large areas (so that only some cells participate in the oscillation), and from averaging multiple oscillatory epochs that are not time-locked to the stimulus and which have different fine structures. In studies of cortical oscillations in vivo, electrodes are often hundreds of microns apart (e.g., Gray et al. 1989 used multiunit and field recording with electrodes about 400 microns apart). In such cases, technical considerations become paramount. These issues have proven to be of less practical concern during oscillations in slices, possibly because local neuronal populations participate in the oscillation in a relatively uniform fashion.

2   Single Hippocampal Pyramidal Cells

In this chapter, we shall consider selective aspects of the electrophysiology of CA1 and CA3 pyramidal neurons, and how some—but far from all—of the physiology can be captured in computer models. The central questions are these: what are the different firing patterns available to these neurons and which combinations of synaptic inputs will evoke which patterns? These questions are relevant to this monograph for several reasons. First, during epileptiform events, pyramidal cells fire single or repeating bursts of action potentials, and one needs to know the role of intrinsic factors in bursting before one can address network factors. Second, during population oscillations, cells fire rhythmically and with little frequency accommodation, despite the pronounced tendency of individual pyramidal cells to accomodate during current injection. How might the brain prime the cells to enter into population oscillations? Finally, either pyramidal cells or interneurons can, during the course of an oscillation and under appropriate stimulation conditions, fire spike doublets or multiplets, which themselves then contribute to shaping the form (in time and space) of the oscillation. As with epilepsy and bursting, one needs to understand in oscillations when intrinsic factors or synaptic factors can induce doublet firing.

As a physical device, a neuron can be viewed as a distributed electrical circuit with these basic elements:

1. The cytoplasm is resistive and linear, with resistivity R_i (in Ω-cm).

2. Current flow from membrane surface to depth of the cytoplasm can be ignored with reasonable accuracy. This means that current flow inside the cell can be modeled with branching chains of resistors. (The three-dimensional nature of real cytoplasm is considered, however, in some models of calcium influx, diffusion, buffering, and uptake.)

3. The cell membrane has distributed linear resistivity R_m (in Ω-cm^2) and capacitance C_m (probably about 1 μF/cm^2, although both lower and higher estimates are in the literature for pyramidal cell C_m).

4. The membrane also contains a variety of ion channels, each characterized by its ionic permeabilities and by the mechanisms that control permeability: membrane potential, chemical ligands in the external milieu, internal [Ca^{2+}], phosphorylation, modulatory binding sites, and so forth. There exists in this vast confluence of molecular biology and biophysics much of the complexity of neurons. In modeling neurons, only a subset of channel types are considered, and the channels are not modeled as such; rather one considers spatially distributed time-, voltage, Ca^{2+}-and ligand-gated conductances. This approach follows the classical work of Hodgkin and Huxley (1952) on the squid giant axon, where the propagating axon potential can be replicated with spatially distributed R_i, R_m, C_m, g_{Na}, and g_k.

Approach to Modeling Neurons

We here present only a brief outline of neuron modeling, referring the reader to other sources (Traub and Miles 1991; Koch and Segev 1998). There are four main elements to such modeling:

1. Describing the so-called passive properties, that is, consequences of R_m, R_i, and C_m, as embodied in the cell of interest;

2. Describing the voltage (and Ca^{2+}-, ligand-, etc.) dependent kinetics of the relevant channel types under conditions where spatial nonuniformities can be neglected during space-clamp or in outside-out patches containing small numbers of channels in a tiny piece of membrane;

3. Determining, as best one can, the density over the membrane of the different channel types. Several sorts of channels, including g_{Na}, g_{Ca} and $g_{K(AHP)}$, appear to have densities that vary with location on the membrane;

4. Analyzing how the resultant model responds, either electrically or with internal Ca^{2+} signals, to current pulses and synaptic inputs directed toward particular parts of the neuron, comparing with experiment.

Modeling spatially distributed neurons in this way was begun by Rall and Shepherd (1968), Dodge and Cooley (1973), Traub (1977), and later by many others.

Passive Properties

The sensible description of passive memebrane properties was pioneered by Wilfrid Rall and expanded by his colleagues (Rall 1962, 1989; Rall and Rinzel 1973). Rall introduced a number of important ideas. First, a segment of dendrite—ignoring active channels—is physically just a leaky coaxial cable, the mathematical physics of which has been studied extensively. The distribution of voltage (V) in space (x) and time (t) is described by a partial differential equation, the cable equation:

$$(r/2R_i)\,(\partial^2 V/\partial x^2) = I_m = C_m \partial V/\partial t + I_{ionic},$$

where r is dendritic radius, I_m is membrane current density, and I_{ionic} is the transmembrane current flowing through channels (includes the leak current corresponding to R_m).

Second, the distribution of voltage in space and time, in certain idealized dendritic trees, is mathematically equivalent (with appropriate change of coordinates) to the distribution of voltage in an unbranched leaky cable of constant radius, called an equivalent cylinder. An example of such a transformable dendritic tree is one in which (a) dendritic radius is constant between branch points; in which (b) at branch points, $r^{3/2} = r_1^{3/2} + r_2^{3/2}$, where r is the radius of the parent branch and r_1 and r_2 are radii of the daughter branches, and in which (c) the total electrotonic length from soma to each of the dendritic tips is constant.

Electrotonic length is defined as follows: define the space constant λ of a cylindrical cable as $\lambda = (aR_m/2R_i)^{1/2}$, where a is the radius. λ defines the spatial scale of decay of voltage in space under temporal steady state when voltage at one point is perturbed by a steady current, in an infinitely long cable. Two major points are often forgotten: λ does not define such a spatial scale, at least not precisely, in a finite cable, and the spatial decay of a time-varying voltage, induced at one point, is steeper than indicated by λ. Thus if an applied current is sinusoidal in time, $e^{i\omega t}$, then the frequency-dependent space constant is actually $\lambda / (0.5(1 + (1 + \omega^2\tau_m^2)^{1/2}))^{1/2}$, derived in Traub and Miles (1991, page 82). The electrotonic length of an unbranched cable of length L then is defined to be L / λ. Finally, the electrotonic distance between two branch points, A and B, in a dendritic tree is $\Sigma_i - {}_1L_i/\lambda_i$, where L_i and λ_i are, respectively, the physical lengths and space constants of the segments intervening between A and B.

This transformation to an equivalent cylinder is important for two reasons. First, some real neurons (e.g., cat spinal motorneurons) have dendritic trees that can be approximated as equivalent cylinders, leading to an appreciation of the practical usefulness of Rall's approach by experimentalists. Second, the cable equation in a uniform cylinder—by a further change of coordinates and then a change of variables—can be transformed into the heat equation and solved explicitly for many interesting sets of boundary conditions (Carslaw and Jaeger 1959). In particular, one can show that the voltage response to a transient perturbation is not well described by exponential decay to steady state with a single time constant $\tau_m = R_m C_m$, such as would occur in a point neuron. Rather, there is an infinite series of exponential terms, corresponding to the spatial redistribution of the voltage with different time constants, and the first several of these time constants may be of practical importance.

There are many other important insights, not discussed here, from the Rall analysis. Perhaps of greatest significance is that, through the use of analytical methods and simulations, investigators have developed a feel for how EPSPs and IPSPs evolve in space and time and interact with each other in idealized systems of simple geometry and negligible active currents. Nowadays, neuron models are often based on anatomically reconstructed neurons, in which the assumptions necessary for the equivalent cylinder transformation fail. The neuron is represented by a set of discrete compartments— perhaps thousands of them—each consisting of a few discrete electrical elements, and properties of the model neuron are studied by computer simulations. Nevertheless, the Rall approach is the starting point for examining synaptic potentials in real neurons.

Channel Kinetics

Equations are needed to model channel behavior in order to predict how membrane currents evolve in time and to predict how such currents are influenced by membrane potential and other factors. There are two approaches for modeling channel behavior. One is appropriate for the study of the biophysics of channel molecules and how molecular alterations can affect channel function. One imagines the channel to be able to exist in any of a finite number of states, each state characterized by its own conductance. In addition, there is a matrix of probabilities (per unit time) for transition from one state to another, with these probabilities, in general, being functions of voltage. Such a model can be used to interpret fluctuations in conductance states in single channel recordings.

In principle, macroscopic currents (caused by currents flowing through large numbers of channels) can be simulated from such a model, but in practice, one usually employs a phenomenological model of the Hodgkin-Huxley type. (The latter model was developed as an explanation of membrane currents well before channel recording was possible, and the model is still useful in electrophysiology.) If the membrane behaves linearly for a particular ion, say Na^+), its behavior is described by a version of Ohm's law, $I_{Na} = g_{Na}$ $(V - V_{Na})$, where I_{Na} is the Na current through a small piece of membrane and where V_{Na} is presumed to be a constant (the equilibrium potential for Na^+) that is determined by the distribution of Na^+ ions on either side of the membrane. The problem is then to describe the time evolution of g_{Na}. Following Hodgkin and Huxley (1952), one writes $g_{Na} = G_{Na}m^3h$, where G_{Na} is a constant determined by the local density of Na channels and where m and h are *state variables*, varying in time and subject to the constraint that $0 \leq m, h \leq 1$. With other types of conductance, h may not be used, and the power of m is some integer other than 3; alternatively, one may have $m(h_1 + h_2)$ and so forth. The symbol m is called the *activation variable* and h the *inactivation variable*: Thus, m increases as V increases, while h decreases as V increases, and m has faster kinetics than h when V is near the resting potential.

Now, one must define the time evolution of m and h. We will illustrate this just for m, whose behavior is governed by the differential equation

$$dm/dt = \alpha_m(V) \times (1-m) - \beta_m(V) \times m,$$

where α_m and β_m are, respectively, the forward and backward rate functions. The α and β processes are also called activation and deactivation, respectively, and have units of time^{-1}.) A way to picture the dynamics of this system, which is particularly useful for interpreting voltage-clamp experiments but of general intuitive value, is that m "tries" to move toward its steady-state value m_∞ (for the present voltage), with a time constant τ_m characteristic of the present voltage. Of course, in general, V keeps changing, although it can be held constant in voltage clamp. To find m_∞, simply set $dm / dt = 0$: thus, $m_\infty = \alpha_m(V)/(\alpha_m(V) + \beta_m(V))$. To find τ_m suppose that V is kept constant, so that α_m and β_m become constants. Then, $dm/dt = 1 - m \times (\alpha + \beta)$, a first-order linear differential equation, in which m relaxes to m_∞ with the time constant $\tau_m = 1 / (\alpha + \beta)$. These equations constitute the formalism used in the cell models and hence in the network models in this book. Further details, for example of the specific rate functions, can be found in these papers, Traub et al. 1991 and 1994.

   Certain additional complexities enter into the description of selected channel types. For example, the C and AHP types of K conductances are gated by $[Ca^{2+}]_i$, with additional strong and weak voltage-dependence (respectively) as well. The NMDA type of glutamate-operated channel is not only ligand-gated but also depends on V and on Mg^{2+} concentration (Jahr and Stevens 1990). Channels may develop slow (seconds) inactivation and even slower recovery from inactivation and are regulated by any number of biochemical processes, including phosphorylation of selected amino acids in the protein. Many sorts of gamma oscillations typically last 1 or 2 seconds, or less, so that their simulation does not require modeling slower membrane processes. Seizures, of course, can last much longer, and slower processes are doubtless relevant, although rarely worked out in detail.

   Even within a spatially limited bit of membrane, complex behavior can emerge through the interaction between different ionic conductances. This process can happen because different conductances may have different equilibrium potentials and /or different kinetics. The resulting possible interplay was first demonstrated by Hodgkin and Huxley, who showed that an action potential originated from the combined actions of g_{Na}, g_K, and g_L (the leak conductance), in part because the activation of g_{Na} was considerably faster than its inactivation and also faster than the activation of g_K. A second example concerns the interactions between g_L, a low-threshold inactivating g_{Ca}, and the h (hyperpolarization-activated) conductance in thalamocortical relay cells. Rhythmic Ca spikes, such as these cells exhibit within a defined range of membrane potential, can be replicated in single-compartment models through the interaction of these conductances (Wang, Rinzel, and Rogawski 1991; Huguenard and McCormick 1992). A final example, pertinent to pyramidal cell dendrites, concerns the interaction between g_{Na} (perhaps at insufficient density to give full-sized action potentials) and one or more types of high-threshold g_{Ca}. In such a case, m_∞ (V) for this g_{Ca} is shifted to the right relative to m_∞ of g_{Na}, and $\tau_m(g_{Ca}) > \tau_m(g_{Na})$. As a result, a single Na action potential might evoke limited Ca influx from a small degree of Ca channel opening, but the repeated depolarizations produced by a rapid series of Na spikes may induce a large Ca-mediated action potential with much greater Ca influx (see later).

Spatial Distribution of Channels

Channel kinetics are conveniently studied in acutely isolated neurons, which lose most of the dendritic tree (Kay and Wong 1986) or in small isolated patches. The idea is to prevent spread of current along the inside of the cell so that currents measured by the electrode actually reflect transmembrane currents, preferably only through the channel(s) of interest. On the other hand, in real neurons under physiological conditions, currents flow within the cell, as well as through multiple types of transmembrane channels. To understand the neuron, one therefore needs, in addition to channel kinetics, information on the spatial distribution of channels.

There are several experimental methods that provide information —usually qualitative—about the spatial distribution of channels:

1. Antibody binding studies (Westenbroek et al. 1989, 1990; Baude et al. 1995). There is the difficulty, however, that antigenically specific channels may not all be functionally active.

2. Measurements of the amplitude of Na and Ca spikes at different locations of the cell (axon initial segment, soma, and dendrites), on occasion with two electrodes at different sites (Wong and Stewart 1992; Spruston, Schiller, et al. 1995). Thus, for example, presumed Ca spikes were found to be of larger amplitude in the apical dendrites of hippocampal pyramidal cells than at the soma (Wong, Prince, and Basbaum 1979). These data can be difficult to interpret sometimes because of interactions between different ionic conductances: for example, a slowly activating K conductance might, in principle, attenuate a Ca^{2+} spike, which is slow, more than it would attenuate a Na^+ spike, which is fast. Such complexities can be studied by selective blockade of some of the ionic conductances with TTX, TEA, 4AP, divalent cations, spider toxins, etc. In addition, pieces of the cell can be studied in physical isolation from each other: in acutely isolated cells (Kay and Wong 1986) or after surgical cuts across the proximal dendrites (Benardo, Masukawa, and Prince 1982). Information can also be obtained with extracellular electrodes (Jefferys 1979).

3. Time-dependent imaging of $[Na^+]_i$ and $[Ca^{2+}]_i$, again taking care to interpret the data in light of interaction between different ionic conductances (Jaffe et al. 1992).

4. Patching onto different cell membrane locations, and estimating the number of channels of various types per patch as a function of location (Johnston, Magee et al. 1996). One such map, for a CA1 pyramidal neuron, based on ionic imaging and multiple patches, is shown in figure 2.1. This map does not give the absolute density of

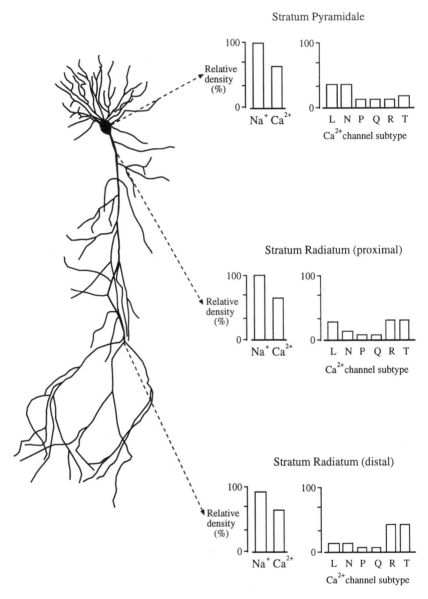

Figure 2.1
Estimated distribution of Na⁺ and Ca²⁺ channels in CA1 pyramidal cells, based on
fluoresence imaging and patch-clamp studies (From Johnston et al., 1996. With permission, from the *Annual Review of Neuroscience*, vol. 19 © 1996 by Annual Reviews.)

channels but does indicate that Na and Ca channels exist over wide regions of the membrane. Imaging data and intracellular recording suggest that Na and Ca channels extend well out into the distal dendrites (Jaffe et al. 1992; see also figure 2.5 and referenced papers). In addition, the subtype distribution of Ca channels is not homogeneous. (For review of the properties of Ca channel subtypes, see Magee and Johnston 1995; Christie, Eliot, et al. 1995).

Some models of hippocampal and neocortical pyramidal cells that have been constructed include—but are not limited to—the following: Traub et al. 1991 and 1994 (which are the ones used in simulations in this book); Jaffe et al. (1994); Migliore et al. (1995); Mainen et al. (1995); Rhodes and Gray (1994); Warman et al. (1994). We shall review here some specific details from one of our CA3 pyramidal cell models (Traub et al. 1994). The compartmental structure consists of a soma and 63 additional compartments that represent a simplified branching dendritic tree (basilar and apical). In addition, there is a 5-compartment, truncated, unmyelinated piece of axon, with the axon initial segment flared, thus allowing simulation of antidromic spikes and of the transduction from somatodendritic electrogenesis to axonal output. The active ionic conductances consist of g_{Na} to generate fast spikes, a high-threshold g_{Ca} (Kay and Wong 1987), and four types of K conductance, delayed rectifier, the transient A conductance, the fast C conductance (gated by both membrane potential and intracellular Ca^{2+}), and the slow Ca^{2+}-gated AHP (afterhyperpolarization) conductance. Kinetics were determined by voltage-clamp data where possible, but the spatial distribution of ionic conductances was manipulated by trial and error in order to replicate as many current-clamp experimental data as possible. Needless to say, the resulting conductance distribution is in no way unique.

An example of a critical current-clamp experiment is the burst that can be induced by a brief somatic current pulse; while the same current pulse, followed immediately by a hyperpolarizing pulse, leads to a single somatic action potential, followed by a (partly) Ca^{2+}-dependent depolarizing afterpotential (Wong and Prince 1978, 1981). The model replicated this experiment as follows. Action potentials are initiated in the axon initial segment and propagate retrograde into the dendrites, actively but with diminishing amplitude (as subsequently demonstrated experimentally in CA1 pyramidal cells: Spruston et al. 1995). When synaptic inhibition is suppressed, a single action potential, even an antidromic one, as also confirmed experimentally, initiates a burst by evoking a dendritic Ca spike. In other cases, two or three somatic spikes in succession might be required to trigger the Ca spike. The dendritic Ca spike in turn leads to a slow depolarizing envelope at the soma, possibly with additional Na spikes. Much of this type of behavior can be captured in a 2-compartment model, in which g_{Na} and g_{Ca} are spatially separated (Pinsky and Rinzel 1994).

The Firing Pattern of Pyramidal Cells Is Determined by the Site—As Well As the Intensity—of Stimulation

In vivo hippocampal pyramidal cells fire in isolated single spikes or in bursts, so-called complex spikes (Kandel and Spencer 1961; Fox and Ranck 1975, Buzsáki, Penttonen et al. 1996). Spontaneous, isolated, i.e., not synchronized, bursts in CA3 pyramidal cells are also recorded in hippocampal slices, particularly when K^+ is slightly elevated, e.g., to 5 mM, but not too elevated, e.g., 8 mM (Wong and Prince 1981; Chamberlin, Traub, and Dingledine 1990). When CA3 pyramidal cells are slightly depolarized by somatic current injection, rhythmic bursts occur, with frequencies up to 3 or 4 Hz, the frequency increasing with depolarization. Further somatic depolarization then causes the firing pattern to switch to spike doublets and then rhythmic action potentials (figure 2.2), a type of behavior suggestive of what occurs during a tetanically evoked oscillation

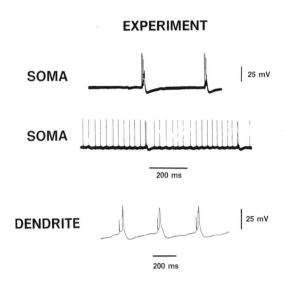

Figure 2.2
Firing patterns in CA3 pyramidal cells depend on membrane potential and on the
site of stimulation. The upper two traces are from the same CA3 pyramidal cell as
it was progressively depolarized by injection of depolarizing current into the soma;
this process switched the firing pattern from bursting (above) to repetitive single
spikes (and occasional doublets) at higher frequency (middle). The bottom trace is
from a different CA3 pyramidal cell; it is a recording taken from the apical dendrite,
in s. radiatum. Injection of current at this site can induce slow (presumed Ca^{2+})
spikes at frequencies up to 8 Hz, faster than bursts that occur during somatic current
injections. (Upper two traces from Wong and Prince, 1981, with permission of American Physiological Society; bottom trace is unpublished data of R. Miles.)

and also reminiscent of a similar transition in thalamocortical relay
cells. Interestingly, somatic depolarization does not lead to bursting
at the 10 Hz and more frequencies, which can be observed during
epileptic afterdischarges (see chapter 5). Of course, somatic depolarization does not accurately reflect synaptic excitation of the neuron, given that excitatory synapses are found almost exclusively on
dendrites.

With this consideration in mind, steady current injections were
made (by R. Miles) into the apical dendrites of CA3 pyramidal cells
(figure 2.2), and it was noted that rhythmic bursts could be evoked

at frequencies of at least 8 Hz, provided that the current was large enough, greater than about 1 nA. The burst morphology in the dendrite was different than at the soma, with dendritic fast (presumed Na) spikes usually of lower amplitude than slower (presumed Ca) spikes, probably reflecting either a greater distance of the dendrite from the axon initial segment or a low density of Na channels in the dendrites, or both.

These firing patterns are replicated—in the steady state, in any case—in the CA3 pyramidal cell model (figure 2.3). The left panels show how increasing levels of current injection into the soma produce the transition bursting → spike doublets and triplets → single rhythmic spikes. The mechanism for this transition is as follows. As dendritic calcium influx becomes larger with repetitive bursting, a large AHP develops that shunts the membrane. A 1 nA current injected into the soma does not lead to enough dendritic depolarization to overcome this shunt and to evoke a dendritic Ca spike. Instead, a stable behavior is reached in which each somatic fast spike propagates to the dendrite as a smaller fast spike and, in turn, causes a small Ca influx. With these spikes occurring rhythmically, a steady AHP shunt is maintained. On the other hand, injection of a large current directly into the dendrite can lead to the necessary depolarization to generate Ca spikes at frequencies > 5 Hz (figure 2.3, right).

Certain aspects of the firing behavior of pyramidal cells are especially relevant for the spatiotemporal structure of gamma oscillations and for the synaptic plasticity associated with gamma. An accurate model of the neuron helps to shed light on these issues and to suggest experiments. Some of the germane issues are the following:

1. Pyramidal cells fire bursts during seizures, but during gamma oscillations, they fire rhythmically, although spike doublets can occur during beta oscillations. How do intrinsic membrane properties

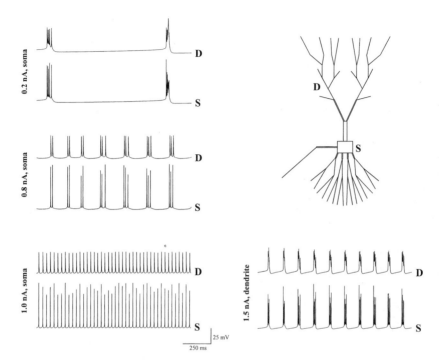

Figure 2.3
Firing patterns in model CA3 pyramidal cell also depend on membrane potential and on the site of stimulation. The inset (upper right) shows the structure of the model, with the axon projecting down from the soma (*S*), and *D* the apical dendritic site from which the dendritic potentials derive in the figure. Left panels (top to bottom): injection of progressively larger currents into the soma leads first to bursts, then spike doublets and triplets, then repetitive single action potentials. Lower right: injection of a large current into the apical dendrite leads to repetitive Ca^{2+} spikes at the dendritic site and to bursts at the soma. The frequency of bursts obtained in this way is higher than when current is injected into the soma. (R. D. Traub, unpublished data, using the simulation model of Traub, Jefferys, Miles et al. 1994.)

contribute to bursting versus nonbursting? (This issue was introduced in figures 2.2 and 2.3 in considering the effects of membrane potential on bursting.) How might the tendency to fire in bursts be regulated by synaptic inputs?

2. Synaptic plasticity appears to be controlled by the magnitude and time course of intracellular Ca^{2+} transients. Ca^{2+} fluxes through either NMDA receptor-channels or through voltage-gated Ca channels will be influenced by Na electrogenesis because of the induced dendritic depolarization. How, then, are Na spikes initiated, and how do they propagate throughout the neuron?

3. Steady injection of current into pyramidal cells, particularly CA1 pyramidal cells, leads to spike trains that exhibit strong frequency accomodation, that is, slowing of the frequency with time (Schwartzkroin 1978; Madison and Nicoll 1984; see also chapter 9). How can pyramidal neurons be primed to fire rhythmically, as they must do during a population oscillation?

The remainder of this chapter will be directed toward these questions.

The data on injection of steady currents into the apical dendrites of pyramidal cells indicate that Ca^{2+} spikes are readily initiated by dendritic depolarization. Figure 2.4A (Traub et. al. 1994, recordings by R. Miles) provides another example of this phenomenon in a CA3 pyramidal cell. Using a briefer current injection, a mixture of fast (presumed Na) and slow (presumed Ca) spikes is evoked. Local extracellular stimulation in stratum radiatum, which is expected to activate dendritic $GABA_A$ receptor-mediated IPSPs, can, if timed appropriately, suppress the presumed Ca spike(s), a result that was actually predicted by the model (figure 2.4, right). The suppression of apical Ca spikes by dendritic inhibition was then confirmed in experiments in which a cut was made to avoid activation of perisomatic inhibition (Miles et al. 1996). This latter study also showed that activation of perisomatic inhibition, even by stimulation of sin-

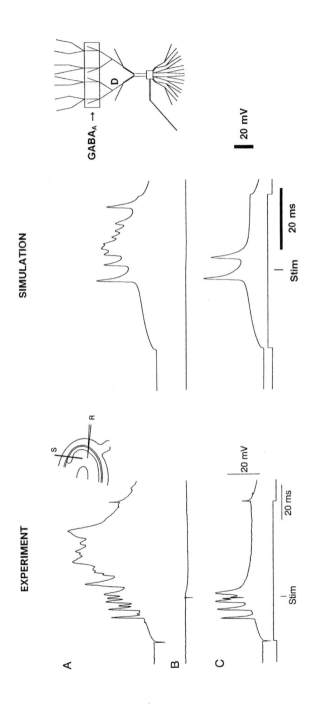

Figure 2.4
Apical dendritic IPSPs can suppress slow spikes (putative Ca²⁺ spikes) in CA3 pyramidal neurons. The insets show, for the experiment, the location of extracellular stimulus and intracellular recording electrodes in s. radiatum and, for the simulation, the site of the dendritic potential plotted (*D*) and the sites at which dendritic IPSPs develop. In the experiment, ionotropic glutamate receptors were blocked with CNQX and APV. (A) Fast and slow spikes are generated in the dendrites by a current pulse (0.5 nA in experiment, 0.6 nA in simulation). (B) Dendritic IPSP, induced by a focal stimulus in the experiment and by a 20 nS conductance pulse decaying with $\tau = 50$ ms in the simulation. (C) The current pulse and dendritic IPSP were combined, resulting in suppression of the slow spike(s) but not the faster ones. (From Traub, Jefferys, Miles et al. 1994.)

gle interneurons, could suppress the full-sized action potentials generated in, or near to, the soma. An implication of this result is that sustained dendritic synaptic inhibition could, in principle, be used by the brain to prevent cell bursting during population oscillations. Dendritic inhibition also, not surprisingly, limits the propagation of fast spikes into the dendrites (Tsubokawa and Ross 1996).

The smaller amplitude of fast spikes in the dendrites as compared to the soma suggests that the density of Na channels is reduced in the dendrites as compared to the soma itself or at least as compared to the axon initial segment. In such a case, computer simulations predict that EPSPs impinging in the apical dendrites can, if not excessively large, depolarize the soma-dendritic membrane and cause a spike that begins first in or near the soma and then back-propagates into the dendrites (Traub et al. 1991, 1994). In a remarkable series of experiments, using simultaneous patch electrodes at soma and dendrites of the same neuron, this prediction has been verified both for neocortical and for CA1 pyramidal neurons, at least under certain conditions (Stuart and Sakmann 1994; Spruston, Schiller, et al. 1995; figure 2.5). Figure 2.5 illustrates two additional points. First there is a significant increase in spike latency—and of the probability of propagation failure—at distal branch points, and second, during repetitive firing at frequencies of about 20 Hz, there is rapid attenuation of the amplitude of dendritic Na spikes, most pronounced in the distal dendrites (see also Callaway and Ross 1995). One possible explanation for this effect is an accumulating voltage-dependent inactivation of dendritic Na channels (Jung, Mickus, and Spruston 1997), a phenomenon not incorporated into the original Hodgkin-Huxley or into our pyramidal cell models. This type of observation demonstrates the future importance of measurements of dendritic potential and Ca^{2+} signals during gamma oscillations.

CA1 pyramidal cells have interesting properties that distinguish them from CA3 pyramidal cells. Injection of steady current into the soma of CA1 cells usually evokes repetitive firing of fast spikes in an accomodating pattern; while current-induced depolarization of the dendrites—and also orthdromic stimulation when $GABA_A$ receptors are blocked—evokes bursts that, in most studies, appear to consist of a mixture of Na and Ca spikes (Wong, Prince, and Basbaum 1979; Wong and Stewart 1992; Masukawa and Prince 1984; Mesher and Schwartzkroin 1980).

Andreasen and Lambert (1995) (see figure 2.6) injected depolarizing current into the dendrites of CA1 pyramidal neurons and described three firing patterns:

1. repetitive fast spikes of declining amplitude; It is possible that these spikes are actually initiated at the soma (figure 2.5) and backpropagate to the dendritic stimulating/recording electrode;

2. compound spikes resembling what other authors have called bursts and appearing to consist of a mixture of Na and Ca spikes;

3. bursting in a form that appears to consist solely of Na spikes. Bursts with similar pattern have been studied in the somata of CA1 pyramidal cells in high $[K^+]_o$ (Jensen et al. 1996; Azouz and Jensen 1996). In the latter case, g_{Ca} is not required for bursting to occur. Instead, a persistent g_{Na} ($g_{Na(P)}$) plays the necessary role of a slower depolarizing conductance that generates the depolarizing envelope of the burst. The muscarinic receptor-modulated M type of K conductance was suggested, by virtue of its appropriate kinetics, to contribute to burst termination. It is possible that the dendritic bursts recorded by Andreasen and Lambert have a similar mechanism. Why there should be differences in g_{Ca} versus $g_{Na(P)}$ in the dendrites of different pyramidal cells is not known, but both types of conductances can be modulated by neurotransmitters (g_{Ca} by metabotropic glutamate receptors) or by biochemical factors ($g_{Na(P)}$ by protein kinase C, in turn influenced by cholinergic receptors; see Fleidervish, Astman, and Gutnick 1997).

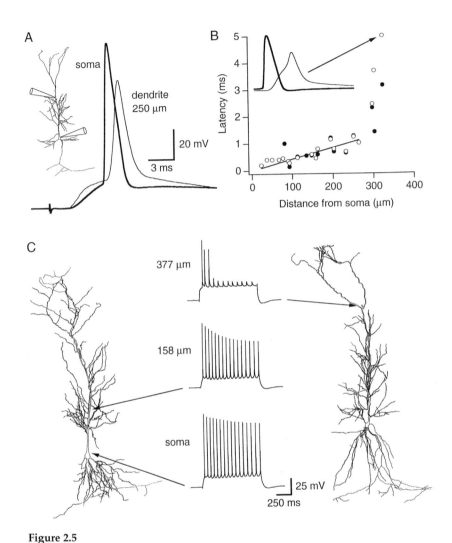

Figure 2.5
Action potentials in CA1 pyramidal cells, elicited by synaptic stimulation, can originate near the soma; action potentials propagate into the dendrites in activity-
dependent fashion. (A) Two simultaneous recordings (as in the inset) during
synaptic excitation of the dendrites; the action potential occurs earlier in the soma
than in the dendrite. (B) Data were pooled from numerous dual recordings to yield
a plot of latency (peak of somatic spike to peak of dendritic spike) versus distance
of the dendritic site from the soma. Action potentials were evoked by synaptic excitation (●) or by current pulses (○). Mean conduction velocity over the first 264 μm

These different sorts of dendritic bursts can be simulated as follows. It is not practical to perform large network simulations using anatomically precise neuron models with hundreds of compartments. A simple modification of the CA3 model, however, renders the cell more CA1-like. This modification requires a narrowing of the three most proximal apical dendritic compartments (by 60% for the apical shaft and by 37% for the first branch segments; cf. Lorente de Nó 1934). In addition, the A conductance density was increased to 1 mS/cm^2 uniformly, it having been shown that this conductance is significant in pyramidal cell dendrites (Hoffman, Magee et al. 1997). In order to replicate Ca-independent bursts (figure 2.7A), g_{Ca} channel density was reduced 80%, and all g_{Na} in the proximal dendrites, but not the soma, was made persistent, that is h_{Na} was constrained to be 1. Finally, the M type of K conductance was inserted into the cell at 0.1 ×, the density of $g_{K(DR)}$ (kinetics as in Traub, Knowles, Miles, and Wong 1984).

With these parameters, dendritic current pulses evoke bursts resembling the recordings of Andreasen and Lambert (1995) (figure 2.7A), as well as those of Azouz et al. (1996). On the other hand, with the original CA3 conductance densities, dendritic current pulses subthreshold for Ca spikes evoke fast spikes that are initiated in the initial segment (figure 2.7B), while larger current pulses evoke compound spikes with a Ca^{2+} action potential (figure 2.7C). The simultaneously recorded somatic potentials also resemble experimental traces (figure 2.8; see also Wong and Stewart 1992).

was 0.24 mm/ms. Inset (somatic spike 105 mV) shows 20 ms of data for the indicated point, somatic spike shown in thick line. (C) repetitive spikes in soma and dendrites. For the cell at the left, simultaneous recordings were made in soma and dendrites, while a 0.2 nA current was injected into the soma. For the cell at right, a 0.2 nA current was injected into the dendrite. Spikes in proximal dendrites attenuate more gradually than in the distal dendrites and attenuate to a lesser degree. (From Traub, Spruston et al., 1998 with permission; the data in A and B are from Spruston, Schiller et al., 1995, and from C, N. Spruston, unpublished data.)

How else, besides synaptic inhibition, could bursting be suppressed? One possible means is through activation of metabotropic glutamate receptors (figure 2.9). This experimental observation is directly relevant to in vitro gamma oscillations evoked by tetanic stimulation as a large metabotropic EPSP follows the tetanus (see chapter 9). The mechanism of switch from bursting to repetitive firing may simply be membrane depolarization (Figures 2.2 and 2.9). The depolarization results because metabotropic glutamate receptors suppress a number of K conductances and also induce at least one inward current (Charpak et al. 1990; Charpak and Gähwiler 1991; Guérineau et al. 1994, 1995). These effects are probably mediated by Group I metabotropic glutamate receptors, mGluR1 and mGluR5 (Gereau and Conn 1995a). Metabotropic glutamate receptors have also been shown to suppress the L type of Ca^{2+} conductance (Sayer, Schwindt, and Crill 1992).

A complicating, and apparently contradictory, observation is that Group I metabotropic receptors are capable of prolonging epileptiform discharges, that is, of inducing additional bursts (Merlin and Wong 1997). A likely resolution of this apparent paradox is that the epilepsy experiments were performed during blockade of $GABA_A$ receptors. In this case, the metabotropically induced inward current may predominate over other effects of metabotropic receptors, including the reduction of g_{Ca}. Notably, $GABA_A$ receptor function is critical for gamma oscillations to occur (see later chapters). This issue of apparently opposite effects of metabotropic receptors demands further study, however. Muscarinic receptors also suppress pyramidal cell bursting; this effect, however, may be independent of the reduction of K conductances, as 8—bromo-cAMP suppresses K conductances but does not suppress intrinsic bursting (Azouz, Jensen, and Yaari 1994).

Intrinsic Oscillatory Membrane Properties

Subthreshold membrane potential oscillations at theta frequency (4–12 Hz) have been found in CA1 pyramidal cells (Leung and Yim 1991; Cobb et al. 1995), in spiny stellate cells of layer 2 entorhinal cortex (Alonso and Llinás 1989), and in neocortical cells (Gutfreund, Yarom, and Segev 1995). Higher frequency, generally subthreshold oscillations—typically appearing within a specific range of membrane potentials—have also been described in a number of cell types, including intralaminar thalamic neurons (Steriade, Curró Dossi, and Contreras 1993); thalamocortical relay cells, in which the oscillation is generated in dendrites by P/Q Ca^{2+} channels (Pedroarena and Llinás 1997); nucleus reticularis thalami neurons (Pinault and Deschênes 1992a,b); aspiny neocortical cells (Llinás, Grace, and Yarom 1991); and long-axoned neocortical cells (Nuñez, Amzica, and Steriade 1992a).

In the latter study, oscillating cells were found in 26 out of 158 cases in cat cortical areas 4, 5, 6, and 7. Oscillations appeared at membrane potentials that were depolarized beyond -62 mV. The frequency ranged from 10–15 Hz up to about 30 Hz. The oscillating cells were regular spiking, and action potentials could ride on the crests of the waves. Modeling studies (Wang 1993) have shown that intrinsic gamma oscillations could, in principle, arise from an interaction between $g_{Na(P)}$ and $g_{K(S)}$, the latter a slowly inactivating K conductance that has been described in cortical neurons (Spain, Schwindt, and Crill 1991). The data of Leung and Yim (1991) suggest that intrinsic theta oscillations depend on g_{Na} and one or more K currents, as do the data of Alonso and Llinás (1989) in hippocampal and entorhinal cortical cells, respectively. To our knowledge, intrinsic gamma oscillations have not been described in CA1 pyramidal cells.

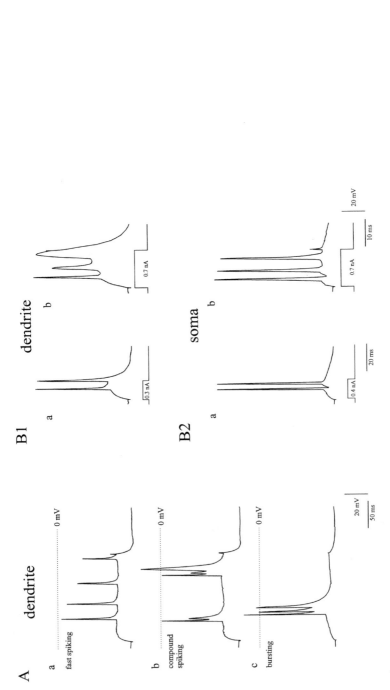

Figure 2.6
Different firing patterns in soma and dendrites of CA1 pyramidal cells. (A) 200 ms current pulses were injected into the distal apical dendrites of different cells. Symbol *a* shows repetitive fast spikes that decrease in amplitude (cf figure 2.5); *b* shows bursts, some of which contain slow (presumed Ca²⁺) spikes; and *c* shows a burst without slow spikes. Such bursts may depend on a persistent Na⁺ current. (B1) smaller depolarizations of a dendrite can evoke a spike doublet, while a larger depolarization evokes a burst containing a slow spike. (B2) comparable depolarizations of the soma evoke spike doublets and brief bursts, generally without slow spikes.
(From Andreasen and Lambert, 1995)

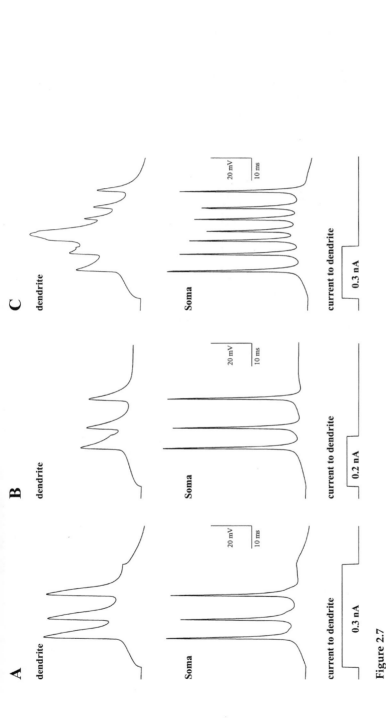

Figure 2.7
Simultaneous dendritic and somatic firing patterns in model CA1 pyramidal neuron. We used the CA3 pyramidal cell model of Traub et al. (1994), modified by addition of a persistent Na^+ conductance and an M type of K^+ conductance (A) or by narrowing of the proximal apical dendrite (B). (A) Burst without slow spikes. (B) Triplet of dendritic fast spikes of declining amplitude, corresponding to full somatic spikes. (C) Dendritic burst with slow Ca^{2+}-dependent) spike. Note the absence of a slow spike in the corresponding somatic burst, the small underlying somatic depolarization, and the somatic spikes back-propagating into the dendrites. (R. D. Traub, unpublished data).

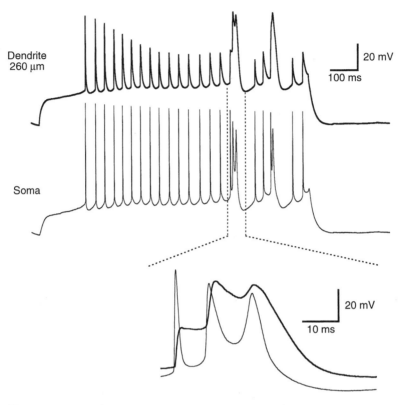

Figure 2.8
Simultaneous somatic/dendritic recordings in a CA1 pyramidal cell of an adult rat. The cell was morphologically identified after biocytin injection, and 0.55 nA tonic current was injected into the dendritic site. Resting membrane potential −68 mV, temperature 35°C. Compare with figure 2.7 (N. Golding and N. Spruston, unpublished data).

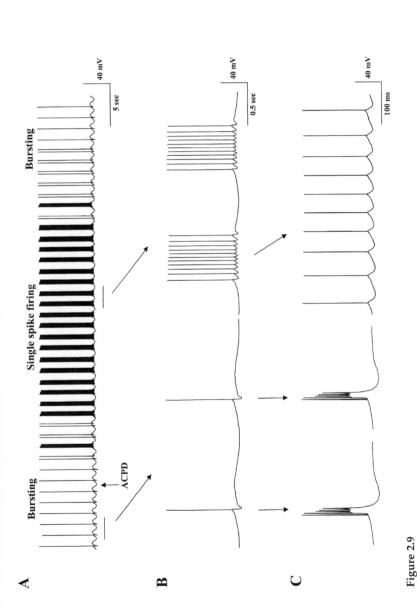

Figure 2.9
Metabotropic glutamate receptor activation can convert burst-firing into rhythmic spiking. The cell illustrated is a bursting layer-5 neocortical neuron, injected with an 0.8 Hz sinusoidal current. The metabotropic glutamate receptor agonist ACPD was applied at the time of the vertical arrow. (From McCormick, Wang, and Huguenard, 1993 with permission).

3   Single Hippocampal Interneurons

The rhythmic firing of interneurons, either in single spikes or spike doublets, is crucial for the organization of gamma rhythms in vitro and in the hippocampus in vivo. In the rat hippocampus in vivo, anatomically identified basket cells are known to participate in gamma rhythms (figure 3.1). In vitro, interneurons, physiologically identified, in strata pyramidale and oriens consistently participate in gamma oscillations. While morphological identification of these interneurons is lacking, it is likely that participating interneurons include basket cells and perhaps also chandelier (axo-axonic) cells.

Within the hippocampus, and neocortex as well, a large variety of interneurons have been identified. They differ in their morphology and position: where is the cell body located, where do the dendrites go, into what layers does the axon extend, how far, and contacting which cell types? They also differ in their physiological properties, with some firing narrow action potentials that are rhythmic and with others firing broader action potentials, sometimes in bursts (Kawaguchi and Hama 1987). They vary further in calcium-binding proteins, parvalbumin, calbindin, calretinin; in staining for neuromodulatory peptides, somatostatin, Neuropeptide Y, cholecystokinin, etc.; in the response to modulatory substances such as acetylcholine and serotonin (Parra et al. 1998); in the function of presynaptic terminals (Poncer et al. 1997; Pearce et al. 1995); and in

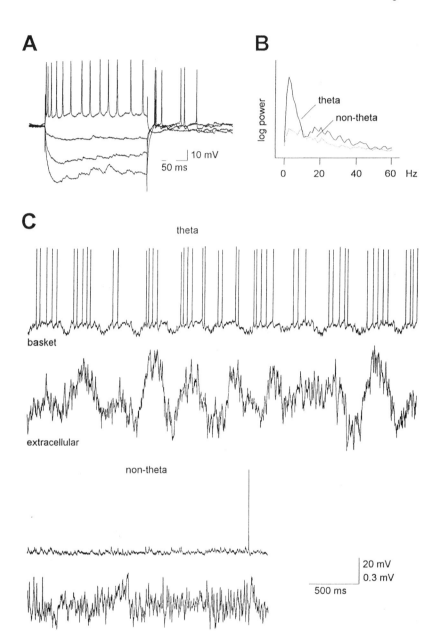

the extent to which the cells can be activated by recurrent excitation and by particular afferent pathways, as well as by other interneurons. Much of this information for the hippocampus is reviewed in the monograph of Freund and Buzsáki (1996).

Here, we shall confine our attention to the physiological properties of those interneurons most likely to be critical for generation of gamma oscillations. We shall present some rather detailed information about these cells. At this stage of our knowledge, many of the important principles of brain oscillations are not yet clear enough that we can be completely confident in purely mathematical, analytically tractable models: it is still necessary to construct detailed simulation models that either actually incorporate known specific facts or else allow researchers to be aware of discrepancies between cell models and real neurons, so as to consider possible consequences of the discrepancies.

Our attention will be directed most especially toward mechanisms relevant to the generation of gamma oscillations. During experimental gamma oscillations in the hippocampal slice (as described in later chapters), interneurons "feel" three major synaptic transmitter-gated inputs. First is a tonic excitatory conductance that tends to make them fire repetitively, deriving from metabotropic receptors. Notably, current injection into basket cells and axo-axonic cells is capable of forcing them to fire at frequencies of several hundred Hz (e.g., Buhl, Han et al. 1994), far faster than is required to generate gamma oscillations. Second are $GABA_A$ re-

Figure 3.1
CA1 basket cells in vivo participate in both theta and gamma rhythms. The recordings illustrated were taken from a single CA1 basket cell in a urethane-anesthetized rat. (A) response of the neuron to depolarizing and hyperpolarizing current pulses. (B) power spectra (note logarithmic vertical scale) of cellular activity (with spikes removed) during theta and non-theta states. (C) simultaneous intracellular and extracellular recording, showing participation of the neuron in both rhythms. Note that action potentials occur during the theta-modulated depolarizations. In the non-theta state (below), the cell fires only rarely. (From Sik et al., 1995 with permission)

ceptor-mediated IPSPs impinging from other interneurons (a topic addressed in the next chapter). Third are synchronized EPSPs impinging from the nearly simultaneous firing of connecting pyramidal cells. The EPSPs have the property that, if sufficiently large, they can evoke an action potential during a period when the interneuron, owing to its post-spike AHP, would normally be refractory. The ability of interneurons to behave in this way is crucial for long-range synchronization (chapter 9); hence, the underlying electrophysiological issues are important to define.

Specific Properties of Basket Cells and Axo-axonic Cells

CA1 basket cells have been investigated by Buhl, Halasy, and Somogyi (1994) and by Buhl, Szilagyi et al. (1996). Basket cells (at least in s. radiatum) and axo-axonic cells contain the calcium-binding protein parvalbumin. For CA1 basket cells, the following physiological parameters were adduced: the action potential width was 0.4 ms at ½ amplitude; the spikes were non-overshooting (unlike pyramidal cells); R_{input} was 31.3 ± 10.9 MΩ; τ_m was 9.8 ± 4.5 ms; the AHP amplitude was large, 13.5 ± 6.7 mV; the mean decrease in firing rate (accomodation) during a steady depolarizing pulse was 42 ± 31%. In the rat, 39% of CA1 basket cells have a spike depolarizing afterpotential (DAP), and the presence of a DAP correlates with the presence of a slow AHP. One possible interpretation of this latter observation is that both the DAP and the AHP are, at least partially, dependent on one or more types of g_{Ca}. A likely result of this heterogeneity of spike DAPs in basket cells is that, while many basket cells show little accomodation in response to steady injected current, others do accomodate or even generate bursts (figure 3.2). Similar variability in firing patterns can be seen in bistratified interneurons (figure 3.2).

Concerning the synaptic activation of CA1 basket cells: the Schaffer collateral-evoked EPSP is largely, but not completely, AMPA re-

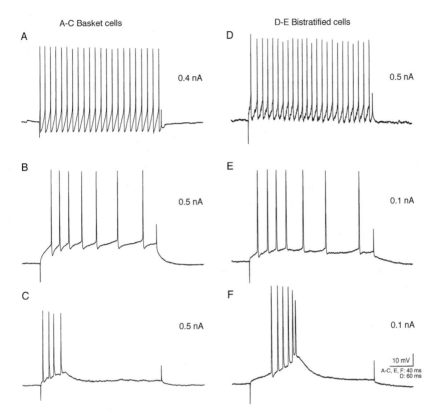

Figure 3.2
Variability in firing patterns of basket cells and bistratified cells. While some cells demonstrate almost no adaptation, other cells do adapt or even fire in bursts. The bistratified cell in (E) and (F) is the same one, held at −57 mV in (E) and at −62 mV in (F). (Figure courtesy of E. H. Buhl, from Buhl, Szilágyi et al., 1996 with permission)

ceptor-mediated. This EPSP has an average rise time of 1.9 ± 0.5 ms and a mean duration of 10.7 ± 5.7 ms. There is also a Schaffer collateral-evoked IPSP in CA1 basket cells, having a latency of 21.4 ms to the peak of the fast IPSP. The reason for this long latency to peak is not clear, given that afferent stimuli cause interneurons to fire with short latency often before principal cells fire (e.g., Miles 1990a). Perhaps high-threshold interneurons also contribute to the IPSP in basket cells, or possibly pyramidal cell firing augments the

IPSP by recruiting additional interneurons to fire. A high-intensity stimulus is needed to evoke the IPSP in CA1 basket cells. A slow IPSP exists as well. The evoked IPSP suppresses firing in a tonically depolarized basket cell for at least 50 ms. CA1 basket cells are additionally (and importantly, for our purposes, as will be seen later) recurrently excited by CA1 pyramidal cells.

The physiological properties of CA1 axo-axonic cells have been investigated by Buhl, Han et al. (1994). These neurons had a resting membrane potential of -65.1 mV, an R_{input} 73.9 MΩ, a mean τ_m of only 7.7 ms (with sharp recording electrodes), and an action potential width of only 0.39 ms at ½ amplitude. The action potential was small, only 64 mV. In most cells, there was a pronounced fast AHP, having a mean duration of 28 ms. There was variability in the degree of spike-frequency adaptation and in the existence of a slow AHP (τ in seconds, as in pyramidal cells). Some cells exhibited a spike DAP (the ionic basis of which is unknown) and even intrinsically generated spike doublets (figure 3.3). The intrinsic doublets are reminiscent of chattering/fast rhythmic bursting cells (see later). Afferent stimulation can evoke a large IPSP that suppresses current-induced firing for at least 50 ms, as is the case for basket cells.

For comparison with these basket and axo-axonic cell data, Whittington, Stanford et al (1997) made some similar measurements in physiologically identified interneurons in rat CA1 s. pyramidale and oriens; most likely, these cells were basket cells and axo-axonic cells. The action potentials lasted 0.6 ms at half amplitude; R_{input} was 38 ± 4 MΩ, the fast AHP amplitude was 9.8 $\pm$ 1.0 mV, and the mean decrease in firing rate, during injection of a steady depolarizing current, was 29%. Intrinsically generated doublets were never observed, so that the interneuronal doublets recorded during population oscillations, by Whittington, Stanford et al. were attributed to a combination of tonic excitation to give the first spike and AMPA receptor-mediated excitation to give the second spike in the doublet (see chapter 9).

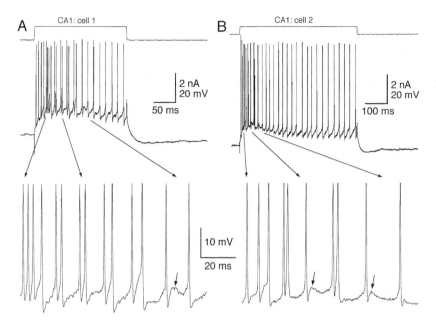

Figure 3.3
CA1 axo-axonic cells sometimes fire spike doublets as an intrinsic property during injection of a steady depolarizing current. The firing pattern of the two cells (A and B) illustrated is generally irregular. Arrows mark spike depolarizing afterpotentials (DAPs) that have failed to reach spike threshold. Only axo-axonic cells with such DAPs fired doublets. The membrane potential of these cells was −70 mV (A) and −71 mV (B). Action potentials are clipped in the bottom traces. (Figure courtesy of E. H. Buhl, from Buhl, Han et al., 1994 with permission)

Are the Dendrites of S. Pyramidale Interneurons Capable of Generating Action Potentials?

The issue of spike initiation in interneurons, as noted above, is critical for understanding interneuron doublets, which in turn, are necessary for one sort of long-range synchronization (chapter 9). We have described how in CA1 pyramidal cells, during orthodromic stimulation of limited amplitude, action potentials are initiated in the soma/IS (or in the axon) and propagate retrograde, even though the synaptic conductance is itself in the dendrites (Spruston, Schiller et al. 1995; figure 2.5 of chapter 2). In contrast, could action potentials be initiated in interneuron dendrites? If so, it might be relevant to the induction of doublet firing. This question has a long history, having been considered, for example, in axotomized motorneurons (Eccles, Libet, and Young 1958; Heyer and Llinás 1977; Kuno and Llinás 1970a,b; Traub and Llinás 1977). Additionally, there are precedents for dendritic action potential generation in mammalian neurons, with careful documentation using dual patch recording from single neurons in mitral cells in the olfactory bulb (Chen, Midtgaard, and Shepherd 1997).

The question of dendritic electrogenesis in hippocampal interneurons arose in the following way. Simultaneous intracellular recordings from pairs of CA3 pyramidal cells revealed in about 30% of cases that an action potential in one cell would evoke an IPSP in the other cell, with a latency as short as 4 or 5 ms or less and a failure rate less than 0.5 (Miles and Wong 1984; see also Traub and Miles 1991). This observation suggested that a single action potential could evoke an action potential in at least some CA3 interneurons. Miles (1990a) recorded from pyramidal cell/interneuron pairs (the interneurons being in s. pyramidale, probably basket cells and axo-axonic cells) and demonstrated directly several important facts: the AMPA receptor-mediated EPSP, produced by a single presynaptic action potential, in interneurons can be as large as 2 mV, has faster rise and decay times than the corresponding EPSP in CA3 pyramidal cells, and can evoke an action potential with latency 2 to 6 ms and probability 0.1 to 0.6. This latter property is called *spike transduction* (figure 3.4).

Spike transduction is rarely observed at synaptic connections between CA3 pyramidal cells (Traub and Miles 1991). Interestingly, it has been reported that Na channels in interneurons and pyramidal cells have similar kinetic properties in terms of activation, although deactivation and inactivation kinetics are different (Huguenard et

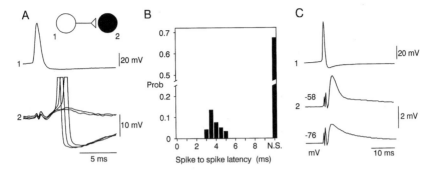

Figure 3.4
Properties of CA3 pyramidal cell → s. pyramidale interneuron synaptic connection: spike → spike transduction. (A) A single action potential in the presynaptic pyramidal cell (1) sometimes (3 instances out of 5 trials in this example) elicits an action potential in the postsynaptic interneuron. Note also the spike AHP in the interneuron. (B) Histogram of the latency from pyramidal cell spike to interneuron spike. The probability of spike transmission was about 0.3 (39 cases in 121 trials, stimulation at 1 Hz), with mean latency (spike peak to spike peak) of 3.1 ± 0.5 ms. N.S means no spike. (C) EPSPs in this particular connection increase in amplitude with depolarization of the interneuron, although at other similar connections the amplitude is decreased with depolarization. (From Traub and Miles, 1995 with permission)

al. 1988; Martina and Jonas 1997). Thus, it seems unlikely that the properties of Na channels per se could explain spike transduction, which would be primarily influenced by Na activation.

It was at first thought that the properties of the interneuron EPSP might be explicable by a somatic location of the synapse, but this assumption turns out to be false (see below). In addition, it is now known that the subunit composition of pentameric AMPA receptors is different in pyramidal cells than in interneurons (see next chapter), giving rise to larger single-channel conductances in interneurons and faster AMPA receptor kinetics, but this finding also by itself—at least in our view—is not sufficient to explain spike transduction in CA3 s. pyramidale interneurons. The problem is one of anatomy. It has been demonstrated in CA3 pyramidal cell/interneuron pairs, in which spike transduction occurs, that the synaptic connection can contain only one or two release sites, occurring on

A

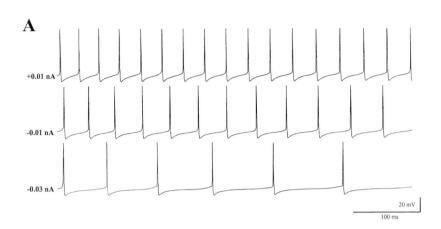

+0.01 nA

-0.01 nA

-0.03 nA

20 mV

100 ms

B

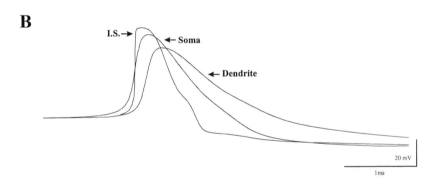

I.S.→   ← Soma

← Dendrite

20 mV

1 ms

C

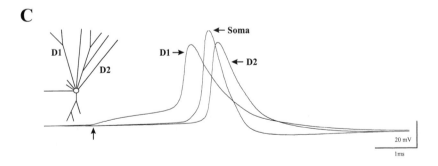

← Soma

D1   D1 →   ← D2

D2

20 mV

1 ms

dendrites, past branch points, and up to 200 μ away from the soma (Gulyás, Miles, Sik et al. 1993; Arancio et al. 1994; figure 3.4). In a compartmental axon/soma/dendritic model, having passive dendrites, with R_m of 50,000 $\Omega-$cm^2 (Thurbon et al. 1994), a huge (24 nS) dendritic EPSC evoked a spike at 6.5 ms latency, far longer than the experimentally observed latency (Traub and Miles 1995).

Spike transduction can be explained by a model in which the density of Na channels in the interneuron dendrites has a patch of 25–50 mS/cm^2 (Traub and Miles 1995). Figure 3.5 illustrates some of the properties of this model. First, the model interneuron fires repetitively in response to somatic current injection, with a small degree of adaptation and with fast-spike AHPs, all in agreement with experiment (figure 3.5A). During somatic current injection, action potentials are initiated in the soma/axon initial segment region and propagate retrograde into the dendrites (figure 3.5B). In contrast, provided the EPSC is large enough, a unitary EPSC into a single dendritic branch can initiate an action potential in that branch, which propagates to the soma and then back out to other branches (figure 3.5C). The threshold EPSC peak conductance was about 1.8 nS. Using somatic patch clamp, Arancio et al. (1994) estimated that the unitary EPSC was 0.2 to 0.5 nS, but the EPSC at the dendritic site is doubtless larger than this. Direct testing of the tenets of this model will probably require simultaneous somatic/dendritic patching in CA3 interneurons.

There are, however, some pieces of indirect evidence that action

Figure 3.5
Interneuron model with active dendritic electrogenesis. (A) The firing rate increases with tonic depolarization. Note also the spike AHP and the minimal adaptation. (B) Spikes induced by tonic somatic current injection are initiated in soma/*IS* and propagate to the dendrites. (*IS* is axon initial segment.) (C) An orthodromic spike is initiated in the dendrite of the EPSP (D1), propagates to the soma, and then to other dendrites (e.g., D2). The inset shows the structure of the model, with the axon projecting horizontally to the left from the soma (circle). (From Traub and Miles, 1995 with permission)

potentials might be initiated in the dendrites of interneurons. First, Freund, and Buzsáki (1996) have noted in a CA1 trilaminar interneuron that action potentials recorded at the soma can take off from different levels of the somatic membrane potential and can be initiated on the trailing phases of EPSPs, as if to indicate intitiation at a site distant from the soma. Second, hyperpolarization of the somata of hilar interneurons can reveal partial spikes, which could in turn be explicable by dendritic action potentials (Michelson and Wong 1994; Traub 1995). This latter issue will be considered further in chapter 6.

In the CA1 region, spike transduction (the causation of a postsynaptic spike by a single presynaptic action potential) is rare (E. Buhl, personal communication), although it can occur (Knowles and Schwartzkroin 1981, figure 4; Ali and Thomson 1998, figure 12). The reasoning above, concerning dendritic electrogenesis, does not, therefore, necessarily apply to CA1.

One critically important point is the following. We have been considering *unitary* EPSCs in interneurons, those evoked by a single action potential in a single presynaptic pyramidal neuron. In the CA1 region, single interneurons may be innervated by as many as 150 presynaptic pyramidal cells (E. Buhl, personal communication). If, as occurs during a synchronized population oscillation, all of these neurons were firing synchronously, the resulting EPSCs in interneurons would be large indeed. It is not unreasonable then to expect an action potential to be induced, even when the EPSCs arrive during the post-spike AHP and even in the absence of significant dendritic electrogenesis.

4

Synaptic Interactions in the Hippocampus

Neither population oscillations at gamma and beta frequencies nor most types of epileptic discharge persist in the absence of synaptic transmission. All of these phenomena emerge from the interactions between neurons, even as the intrinsic properties of the individual neurons contribute in interesting ways. For this reason, it is necessary to review how neurons communicate with each other. We shall concentrate on interactions between pyramidal cells, between interneurons, and between pyramidal cells and interneurons (and vice versa), focusing particularly on basket cells and axo-axonic cells. These are the synaptic interactions that, as of this writing, appear to be most critical for gamma oscillations. An earlier review of synaptic interactions in the hippocampus was included in the monograph of Traub and Miles (1991). The reader can also consult Bernard and Wheal (1994).

CA3 Pyramidal Cell → CA3 Pyramidal Cell

This connection has been analyzed with pair recordings (Miles and Wong 1986, 1987a; Traub and Miles 1991) and with computer simulations (Traub, Jefferys et al. 1994; figure 1). The unitary EPSP produced by a single presynaptic action potential ranges from 0.6 to 1.3 mV, with time to peak of 5–12 ms, significantly slower than the time to peak in s. pyramidale interneurons. The slow time to peak results

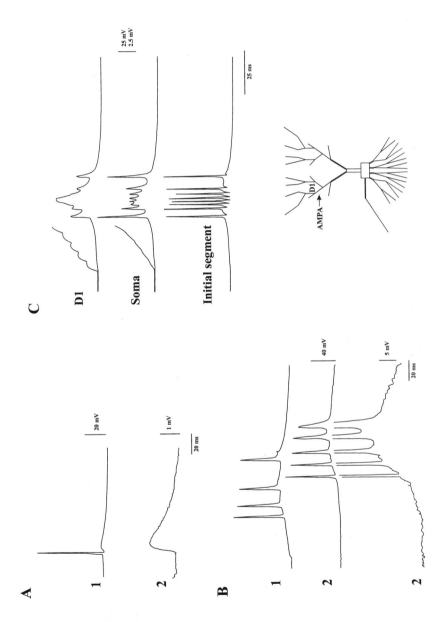

partly from filtering caused by the dendritic location of the synapse and partly because the EPSC itself is probably slower than in interneurons, owing to different subunit subcomposition of the respective AMPA receptors (see below). The probability of spike transduction at this synapse is low, about 5%. In contrast, a presynaptic burst can induce a postsynaptic burst with probability 0.3 to 0.5 and with a rather long latency, 8–30 ms from the first spike in the presynaptic burst to the first spike in the postsynaptic burst. Burst propagation can be explained in that there is a limited density of Na channels in the dendrites. In addition, a single EPSP does not depolarize the soma sufficiently to induce an action potential. Two or three EPSPs in a series, however, can temporally summate (thus giving the latency of tens of ms) and induce a brief series of back-propagating somatic spikes, which eventually induce a dendritic Ca spike and the burst depolarization in the postsynaptic cell (figure 4.1).

The connectivity between CA3 pyramidal neurons in the guinea-pig hippocampal slice has been estimated as about 2% (Traub and Miles 1991). Synaptic contacts are formed on both basal and apical dendrites, the contact site preferred depending on the location of the presynaptic cell (Li et al. 1993). Li et al. estimated that in the rat in vivo, one CA3 pyramidal cell contacted 30,000 to 60,000 other pyramidal cells, most of which, in general, would be CA1 cells. In

Figure 4.1
Properties of synaptic connections between two CA3 pyramidal cells. (A) Averaged EPSP (below) in response to a single presynaptic action potential (above). (B) A burst in a single presynaptic CA3 pyramidal cell (1) can induce a burst in a postsynaptic pyramidal cell (2, shown at two different gains). At this connection, the probability of burst transmission was about 0.3, stimulating at 0.5 Hz, and the latency from first spike to first spike varied from 12 to 30 ms. (C) A simulated presynaptic burst (5 EPSPs into site D1 in the apical dendrites, as in the inset below) leads to a smoothed EPSP at the soma and to action potentials that are initiated in the axon initial segment. These action potentials propagate into the dendrites and induce Ca^{2+} electrogenesis, with a resulting burst in the model pyramidal neuron. (A and B from Traub and Miles, 1991 with permission; C from Traub, Jefferys, Miles et al. 1994)

vivo, CA3 pyramidal cell axons can extend at least one-half the length of the hippocampus along the longitudinal axis (Tamamaki et al. 1984; Ishizuka et al. 1990). Physiological experiments in longitudinal slices indicate that the probability of synaptic contact falls off with distance (Miles, Traub, and Wong 1988).

CA3 Pyramidal Cell → CA3 Interneuron, S. Pyramidale

Spike transduction at this synapse can be explained by dendritic spike generation (see chapter 2), although this mechanism has not been confirmed by patch recording. Miles (1990a) characterized some of the functional properties of this synaptic connection. The unitary EPSP is 1–4 mV, with its peak at 1.5–4 ms. The probability of spike transmission is as high as 0.6, with a latency as short as 2.5 ms. Nevertheless, a high-frequency burst of 7 spikes in a presynaptic pyramidal cell may evoke only a single IPSP in a disynaptically inhibited second pyramidal cell: as if to imply that the pyramidal → interneuron synaptic connection can not sustain high-frequency spike transduction. In spite of this, at the level of subthreshold EPSPs, there is a striking facilitation of EPSP size during the course of a 3-spike presynaptic burst. In other words, facilitation can exist at the subthreshold level, but with depression at the spike level, a matter that could be of significance during population oscillations.

One way of reconciling these apparently contradictory observations is that: facilitation really does exist at the synaptic level, but once the interneuron actually fires, its deep AHP prevents unitary EPSPs from firing the cell again until the AHP wears off (R. Miles, personal communication). Of course, synchronized EPSPs, impinging from multiple pyramidal cells firing simultaneously, might be able to overwhelm the AHP and cause a second action potential at a brief interval. This mechanism would be in accord with the ability of afferent volleys in vivo to induce, at

least sometimes, doublet firing in interneurons (Buzsáki and Eidelberg 1982).

As noted in chapter 2, the local excitatory synaptic connection to
CA3 s. pyramidale interneurons is often mediated by a single dendritic release site. The s. pyramidale interneurons examined were
most often parvalbumin-positive, hence probably basket cells and
axo-axonic cells (Gulyás, Miles, Sik et al. 1993). Sik, Tamamaki, and
Freund (1993) studied the arborization of a single rat CA3 pyramidal cell axon in vivo. They also found that most connections to parvalbumin-positive interneurons were mediated by single contacts,
with 2.1% of the total 15,295 boutons (i.e., about 320) contacting
parvalbumin-positive cells. Although this number is a small percentage, it remains the case that a single pyramidal neuron excites
many parvalbumin-positive interneurons.

CA3 Interneuron → CA3 Pyramidal Cell

Miles (1990b) performed pair recordings of anatomically unidentified s. pyramidale interneurons connecting to nearby pyramidal
cells. Picrotoxin-sensitive, $GABA_A$ receptor-mediated IPSPs were
observed but not $GABA_B$ IPSPs. Unitary IPSPs ranged from 0.3 to
2.6 mV, with time to peak 3–10 ms. Each individual interneuron,
however, produced IPSPs of similar amplitude in different connected pyramidal cells. In retrospect, these findings may be a consequence of each interneuron's contacting particular regions of its
postsynaptic target cells. Connections with small IPSPs were associated with transmission failures but not connections with large
IPSPs. In some cases, repetitive firing of the interneuron was required to induce a consistent IPSP, as has been seen at certain connections in CA1 (Knowles and Schwartzkroin 1981; Lacaille and
Schwartzkroin 1988b). There was little correlation between intrinsic
properties of the interneuron (spike ½-width, AHP duration) and
the IPSP amplitude. Gulyás, Miles, Hajos, and Freund (1993)

showed that, in the CA3 region, s. pyramidale interneurons included basket cells and axo-axonic cells but also on occasion interneurons that innervated the dendrites of nearby pyramidal cells.

Miles et al. (1996) studied the synaptic interactions between single CA3 s. pyramidale interneurons and single CA3 pyramidal cells. The interneurons were classified as *perisomatic*, making synaptic contacts mostly in s. pyramidale, and *dendritic*, making synaptic contacts in basal or apical dendrites, or both. The perisomatic cells would have consisted of basket and possibly axo-axonic cells. The unitary IPSPs from perisomatic interneurons averaged 1.2 ± 0.5 mV, with time to peak 2.8 ± 1.0 ms and with duration at half-amplitude of 27 ± 11 ms. IPSPs produced by dendritic interneurons were slower. They averaged 1.0 ± 0.4 mV in amplitude, with time to peak 7.6 ± 2.2 ms and with duration at half-amplitude of 43 ± 7 ms. Single perisomatic interneurons formed 2–6 terminals on a pyramidal cell, the dendritic cell forming 5–17 terminals. Dendritic interneurons had a narrower horizontal spread of their axons than did interneurons contacting perisomatic regions, an apparent difference from CA1 (see below). A unitary IPSP from a perisomatic interneuron was able to suppress spike generation in a pyramidal cell, and as noted in chapter 2, dendritic inhibition (at least as evoked by extracellular stimulation) could suppress dendritic Ca^{2+} electrogenesis.

CA1 Pyramidal Cell → CA1 Pyramidal Cell

This connection has been examined by Deuchars and Thomson (1996), using pair recordings (figure 4.2). They found 9 monosynaptically connected pairs out of 989 tries, giving an in vitro connectivity of about 1%. At a resting membrane potential of -67 to -70 mV, the EPSP amplitude was 0.7 ± 0.5 mV, with a range 0.17 to 1.5 mV. The mean width at half-amplitude was 16.8 ± 4.1 ms. In one cell pair that was fully reconstructed, there were two synaptic con-

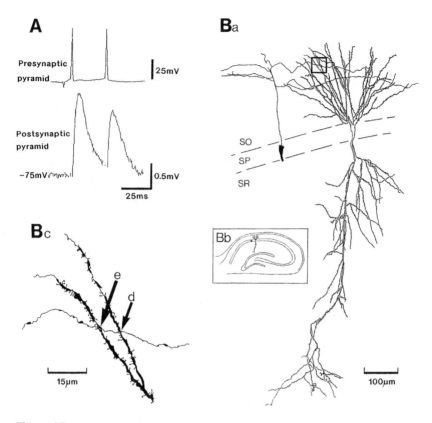

Figure 4.2
Properties of synaptic connections between CA1 pyramidal cells. (A) Average of 100 EPSP pairs in response to pairs of action potentials in the presynaptic neuron. There is paired pulse depression. (Ba) The presynaptic and postsynaptic neurons were filled with biocytin and reconstructed. The soma and axon of the presynaptic cell are shown on the left and the soma/dendrites of the postsynaptic cell on the right (location of the neurons in the slice is shown in Bb insert). Synaptic contacts occurred only in the boxed area. (Bc) There are two synaptic boutons from the presynaptic cell on third-order basal dendrites of the postsynaptic cell. These contacts were confirmed by electron microscopy. (From Deuchars and Thomson, 1996 with permission)

tacts, each on a third-order basal dendrite. The EPSPs had AMPA and NMDA receptor-mediated components. The synaptic connectivity does not appear to be random, in that nearby pyramidal cells can be presynaptic to the same pyramidal cell. Paired-pulse depression was found for EPSP amplitudes of 40–70% when interspike intervals were less than 20 ms, but there was less than 10% depression when the interspike intervals were 30–50 ms. Other investigators have found evidence for CA1 pyramidal cell interconnectivity, using more indirect means (Christian and Dudek 1988; Crépel, Khazipov, and Ben-Ari 1997; Traynelis and Dingledine 1988; Jensen and Yaari 1997; Whittington, Traub et al. 1997; see also chapter 10).

CA1 Pyramidal Cell → CA1 Interneuron

A unitary EPSP onto an anatomically identified CA1 basket cell is illustrated by Buhl, Halasy, and Somogyi (1994). It is rare for a single pyramidal cell action potential in vitro to induce firing in a CA1 s. pyramidale interneuron, unlike the case in CA3 (E. Buhl, personal communication). A disproportionate number of CA1 pyramidal cell synaptic connections are made onto nearby interneurons, about 50%, even though interneurons form only about 10% of the total neuronal population (E. Buhl, personal communication). The anatomy of a CA1 pyramidal cell → basket cell connection has been studied in detail, and only one release site (in the alveus) was found (Buhl, Halasy, and Somogyi 1994), similar to the corresponding situation in CA3 (Gulyás, Miles, Sik et al. 1993).

The properties of the CA1 pyramidal cell → basket cell connection have also been studied in seven cases, with dual intracellular recordings by Ali, Deuchars et al. (1998). These latter authors found a wide range of unitary EPSP sizes, from 0.15 to 3.6 mV; the rise times of the EPSPs were 0.4 to 1.6 ms, with half-widths 2.2 to 9.7 ms. Failure rates ranged from 0 to 49% at different connections; the zero-failure rate that could occur is interesting, in view of the single release site. It was estimated that 1 in 22 nearby CA1 pyramidal cells contacted a given basket cell. The synaptic connection exhibited depression with repetitive firing of the pyramidal neuron when spike intervals were 15 to 30 ms.

CA1 Basket Cell → CA1 Pyramidal Cell

There are about 25 basket cell inputs per CA1 pyramidal cell (Buhl et al. 1994). Further data from Buhl, Cobb, Halasy and Somogyi (1995) on this connection are as follows. About half of the synaptic contacts are on the soma and half on the dendrites (usually < 60 microns from soma). The number of pyramidal cell synapses formed by a single presynaptic basket cell ranged from 10 to 12 in two examples. In the slice, about 7,000 pyramidal cells were estimated to be in the axonal field of a single basket cell, of which about 13% of the pyramidal cells were innervated. It has been estimated that in vivo one basket cell contacts about 1,140 pyramidal cells (Halasy, Buhl et al. 1996). Li et al. (1992) estimated that 1,200 pyramidal cells were contacted in vivo, a similar figure.

An example of a CA1 basket cell → CA1 pyramidal cell pair is shown in figures 4.3 and 4.4. Following Buhl, Cobb et al. (1995), we note that, at the CA1 basket cell → CA1 pyramidal cell connection, failures are rare. The unitary IPSP averages 0.45 mV at -58 mV, with a 10–90% rise time of 4.6 ± 3.2 ms and with a 31.6 ± 18.2 ms duration at half-amplitude (figure 4.3). The IPSPs involve GABA$_A$ receptors, and have a τ_{decay} of the voltage of 32.4 ± 18 ms. Unitary IPSPs can be larger than 2 mV. The IPSPs reverse at -74.9 ± 6.0 mV. The unitary conductance was 0.95 ± 0.29 nS. Up to 4 IPSPs in a rapid train summate, an issue that will be of importance in long-range synchronized gamma oscillations when interneurons fire doublets with short interspike intervals and when both IPSPs must be faithfully transmitted (chapter 9). If the high-frequency IPSP train continues, the summated IPSPs decline to a steady-state value; Buhl

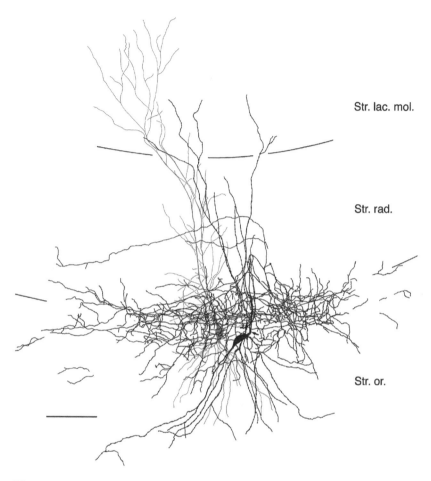

Str. lac. mol.

Str. rad.

Str. or.

Figure 4.3
The CA1 basket cell → pyramidal cell synaptic connection: morphology. Light microscopic reconstruction of a synaptically connected and intracellularly labeled cell pair. Both cells were identified due to their distinctive firing patterns (figure 4.4). The basket cell has soma on the right (spines not shown), and the pyramidal cell soma is on the left. The basket cell axon emerged from the soma (arrow) and ramified densely within the cell body layer and adjacent portions of stratum radiatum (Str. rad.) and stratum oriens (Str. or.). The borders between cell layers are indicated by solid lines. Following analysis with the light microscope, the synaptic target profile of the inhibitory cell was assessed by means of random electron microscopic bouton sampling. From a total of 61 labelled boutons, 29 (48%) were found to be in synaptic contact with somata, 2 (3%) on spines, and the remaining 31 (49%) formed synapses with dendrites. Scale bar: 100 μm. (Figure kindly provided by E. H. Buhl; from Buhl, Cobb et al., 1995 with permission of Blackwell Science)

et al. interpreted this decline to result from presynaptic $GABA_B$ receptors (see also Davies et al. 1990). During repetitive firing of the interneuron at low frequencies, the unitary IPSPs decreased in amplitude, even in a 1–3 Hz frequency range. A post-IPSP depolarization was noted, averaging 0.21 mV and peaking at 130 ± 33 ms after the presynaptic spike (i.e., theta frequency rather than gamma—see also Cobb et al. 1995). A similar post-IPSP overshoot was also described by Miles and Wong (1984) in the CA3 region.

CA1 Axo-axonic Cell → CA1 Pyramidal Cell

One CA1 axo-axonic cell contacts approximately 686 CA1 pyramidal cells in a 400 micron-thick slice (Buhl et al. 1994) and about 1,200 pyramidal cells in vivo (Li et al. 1992). Synaptic contacts are formed exclusively on the axon initial segment and apparently only on the initial segment of pyramidal cells, with interneurons being avoided as targets. There are at least 3 boutons per connection (Buhl et al. 1994). Axo-axonic cells can be feed-forward excited by afferent fibers and can also be synaptically inhibited, exhibiting both $GABA_A$ and $GABA_B$ IPSPs. An anatomically characterized axo-axonic cell → dentate granule cell pair was studied by Buhl, Halasy, and Somogyi (1994). The unitary IPSPs were of rapid onset, average amplitude 0.46 mV, maximum amplitude 2 mV, and reversal at -78 mV.

CA1 Interneuron → CA1 Pyramidal Cell Dendrites

There are many sorts of interneurons besides basket cells and axo-axonic cells (Freund and Buzsáki 1996), including bistratified cells, oriens/lacunosum-moleculare cells (o/lm), and others with cell body in s. radiatum and s. lacunosum-moleculare. The anatomy of bistratified cells has been described by Halasy, Buhl, Lörinczi et al. 1996: at least some of the cell bodies lie in s. pyramidale. The axons contact dendritic shafts and spines of pyramidal cells in s. oriens

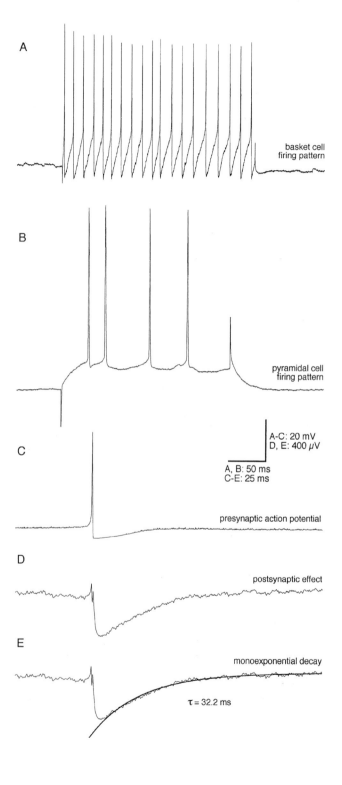

A — basket cell firing pattern

B — pyramidal cell firing pattern

A-C: 20 mV
D, E: 400 µV

A, B: 50 ms
C-E: 25 ms

C — presynaptic action potential

D — postsynaptic effect

E — monoexponential decay

τ = 32.2 ms

and s. radiatum, although a given bistratified cell may prefer one lamina or the other. The axonal field of bistratified cells averages 1,250 microns in the plane of the slice, longer than for basket cells (average 760 microns). Unlike basket cells, the dendrites of bistratified cells rarely reach to s. lacunosum-moleculare; presumably bistratified cells do not receive input from the entorhinal cortex (perforant path), although basket cells do receive such input. This observation could be relevant during the theta rhythm in vivo, which is prominent in the entorhinal cortex. The synaptic boutons of bistratified cells are smaller than the boutons of basket cells, perhaps reflecting a smaller release probability.

Differences in Kinetics of GABA$_A$ IPSCs in Soma Versus Apical Dendrites of CA1 Pyramidal Cells

Using a variety of techniques, including extracellular stimulation in different laminae and focal applications of bicuculline, Pearce (1993) determined that there were two types of GABA$_A$ synaptic responses in CA1 pyramidal neurons, both bicuculline-sensitive: a fast one near the soma (decay time constant 4.0 ± 0.8 ms at -80 to -100 mV) and a slow one in the apical dendrites (decay time constant 39.2 ± 5.8 ms at -80 to -100 mV). Both responses decay more slowly at

Figure 4.4
The CA1 basket cell → pyramidal cell synaptic connection: physiological properties of the cell pair illustrated in Figure 4.3. (A) The presynaptic cell is fast-spiking, firing nonaccommodating trains of action potentials, which are followed by deep, fast AHPs (fAHPs). (B) The postsynaptic neuron exhibits physiological characteristics of pyramidal cells, including a marked spike-frequency adaptation and action potentials followed by comparatively small fAHPs. (C) The presynaptic cell was depolarized until it fired single action potentials. (D) Spike-triggered averaging techniques revealed a short-latency IPSP in the postsynaptic cell. (E) The decay phase of the unitary IPSP could be adequately fitted with a single exponential function, $\tau = 32.2$ ms. Both cells were identified anatomically using biocytin injections and are shown in figure 4.3 (Kindly provided by E. H. Buhl; from Buhl, Cobb et al., 1995 with permission of Blackwell Science)

depolarized potentials. This result is similar, at least qualitatively, to results in CA3 based on interneuron/pyramidal cell pair recordings (Miles et al. 1996), and one interpretation could also be similar: dendritic IPSPs are specialized for suppression of g_{Ca}, while perisomatic IPSPs suppress Na spike generation. It has also been shown, however, that dendritic IPSPs in CA1 pyramidal neurons can regulate the back-propagation of Na spikes into the apical dendrites (Tsubokawa and Ross 1996).

Anatomy of CA1 Interneuron → Interneuron Connections

The anatomy of interneuron → interneuron connections is important for our purposes because pharmacologically isolated networks of interneurons can generate gamma oscillations (chapter 8), and considerable evidence indicates that the oscillation emerges from mutual synaptic inhibition between the interneurons. In vivo, one CA1 basket cell was found to contact 64 parvalbumin-positive (PV) interneurons, mostly via a single bouton on the soma or proximal dendrites (Sik, Penttonen et al. 1995). Using data from these studies (Wang and Buzsáki 1996), the in vivo density of CA1 basket cell/basket cell connectivity (locally) has been estimated to be about 10%. GAD-immunoreactive boutons abut on the somata of PV-immunoreactive cells in CA3 and CA1, mostly in s. pyramidale and oriens (Fukuda, Aika et al. 1996), providing further anatomical evidence for interneuron → interneuron connections. Most of the boutons so abutting were themselves PV immunoreactive. Such boutons are not much reduced in number by disconnection of the septum, so that they probably originate from other hippocampal interneurons. It was concluded that connectivity is particularly dense between parvalbumin-positive cells (especially in CA3), but there is also connectivity to and from other interneuron types. There is, however, one exception: axo-axonic cells do not inhibit other interneurons, according to anatomical studes (Buhl, Han et al. 1994).

One complication in applying these data in a straightforward way to basket cells is that there are probably two types of basket cell, parvalbumin-positive and CCK (cholecystokinin), with PV cells innervating each other, and CCK cells innervating each other. CCK basket cells may have their somata in layers other than in s. pyramidale, especially s. radiatum.

Interneuron Pairs

Cobb, Halasy, et al. (1997) studied the anatomy and physiology of 4 interneuron/interneuron pairs in CA1. In two cases, the presynaptic cell was a basket cell. In the first of these cases, the postsynaptic cell was also a basket cell (figure 4.5). The unitary IPSPs evoked in the postsynaptic basket cell averaged 0.25 mV at −59 mV membrane potential, with 1.3 ms time to peak and duration 27 ms at half-amplitude. In the second case, the postsynaptic interneuron was a bistratified cell (with axonic contacts to basal and apical dendrites of pyramidal neurons). In this case, 12 synaptic contacts were made on the soma and proximal dendrites of the bistratified cell. The unitary IPSPs were 0.37 mV at −55 mV membrane potential, with time to peak 1 ms. The IPSPs lasted only 5.6 ms at half-amplitude.

Autapses on Interneurons

In cat visual cortex, basket cells (as well as dendrite-targeting interneurons) contact synaptically their own dendrites with multiple release sites (12 ± 7 in the case of basket cells) (Tamás, Buhl, and Somogyi 1997). The possibility of such autapses must be considered in the hippocampus as well.

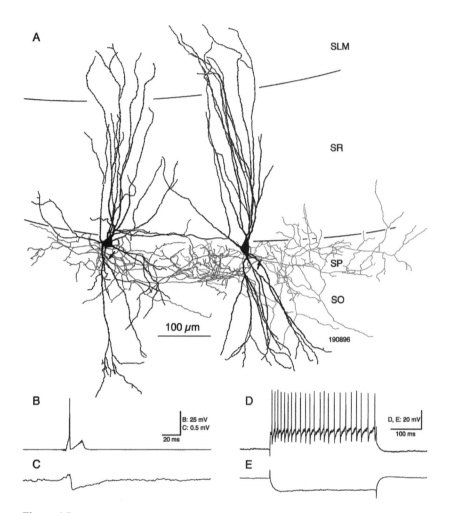

Figure 4.5
The CA1 basket cell → basket cell synaptic connection: light microscopic reconstruction and physiological characterization of a cell pair in the rat. (A) Light microscopic drawing shows two smooth-dendritic local circuit neurons having the characteristic morphological features of basket cells, such as a convoluted axon densely innervating s. pyramidale (SP), as well as portions of adjoining s. radiatum (SR) and s. oriens (SO). The presynaptic cell is on the left. While both dendritic arbors were reconstructed in entirety, the respective axonal arbors are illustrated from only two adjacent 60 μm sections. Furthermore, only those portions of axon are represented that could be followed back to the parent soma. Synaptic coupling was revealed

Further Data on the Kinetics of IPSCs in Interneurons

Whittington et al. (1995b) measured the kinetics of population IPSCs in physiologically identified CA1 interneurons (probably basket cells or axo-axonic cells) during gamma oscillations. The oscillations were evoked by pressure ejection of glutamate during pharmacological blockade of ionotropic glutamate receptors, hence by activation of metabotropic glutamate receptors (see chapter 8). The decay time constant of these synchronized IPSCs was 9.1 ± 0.4 ms, with a range of 8–15 ms.

Molecular and Biophysical Aspects of AMPA Receptors

Different sorts of AMPA receptors vary in a number of properties, including kinetics, rectification, and Ca permeability. There are notable differences between AMPA receptors on principal cells and most AMPA receptors on interneurons. A technical consideration in this field is that synaptic potentials in intact neurons (including AMPA and $GABA_A$ receptor-mediated) often relax with a time constant close to the membrane time constant, a consequence of embedding of the receptors in the extended somatodendritic cables. It is possible to determine the time course of the actual receptor-mediated conductance more accurately in outside-out patches, us-

by evoking single action potentials in the presynaptic basket neuron (B) and concomitantly monitoring the evoked response in the postsynaptic neuron. In the average (C: n = 828 sweeps), it is apparent that presynaptic firing elicited short-latency hyperpolarizing IPSPs with fast kinetics. In response to depolarizing current pulses (D: 300 ms, 1.1 nA), the postsynaptic basket cell fired a weakly accommodating train of short-duration action potentials. Injection of hyperpolarizing current pulses revealed a small degree of time-dependent inward rectification (E). SLM, stratum lacunosum-moleculare. Scale bar: 100 μm. (Figure courtesy of E. Buhl, from Cobb, Halasy, Vida et al., 1997 with permission)

ing fast application of the agonist and possibly also of modulatory drugs. Some disadvantages of this technique are that the receptors studied are likely to be extrasynaptic and that the measurements often are taken at room temperature, leading to overestimates of time constants. Outside-out patches have been combined with single-cell RT-PCR (reverse-transcriptase polymerase chain reaction), often in the same cell, to study correlations between receptor kinetics and receptor subunit composition (Bochet et al. 1994; Geiger et al. 1995; Jonas and Monyer, in press). With outside-out patch, the deactivation time constant of the synaptic current is defined to be the decay τ after a short (e.g., 1 ms) agonist application; the desensitization time constant is the decay τ after a prolonged agonist application (e.g., 100 ms) (figure 4.6 and table 4.1).

Some specific details from these studies (Geiger et al. 1995) are the following. AMPA receptors on interneurons (compared with principal cells) appear to have a larger single-channel conductance (Haverkampf et al. 1997), as well as a larger physiologically activated conductance (Arancio et al. 1994). The upstroke of the EPSC is faster in interneurons, with the EPSC deactivating and desensitizing more rapidly and more completely. AMPA receptors on interneurons tend to be Ca^{2+}-permeable, although one type of interneuron in hippocampal stratum lacunosum-moleculare has been found in which different pathways activate either Ca^{2+}-permeable or Ca^{2+}-impermeable AMPA receptors (Tóth and McBain 1997); in contrast, AMPA receptors in pyramidal cells are Ca^{2+}-impermeable. The current-voltage relation of principal cell AMPA receptors, in Na-rich solutions, is more linear (less rectifying) than for interneurons. Present data suggest that the presence of a single GluR-B subunit (also called GluR-2) in the AMPA receptor pentamer is sufficient to render the receptor impermeable to Ca^{2+}; and the presence of GluR-D (GluR-4) subunit(s) probably results in faster kinetics than when this subunit is absent.

Table 4.1
Properties of AMPA receptors in a principal neuron and in an inhibitory neuron

	Deacti-vation τ	Desensi-tization τ	P_{Ca}/P_{Na}	flip GluR A/B/C/D (%)	flop GluR A/B/C/D (%)
CA3 pyramidal cell	3 ms	15.2 ms	0.10	45/36/ND/0	8/8/ND/0
DG basket cell	1.4 ms	5.5 ms	1.59	6/4/ND/0	59/8/ND/13

Kinetic measurements at 20–24° C; ND, not determined; "flip" and "flop" represent alternate splice variants.
Data from Geiger et al., 1995.

NMDA Receptors

Besides AMPA receptors, both principal neurons (Ascher, Breges-tovski, and Nowak 1988; Hestrin et al. 1990; McBain and Dingledine 1992) and interneurons (Sah, Hestrin, and Nicoll 1990; Traub, Jefferys, and Whittington 1994) contain NMDA receptors. These receptors are notable for their slow kinetics (Forsythe and Westbrook 1988), Ca^{2+} permeability (Alford et al. 1993), gating by transmembrane voltage and Mg^{2+} concentration (Ascher et al. 1988; Mayer, Westbrook, and Guthrie 1984; Jahr and Stevens 1990), and regulation by a number of modulatory substances, including glycine (Forsythe, Westbrook, and Mayer 1988). The 10–90% rise time of the NMDA conductance was measured as 4.5–16 ms in CA1 pyramidal cells (whole-cell recordings), and 9.1 ms in s. moleculare interneurons. The decay time constants were (fast and slow, respectively) 66.5 and 354 ms for CA1 pyramidal cells and 34 and 212 ms for CA1 s. moleculare interneurons, i.e., slower in the pyramidal cells than in the interneurons (Perouansky and Yaari 1993). In outside-out patches taken from CA1 and CA3 pyramidal neurons, recorded at 20–24°C, the NMDA current had an exponential rising phase with

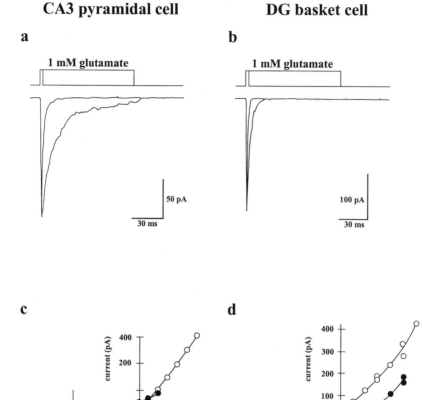

CA3 pyramidal cell   DG basket cell

Figure 4.6
AMPA receptors in principal cells versus interneurons: kinetics, Ca permeability, and rectification. Data are from outside-out patches, pulled from the soma and studied at room temperature. (a, b) 1 ms and 100 ms pulses of glutamate were applied in Na⁺ rich solutions to activate inward currents. Relaxation from the fast pulse indicates deactivation and from the slow pulse desensitization. Both processes are slower in the pyramidal cell than in the interneuron. (c, d) Current-voltage (I-V) curves for peak glutamate-activated currents, recorded in Na⁺–rich extracellular

time constant 7 ms, and the decay time constants were about 200 ms (first 80% of the decay), and 1–3 seconds for the remainder of the decay (Spruston, Jonas, and Sakmann 1995). NMDA receptors do not appear to be critical for the generation of either gamma or beta oscillations but are of course central in certain experimental models of epilepsy. Some of these models will be considered in the next chapter. NMDA receptors are also required for some, but not all, types of synaptic plasticity (Malenka and Nicoll 1993). Molecular aspects of NMDA receptors, including subunit composition and its correlation with functional properties, are reviewed in Jonas and Monyer (in press).

Depolarizing GABA$_A$ Potentials

Both principal neurons (reviewed in Stelzer 1992) and interneurons (Michelson and Wong 1991) sometimes exhibit depolarizing responses mediated by bicuculline-and picrotoxin-sensitive GABA$_A$ receptors. Depolarizing GABA responses are especially likely to occur in neurons from immature animals, as in the first week or so postnatally in the rat hippocampus (Ben-Ari et al. 1989). Hyperpolarizing GABA$_A$ conductances exhibit greater Cl$^-$ permeability than HCO$_3{}^-$ permeability, while the reverse is true for the depolarizing GABA$_A$ conductance (Perkins and Wong 1996). In CA1 pyramidal cells, these responses are more likely to be found in the apical dendrites than at the soma (Lambert, Borroni et al. 1991). Wong and Watkins (1982) were, however, able to

solution (○) and in Ca^{2+}−rich solution (●). In Na$^+$−rich solution, the I-V relation of the pyramidal cell is almost linear but not in the interneuron. Arrows indicate the reversal potential of glutamate-activated current in Ca^{2+}−rich solution. For the pyramidal cell, this reversal potential is not far from the K$^+$ reversal potential, indicating that these AMPA receptors are not permeable to Ca^{2+}. In contrast, in the basket cell, this reversal potential is far from the K$^+$ reversal potential, indicating that these AMPA receptors are permeable to Ca^{2+}. (From Geiger et al., 1995 with permission)

evoke both hyperpolarizing and depolarizing $GABA_A$ responses in hippocampal pyramidal neurons by spritzing GABA onto both soma and dendrites. It is possible, but not proven, that the subunit composition of depolarizing $GABA_A$ receptors is somehow different than the compositions of hyperpolarizing receptors and that the depolarizing $GABA_A$ receptors—as may also be true of metabotropic $GABA_B$ receptors (Dutar and Nicoll 1988a)—are extrasynaptic, at least in mature animals. Notably, single interneurons have so far failed to elicit either depolarizing $GABA_A$ or $GABA_B$ responses in postsynaptic neurons, even after repetitive activation. If the receptors are indeed extrasynaptic, then their activation would be enhanced under conditions when interneurons fire synchronously and so might release sufficient GABA to spill over to extrasynaptic sites, a scenario that appears to occur in the presence of the drug 4–aminopyridine (4–AP) (see later chapters).

More on Metabotropic Glutamate Receptors

In chapter 2, we discussed some of the actions of metabotropic glutamate receptors on pyramidal cells and described how these actions might prime the cells for participation in oscillations. Here, we shall present further data on the effects of metabotropic glutamate receptors on synaptic transmission and on their classification and biochemical mechanisms.

At least eight types of metabotropic glutamate receptor (mGluR) have been described in the mammalian CNS. These receptors exist on excitatory and inhibitory neurons, both pre- and postsynaptically, and on glial cells. Receptor types have been classified into three groups on the basis of effector mechanisms and of pharmacological sensitivity.

Group I mGluRs consist of receptor types mGluR1a and mGluR5. These receptors are coupled to a G-protein (Gq/11), which activates phospholipase C. The resulting production of 1,2–diacylglycerol (DAG) and inositol-(1,4,5)-triphosphate (IP3) activates protein kinase C and releases calcium ions from the endoplasmic reticulum, respectively (Sharon et al. 1997; Abdul-Ghani et al. 1996). Protein kinase C further inhibits potassium channels but may also serve to desensitize group I mGluRs via phosphorylation, so as to prevent excessive receptor activation (Alaluf et al. 1995).

Groups II and III metabotropic glutamate receptors consist of types mGluR2–4 and mGluR6–7. They share a common effector system in G_i/G_o- dependent inhibition of adenyl cyclase activity (Prezeau et al. 1992). Activation of these receptors also dissociates the alpha subunit of G_i/G_o, which may in turn directly inhibit voltage-dependent Ca^{2+} channels (Chavis et al. 1994; Choi and Lovinger 1996).

Location

In the hippocampus, the distribution of types of metabotropic glutamate receptors is highly delineated. The predominantly excitatory Group I receptors are found exclusively on postsynaptic membranes (Martin et al. 1992). The types mGluR1 and mGluR5 are found mainly on dendrites but sometimes also on the somata, of pyramidal cells (Lujan et al. 1996). At the synaptic level, these receptors have a particular distribution around the edge of the postsynaptic membrane specialization, forming an annulus approximately 100 nm wide (Lujan et al. 1997). Group II and III mGluRs are found mainly presynaptically in the hippocampus (Ohishi et al. 1994, 1995). In addition, it has been suggested that there may be a synapse-specific distribution of group III mGluRs. Presynaptic concentrations of mGluR7 have been shown to be somehow related to the postsynaptic concentration of type I mGluRs (Shigemoto et al. 1996). These observations suggest the possibility that metabotropic receptors modulate the ionotropic glutamatergic excitation of hippocampal pyramidal cells and interneurons.

Receptor-Mediated Responses

The spatial distribution of metabotropic glutamate receptors has important implications for the control of synaptic activity. Single EPSPs are attenuated by activation of mGluRs (Manzoni and Bockaert 1995; Kamiya et al. 1996). This effect appears to be mediated by decreased transmitter release caused by activation of presynaptic receptors (Baskys and Malenka 1991). These group II/III mGluRs operate by inhibition of presynaptic voltage-gated Ca^{2+} channels (Takahashi et al. 1996) and by calcium-independent mechanisms (Scanziani et al. 1995). Some researchers, however, have suggested an inhibitory role for presynaptic group I mGluRs (Choi and Lovinger 1996). In contrast, repeated activation of excitatory synapses in the presence of mGluR agonists results in an augmentation of excitatory synaptic transmission. Paired pulse facilitation, or a decrease in paired pulse inhibition of EPSPs, are seen in the presence of the broad-spectrum mGluR agonist (1S,3R)-ACPD. Although postsynaptic mGluRs potentiate EPSPs via a $[Ca^{2+}]_i$-dependent mechanism (Bortolotto and Collingridge 1995), the group I postsynaptic mGluRs appear not to be involved in paired-pulse facilitation (Brown and Reyman 1995).

Similar effects of mGluR agonists are seen on GABAergic IPSPs. Activation of both group I and group II/III mGluRs together results in an increase in the spontaneous activity of interneurons but also attenuates the amplitude of evoked IPSCs (Jouvenceau et al. 1995). The decrease in IPSC amplitude has been reported to be caused by activation of Group II/III receptors located presynaptically on inhibitory terminals, whereas the increase in spontaneous activity is caused by depolarization of interneurons via activation of group I somatodendritic mGluRs (Poncer et al. 1995). The nature of this somatodendritic effect on interneurons is that of a slow depolarization, which can be induced by repetitive (tetanic) synaptic stimulation (Miles and Poncer 1993; Poncer and Miles 1995). The degree of depolarization appears to depend on the type of interneuron stimulated, with some interneurons responding with dramatic depolarization, while others respond more modestly (McBain et al. 1994).

A consequence of these effects on EPSPs and IPSPs is that activation of mGluRs favors postsynaptic responses to repetitive high-frequency synaptic activation over irregular low-frequency activation. In essence, mGluRs filter out occasional synaptic events, while favoring rhythmic activity at frequencies of tens of Hz and higher. It is also interesting to note that this repetitive pattern of excitatory synaptic activity is also far more likely to activate mGluRs in the first place: the annular arrangement of mGluRs at glutamatergic synapses suggests that rapid, repeated activation would be most likely to cause enough glutamate overspill from the synaptic cleft to facilitate binding to mGluRs. Activation of mGluRs in area CA3 of the hippocampus generates rhythmic 8–27 Hz synchronized oscillations in pyramidal cells (Taylor et al. 1995). These oscillations are synchronized by AMPA receptors and occur as a consequence of metabotropic activation facilitating the repetitive engagement of recurrent excitatory synaptic connections. Similar phenomena can be seen with IPSPs after metabotropic stimulation of hippocampal CA1 and the superficial layers of the neocortex (Whittington et al. 1997; see also chapter 8). Strong depolarization of inhibitory interneurons following tetanic stimulation leads to trains of IPSPs that can be synchronized at gamma frequencies (Miles and Poncer 1993; Whittington et al. 1995b).

The relationship between mGluRs and repetitive synaptic activation of neurons has consequences for the effects of these receptors on synaptic plasticity and on epileptiform activity. Activation of mGluRs with ACPD produces a slow-onset, long-term potentiation of excitatory synaptic transmission (Bortolotto and Collingridge 1995), consisting of an augmentation of postsynaptic AMPA receptor-mediated EPSPs. These authors reported no involvement of inhibitory transmission in this phenomenon, but similar activation of mGluRs has been reported to produce long-term depression of GABAergic synaptic transmission (Liu et al. 1993). This long-term enhancement of excitation, together with depression of inhibition, would be expected to favor epileptiform activity. Indeed, intracerebral injection of group I mGluR agonists causes limbic seizures in vivo (Monn et al. 1996), and in disinhibited hippocampal slices, activation of group I mGluRs promotes ictal activity (Merlin and Wong 1997). Monn et al. (1996) found, in contrast, that seizures could be blocked by agonists at mGluR II/III receptors. Somewhat confusingly, in disinhibited hippocampal slices, agonists at mGluR II/III receptors increase the frequency of interictal bursts (Merlin, Taylor, and Wong 1995). In other preparations, including the neocortex in vitro and the isolated perfused brain, a seizure-reducing effect of ACPD has been reported (Burke and Hablitz 1994; Federico and MacVicar 1996).

5

Networks of Pyramidal Cells: Synchronized Bursts

The most compelling reason for studying epilepsy is the relief of human suffering caused by the disorder. Yet, it is also true that research on experimental epilepsy has led to, or at least facilitated, considerable progress in understanding the normal brain. Experiments concerning dendritic burst generation, the roles of excitatory synaptic connections between pyramidal cells, and the structure and function of GABA receptors and NMDA receptors have all been motivated, at least in part, by the need to understand epilepsy.

The temporally extended synchronization of cell firing that occurs during seizures is considered pathological: normal brain function is disrupted; threshold may be lowered for the generation of future seizures; and neuronal injury or death can result. In spite of this pathology, epilepsy serves not only to motivate cellular and molecular studies but also to act as a model system for understanding certain normal brain activities, which require populations to fire synchronously and rhythmically. Such brain activities include the generation of the manifold sorts of population oscillations of which the brain is capable, including gamma and beta waves. Furthermore, seizures—or at least one sort of experimental seizure—are easier to analyze than other population oscillations because of the absence of synaptic inhibition in the experiments, so that only excitatory synaptic interactions (and intrinsic cell properties) need be addressed.

As will be discussed in later chapters, repetitive (tetanic) stimulation of the hippocampal slice can induce an epoch of gamma oscillation. Tetanic stimulation at higher intensity can evoke an epoch of gamma followed by an epoch of beta (10–25 Hz) oscillations, and still higher intensity can evoke the sequence $\gamma \to \beta \to$ {one or more synchronized bursts}, that is, an epileptiform event (see figure P.2). Clearly, these various phenomena are related, and we can not hope to understand one without understanding the others.

One of the most important aspects of epileptogenesis is that the form of cortical seizures is usually stereotyped, even though many different sorts of network parameter alterations can be used experimentally to induce the seizure. Thus, one can block $GABA_A$ receptors, unblock NMDA receptors (by reducing extracellular Mg^{2+}), or increase nonspecifically action-potential-induced transmitter release and spontaneous synaptic noise (as happens in 4AP and elevated $[K^+]_o$). We have previously analyzed diverse experimental epilepsies in order to highlight the underlying physical principles that these (and perhaps other) experimental models share (Traub, Borck et al. 1996). Probably, none of these models perfectly captures what happens in the one or two seconds after strong tetanus. The enhancement of EPSPs that occurs after a strong tetanus, together with the persistence of IPSPs, might suggest that the 4AP and high $[K^+]_o$ models are the most relevant ones for a book on oscillations (Rutecki et al. 1985, 1987; Korn et al. 1987; Chamberlin et al. 1990; Perreault and Avoli 1991, 1992). Caution is in order, however, as almost all of this epilepsy work was done in CA3, wherein EPSPs are, under baseline conditions, relatively large and the pyramidal/ pyramidal connectivity extensive, whereas in vitro hippocampal gamma oscillations are most often studied in CA1, where baseline EPSPs are smaller and less plentiful.

We shall consider in this chapter a range of epilepsy models that we believe are relevant to the epileptogenesis that can arise shortly after tetanic stimulation: the disinhibition model because it is the best understood and because different types of synchronization are expressed within this single model; changes in polysynaptic circuitry produced by tetanic stimulation; certain features of 4AP epileptogenesis; synchronized oscillations produced in CA3 by metabotropic receptor activation, either glutamate or muscarinic. These epilepsy models are defined in terms of the pharmacological or other manipulations that are brought to bear on neuronal tissue, so as to induce one or more synchronized bursts in series. But synchronized bursts are not all identical in the details of their structure or in their mechanisms of generation. We need to consider three sorts of synchronized burst:

1. bursts that arise in a population of pyramidal cells that are in a resting state, wherein bursting in one or a few cells sets off a chain reaction of bursting that spreads throughout the population;

2. bursts that arise in a population of neurons whose dendrites are intensively depolarized, and so are prone to generate trains of intrinsic dendritic bursts (chapter 2, figures 2.2 and 2.3);

3. bursts that arise in a population of neurons, at rest or hyperpolarized, in which there is a continuous barrage of spontaneous EPSPs, but in which inhibitory interneurons are also functional.

The Epileptic Chain Reaction

We know that monosynaptically connnected CA3 pyramidal cells exhibit burst transduction, the ability of a burst in the presynaptic cell to induce a burst in the postsynaptic cell, with latency in the tens of ms and probability 0.3 to 0.5 (Miles and Wong 1986, 1987a; Traub and Miles 1991; chapter 4). In addition, the probability of connection between two CA3 pyramidal cells is in the slice about 2%, so that within a population of thousands of pyramidal cells, any given pyramidal should contact scores of others. With a burst transduction probability of about ½, bursting in one pyramidal cell should induce bursting in some tens of other cells. At the same time, however, under resting conditions in the slice, firing in any one CA3 pyramidal cell will recruit firing in multiple interneurons, including cells producing inhibition perisomatically and in the dendrites of many pyramidal cells (but not all, because disynaptic inhibition is not observed in all pyramidal cell pairs). This inhibition should suppress cell firing and dendritic calcium spikes, respectively, in post-synaptic pyramidal cells (Miles et al. 1996) via $GABA_A$ receptors.

In the presence of drugs (e.g., picrotoxin or bicuculline) that block $GABA_A$ receptors, however, bursting can spread from one cell to multiple cells, and so, in a series of steps of exponentially increasing amplitude, recruit the entire population—a chain reaction. This concept predicts that a synchronized epileptic burst will occur concurrently with a large EPSC in any given pyramidal cell, owing to the near simultaneous firing of all of that cell's synaptic precursors and that stimulation of a single cell should be able to recruit the entire population. Both of these predictions have been verified (Johnston and Brown 1981; Miles and Wong 1983, 1987a). Yet, it is the case that not *all* individual CA3 pyramidal cells can recruit the entire population, rather only about ⅓ of them (Miles and Wong 1983).

Some of the more subtle predictions of this theory are illustrated in figure 5.1, taken from Traub and Wong (1982). Column *A* shows the results of a model of 100 pyramidal cells, with 5% connectivity and with pyramidal/pyramidal synapses strong enough for burst transduction; synaptic inhibition was not present. Column *B* shows the results of focal stimulation (a small shock to the fimbria) of the CA2 region in vitro (a region resembling CA3 in its properties) in the presence of the $GABA_A$ receptor-blocking drug penicillin. Line by line, the figure shows:

1. the stages of growth of firing in the model. This quantity was not accessible experimentally at the time, although present optical methods now allow one to estimate it. The population discharge in

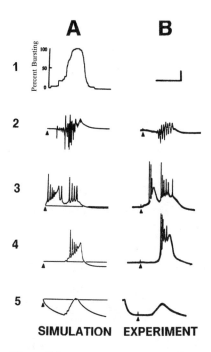

Figure 5.1
With blockade of GABA$_A$ receptors in the CA2/CA3 region, small stimuli evoke synchronized bursting of pyramidal cells with long latency (about 100 ms). (A) Simulation of 100 pyramidal cell network, with each cell connected to an average of 5 others via synapses that permit burst transmission. At ▲ four cells were stimulated, the growth of activity being shown in line 1. (B) Experiment in the disinhibited CA2 region of a guinea-pig hippocampal slice. At ▲ a shock was given to the fimbria. Line 2 shows field potentials, lines 3–5, intracellular recordings (same cell in lines 4 and 5, but hyperpolarized in line 5 to reveal the giant EPSP during the epileptiform event). Further details in text. Calibrations: 50 ms (simulation), 60 ms (experiment); 4 mV (A2 and B2), 25 mV (A3, A4, A5), 20 mV (B3, B4, B5). (From Traub and Wong, 1982, with permission of the American Association for the Advancement of Science)

the model is terminated by intrinsic conductances, such as the Ca^{2+}-activated AHP. $GABA_B$ conductances might also contribute.

2. the epileptiform field potential. The important point here is the long latency (many tens of ms) from onset of the stimulus to the peak of this potential. The underlying physical idea is that several stages of growth are required before enough cells are firing to produce a measurable field potential, and the first stages (at least) each take tens of ms, the time required for burst transduction. As one would expect, increasing the intensity, which will recruit more neurons at the start, reduces the latency to the epileptiform field potential (Wong and Traub 1983). Note that there is a fine structure in the experimental epileptiform field potential that is not present in the simulation. This fine structure represents correlations in firing times on a sub-millisecond time scale between different pyramidal cells and may be a result of currents flowing in the extracellular medium, an effect not incorporated into this particular model (Snow and Dudek 1984; Traub, Dudek et al. 1985). The fine structure might also, in principle, depend on gap junctions (Draguhn et al. 1998).

3. those rare pyramidal neurons that fire early in the event can be reexcited by the full population burst, so as to generate a double burst.

4. much more commonly, pyramidal cells show little disturbance of their resting membrane potential until they burst suddenly. This observation again is a reflection of the exponential growth of the bursting process in the population.

5. consistent with the data of Johnston and Brown (1981), hyperpolarization of a pyramidal cell uncovers a large EPSP, coincident with the main population burst.

The chain-reaction type of synchronized burst, occurring in a localized population of neurons (say, thousands of cells) is conceptually simple enough, that it serves as a archetype with which other sorts of epileptic phenomena can be compared. We shall next consider two variations of the theme: partial disinhibition and spatially nonuniform inhibition.

The Epileptic Chain Reaction Modified by Synaptic Inhibition

Synaptic inhibition acts in a manner somewhat analogous to the control rods in a nuclear reactor: it prevents enough burst transduction (analogous to induced fissions) so that the full chain reaction can not proceed. This mechanism was demonstrated experimentally by Miles and Wong (1987a) (figure 5.2). Two CA3 pyramidal cells were recorded while picrotoxin (a blocker of $GABA_A$ receptors) was washed into the bath. The presynaptic cell was induced to burst at 0.5 Hz by current pulses. Under resting conditions, with the two pyramidal cells not being monosynaptically connected, bursting in the presynaptic cell had no apparent effect on the postsynaptic cell. And eventually, when the concentration of picrotoxin was high enough, stimulation of the presynaptic cell evoked a population burst, which of course, engaged the recorded postsynaptic cell. But in between, one could see polysynaptic pathways opening up, first a single one (i.e., the postsynaptic cell exhibited an EPSP of the sort one would expect were a single intercalated pyramidal cell to burst), then a dual pathway, and finally and suddenly, many pathways. The switch from one → two → many pathways has been analyzed in models (Traub et al. 1987a, 1987b; Traub and Miles 1991). The most critical idea for our purposes is the threshold nature of the transition—as synaptic inhibition is progressively reduced—from limited bursts in a fraction of the population to bursts involving the entire population. It has recently been shown in the subiculum that $GABA_B$ receptors also regulate the ability of a small stimulus to induce a synchronized epileptiform burst (Stanford et al., in 1998).

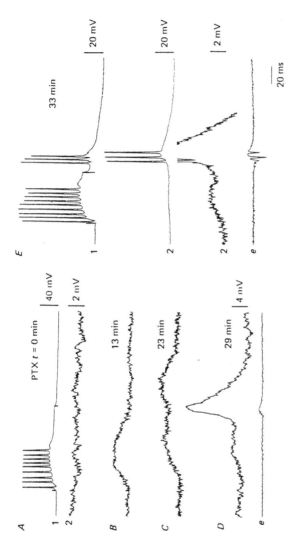

Figure 5.2
GABA$_A$ receptor-mediated IPSPs regulate propagation of firing between CA3 pyramidal cells. Bursting
was repeatedly induced in a presynaptic pyramidal cell (1), and the effects were observed in a different
pyramidal cell (2), not monosynaptically connected to the first one. (A) Under control conditions, a
burst in cell 1 produces no effect on cell 2 (B–E) Picrotoxin (PTX) was washed in, progressively blocking
GABA$_A$ receptors. First, a broad EPSP appears (B); next, a double EPSP (C); then, a double EPSP (D),
in which the second EPSP is large and associated with a small field potential (e, trace below), indicative
of partial synchronization of the population; and finally, synchronization of the population (E), with
cells 1 and 2 both firing bursts and with a larger field potential (e, trace below). Experiment performed
in isolated CA3 segment in vitro. (From Miles and Wong, 1987a).

Synaptic Inhibition That Is Spatially Nonuniform

We have mentioned that, in a statistical sense, excitatory contacts made by CA3 pyramidal cells on other CA3 pyramidal cells are spatially localized: the probability of contact falls off with a characteristic length of 0.6 to 1.0 mm (chapter 4; Miles, Traub, and Wong 1988). It is reasonable to assume that the same fall-off in connection probability with distance applies to synaptic connections made by pyramidal cells onto interneurons. If this assumption is correct, and given established data on the kinetics of synaptic interactions (chapter 4), then one can understand a phenomenon known as the *inhibitory surround* (Prince and Wilder 1967). If inhibition is blocked locally, in a region some mm in lateral extent, then synchronized bursts appear in pyramidal cells within the region, but some mm away pyramidal cells exhibit large IPSPs that may be admixed with EPSPs (figure 5.2; Dichter and Spencer 1969).

The way that this phenomenon comes about appears to be that, for synchrony to develop within the disinhibited region, the same principles as described above will apply, provided that the region is large enough to contain a critical degree of synaptic connectivity. In the guinea-pig dorsal hippocampal slice, for instance, the minimum aggregate is estimated to contain about 1,000 CA3 pyramidal cells: Miles, Wong, and Traub 1984; Traub and Miles 1991. Into neighboring regions, a few mm away, some of the axons—from bursting pyramidal cells in the disinhibited region—will contact both pyramidal cells and interneurons, with comparable conduction delays. But the interneurons will fire and produce IPSPs in nearby pyramidal cells before the EPSPs reach their peak because disynaptic inhibition outruns monosynaptic excitation (see chapter 4), so that, in general, the pyramidal cells in the surround region will not fire immediately and instead will be hyperpolarized. After that, the issue devolves into the balance between the total amount of excitation emerging from the disinhibited zone, and the total inhibition produced by interneurons in the surround zone, a balance determined by connection probabilities, unitary conductance parameters, receptor desensitization, and so forth.

In experiments and in models (using reasonable estimates of these parameters), prolonged hyperpolarization develops in most of the pyramidal neurons in the surround (figure 5.3). The significance of these results for the understanding of oscillations is that: it highlights the essential role that timing can play in emergent population phenomena. It also emphasizes the importance of being able to reconstruct neuronal circuitry in detail for certain population phenomena to become intelligible.

Epileptiform Events Following Minutes after a Tetanic Stimulus

Miles and Wong (1987b) showed that, after tetanic stimulation (50 Hz for 5 s, perhaps multiple times) of CA3, following a latent period of minutes or tens of minutes, synchronized bursts could be elicited following stimulation of a single pyramidal cell, even without pharmacological blockade of synaptic inhibition. Sometimes, this synchronized activity had an unusual appearance, that of an oscillation at about 10 Hz of increasing amplitude. Additionally, it was found that in a period of minutes to tens of minutes after a tetanus, not only did polysynaptic excitatory circuitry open up as with partial blockade of inhibition postsynaptically (figure 5.2; Miles and Wong 1987a), but also the properties of disynaptic inhibition between pyramidal cells were altered. In addition to mean IPSPs becoming smaller, IPSP failures began to occur.

One possible interpretation of these results (not yet proven) is that some minutes after tetanic stimulation, synaptic depression develops at (for at least some) pyramidal cell→interneuron connections to produce a novel form of partial disinhibition. We should note

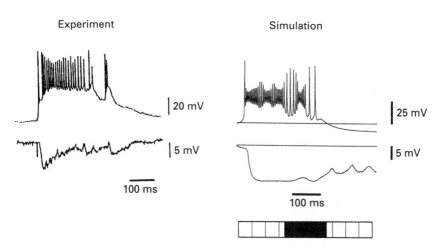

Figure 5.3
The inhibitory surround can be explained by the wider spread of pyramidal cell axons than of interneuron axons. The experiment was performed in a longitudinal CA3 slice, with picrotoxin applied focally at one end. A neuron in the disinhibited region (upper trace) exhibited a burst riding on a large depolarizing wave with a secondary burst, while another neuron (lower trace), recorded 2–3 mm away, exhibited large IPSPs. The simulation was of a network of 8,000 pyramidal cells in a 20 × 400 array and 800 inhibitory cells in a 2 × 400 array, with GABA$_A$ receptors blocked in the central region (shown in the inset). A pyramidal cell in the disinhibited region (upper trace) exhibits an epileptiform burst with a secondary burst, while a pyramidal cell 3.2 mm from the center of the array is inhibited (lower trace). In the model, contacts of pyramidal cells are distributed with probability that declines with space constant 1 mm along the 8 mm extent of the array, while outputs of interneurons are constrained to extend no more than 300 μm from the cell. (From Traub, Jefferys, and Miles, 1993.)

that gamma oscillations in CA1 follow the tetanic stimulus within 150 ms, not minutes and that indirect evidence suggests that, on this much shorter time scale, the pyramidal cell→interneuron connections, at least locally, are not suppressed. Indeed, these connections may even be enhanced (chapter 9). On the other hand, a role for synaptic depression at pyramidal cell→interneuron connections does appear likely in explaining some of the plastic changes observed after gamma oscillations induced by intense tetanic stimuli (chapter 10).

Secondary Bursts: A Rapid Series of Synchronized Bursts During Strong Dendritic Excitation

Disinhibition of hippocampal slices from mature animals sometimes results in an initial synchronized burst, as described above
(the 1º, or primary burst) and also in a succeeding series of 1–10
secondary (2º) synchronized bursts, at frequencies about 8–15 Hz
(Hablitz 1984; Miles, Wong, and Traub 1984; figure 5.4). These events
are of clinical interest: just as the single synchronized burst resembles an interictal spike in the EEG, so a brief afterdischarge with 2º
bursts resembles a polyspike in the EEG. Furthermore, 2º bursts
seem to represent a transitional state between the interictal burst
and a sustained seizure. This relationship is especially true because,
in slices from immature animals, 2º bursts can continue for tens of
seconds (Swann, Smith, and Brady 1993). Both 1º and 2º bursts can
arise in small bits of CA3 containing an estimated 1,000–2,000 pyramidal cells, so that thalamocortical circuits are not required for
their generation (Miles, Wong, and Traub 1984).

The clue to the mechanism of 2º bursts came from examining series of bursts in Purkinje cells. These bursts were generated entirely
by intrinsic mechanisms: sustained inward currents (as might be
produced by $g_{Na(P)}$) induce a series of dendritic Ca^{2+} spikes (Llinás
and Sugimori 1980a, b). These events resemble 1º and 2º bursts of
the sort illustrated in figure 5.4. Hippocampal pyramidal cells generate series of Ca^{2+} spikes in response to intense dendritic current
injection (chapter 2, figures 2.2 and 2.3). This production suggested
that the disinhibited CA3 network could itself produce the necessary dendritic current injection via excitatory synaptic conductances, rather than, or in addition to, intrinsic conductances (Traub,
Miles, and Jefferys 1993).

One way this process might happen is that, during the initial 1º
burst, all the pyramidal cells are firing at high rates, hence are re-

EXPERIMENT

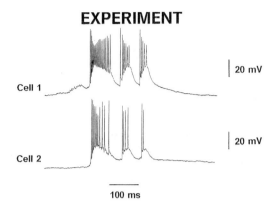

SIMULATION

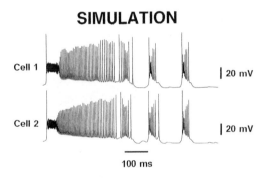

Figure 5.4
Epileptiform events can consist of an initial primary (1°) burst followed by secondary (2°) bursts. Experiment shows dual intracellular recordings from the CA3 region
in vitro with $GABA_A$ receptors blocked by picrotoxin. The simulation shows two
pyramidal cell somatic potentials from a model of 128 pyramidal cells (each as in
Traub, Jefferys, Miles et al. 1994), each connected to 20 others. Synaptic connections
utilize AMPA and NMDA receptors, the latter desensitizing with time constant 350
ms (see Traub, Miles, and Jefferys, 1993; Traub, Jeffeys, and Whittington, 1994).
(Experiment by R. Miles, unpublished data; from Traub and Jefferys, 1997.)

leasing glutamate. The induced activation of NMDA receptors would produce synaptic conductances with long relaxation time constants (> 100 ms, Forsythe and Westbrook 1988). These conductances would induce 2° bursts by producing series of dendritic Ca^{2+} spikes. Blockade of AMPA receptors aborts 1° bursts entirely (Lee and Hablitz 1989), suggesting that AMPA receptors are the fundamental mediators of burst transduction, at least in media with normal $[Mg^{2+}]$. However, the role of AMPA receptors in the 2° bursts is predicted to be different: to provide synchrony by phase-advancing bursting in some of the cells, rather than to spread bursting from cell to cell. In other words, pyramidal cells are strongly coupled during the initial burst but weakly coupled during the secondary bursts.

Of course, once 2° bursts begin, NMDA receptors will continue to be activated, so that, in principle, 2° bursts could continue indefinitely. Desensitization of NMDA receptors is known to occur, however (Vyklicky et al. 1990) and could contribute to terminating the series of 2° bursts (Traub, Jefferys, and Whittington 1994).

Propagation in Space of Primary and Secondary Bursts

There are two experimental implications of our hypothesis that 1° and 2° bursts are not synchronized by identical mechanisms. First, NMDA blockers should differentially suppress the 2° bursts more than the 1° burst; we will return to this issue later in the chapter. Second, the 1° burst should be more robust than the 2° bursts to inhomogeneities in the tissue, provided enough connections exist to allow synchronization in the first place.

This latter issue can be addressed by analyzing the propagation of epileptiform events in longitudinal CA3 slices. Such slices can be cut so as to be almost 1 cm long, a large distance compared with the average spread of pyramidal-pyramidal connections (of the order of 1 mm). Pyramidal cell axon conduction velocity in this preparation is about 0.5 m/s (Andersen et al. 1978; Miles et al. 1988), providing an upper limit to how fast epileptic discharges might spread. What actually happens is that 1° bursts develop near to a focal stimulus and then spread at about 0.1 to 0.2 m/s, significantly slower than axon conduction velocity (Knowles et al. 1987; Miles et al. 1988; Traub, Jefferys, and Miles 1993; figure 5.5). The reason is that the synaptic connections are, on average, localized; and development of the discharge requires that bursting propagate from neurons to neurons, this synaptic integration process taking finite time.

In contrast, 2° bursts may either propagate from one end of the slice to the other at about the same velocity as the 1° burst; propagate only part of the length of the slice; or propagate in the reverse direction to the initial burst (Knowles et al. 1987; Traub, Jefferys, and Miles 1993; figure 5.5). In simulations of the longitudinal slice, using 8,000 pyramidal cells, all three of these patterns can be observed (Traub et al. 1993). When NMDA conductance is high enough and all parameters are distributed uniformly, the 2° bursts propagate in the same direction as the initial burst. In contrast, when some parameter is nonuniform (e.g., g_{NMDA} or $g_{K(AHP)}$), 2° bursts are initiated preferentially in the most excitable region (possibly at the end of the slice opposite to the stimulus), and the bursts may fail to propagate the entire length of the array (figure 5.6). The initial burst, as in experiments, always developed around the site of stimulation.

An unexpected model prediction in the study of Traub, Jefferys, and Miles (1993) (verified experimentally) was that blockade of NMDA receptors would slow the propagation of the 1° burst. This result is interesting: it provides further evidence that NMDA receptors occur in recurrent excitatory connections in the first place. Studies in low Mg^{2+} provide still more evidence for this crucial notion (Traub, Jefferys, and Whittington 1994), as do pair recordings (Deuchars and Thomson 1996). The propagation result also shows that NMDA receptors become engaged even during the initial burst and even in normal Mg^{2+}.

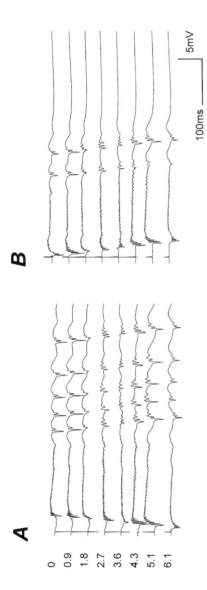

Figure 5.5
Experimental evidence that primary and secondary bursts have different properties: the secondary bursts may propagate in the *same* or in the *opposite* direction as the primary burst. The experiments were performed in longitudinal CA3 slices from the guinea pig with GABA$_A$ receptors blocked by bicuculline. Field potentials were obtained simultaneously from 8 electrodes, at distances (from the temporal end of the slice) in mm given by the numbers on the left. Epileptiform events were triggered by a local shock. (A) A shock to the septal end of the slice produces a 1° burst that propagates away from the stimulated end but 2° bursts that propagate toward the stimulated end. (B) In contrast, a shock to the temporal end produces a 1° burst that again propagates away from the stimulated end, but 2° bursts that also propagate away from the stimulated end. (From Traub, Jefferys, and Miles, 1993.)

The behavior of epileptiform bursts in space provides an interesting contrast to gamma oscillations in the slice. In the latter case, there can exist phase lags along the preparation that are less than expected from axon conduction delays, rather than more, as is the case with epileptiform bursts. One difference between the two situations is that, in the gamma oscillation case, but not in the epilepsy case, the output of interneurons is available to act as a timing device.

Tertiary Bursts: A Sustained Seizure-like Event

In some disinhibited preparations, the 2° bursts are succeeded by a series of synchronized tertiary (3°) bursts, at frequencies of about 1–5 Hz and lasting for seconds, tens of seconds, or even longer (figure 5.7; Traub, Borck et al. 1996). Tertiary bursts are more likely to occur in ventral hippocampal slices than dorsal ones and are also more likely to occur when $[K^+]_o$ is somewhat elevated (Anderson and Jefferys 1997). Note that between the 3° bursts, somatic membrane potential is near to its resting value, although the dendrites could be depolarized. Also, the potential is noisier than before the epileptic event begins; this noise is presumably spontaneous synaptic noise and may be caused by additional elevations in $[K^+]_o$ that are induced by the first series of bursts (C. Borck and J. G. R. Jefferys, unpublished data). After the last 3° burst, there is some additional membrane activity suggestive of partially synchronized bursting in the population (cf. Figure 5.2D). The overall structure of this in vitro population event is similar to that of at least some clinical electrographic seizures.

We have described how 1° and 2° bursts can be simulated in networks of pyramidal cells with recurrent excitatory connections, utilizing AMPA and NMDA receptors (figure 5.4; Traub, Miles, and Jefferys 1993), and we have mentioned how NMDA receptor desensitization can act to limit the number of 2° bursts (Traub, Jefferys, and Whittington 1994). Adding one single new structural element

A)

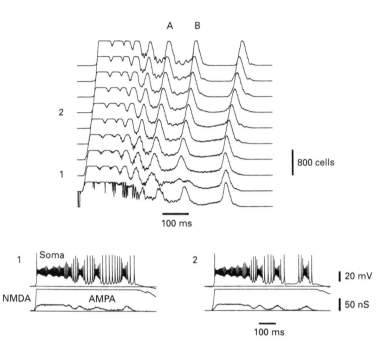

B)

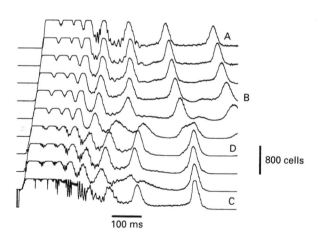

to the model permits the simulation of 1°, 2°, and 3° bursts as well: spontaneous EPSPs at sufficiently high frequency (figure 5.8). Such EPSPs can, in principle, represent spontaneous transmitter release and/or ectopic action potentials arising in axons or presynaptic terminals, a phenomenon that appears to occur in the post-tetanic-stimulation and in the 4AP epilepsy models (Stasheff, Hines, and Wilson 1993; Stasheff, Mott, and Wilson 1993; Traub, Colling, and Jefferys 1995). Spontaneous EPSPs produce membrane noise, as seen in the experimental records, and provide a background exci-tatory bombardment, such that once a few pyramidal cells are firing and once AHPs have decayed sufficiently, a burst can be initiated through strong coupling, that is to say, recurrent EPSPs.

Synchronization in the Presence of Spontaneous EPSPs

Our hypothesis on the origin of 3° bursts is based on studies of synchronous discharges that occur in the presence of spontaneous EPSPs in elevated $[K^{+}]_{o}$ (Chamberlin et al. 1990; Traub and Dingle-dine 1990) and in 4AP (Traub, Colling, and Jefferys 1995). In both of these models, synaptic inhibition is present, at least to some de-

Figure 5.6
Simulations of propagating primary and secondary bursts. Simulations were per-formed in a 20×400 array of pyramidal cells; GABA$_B$ receptor-mediated inhibition was present (although not relevant to the propagation shown), but GABA$_A$ receptor-mediated inhibition was blocked. Epileptiform events were evoked by stimulating 500 cells at one end of the array. Signals plotted are the number of pyramidal cells in each of ten 20×40 blocks that are depolarized more than 20 mV from rest. (A) When conductance densities are distributed uniformly, 1° and 2° bursts propagate in the same direction. Below: for two cells, one at each of the locations designated, we show the somatic membrane potential and total AMPA and NMDA conduc-tances received by the cell. Note the delay in onset of the conductance in cell 2 and the saturation of the NMDA conductance. (B) When NMDA conductance density is nonuniform (less in the middle of the array than at the ends), then 2° bursts can propagate in the reverse direction to the 1° burst. (From Traub, Jefferys, and Miles, 1993).

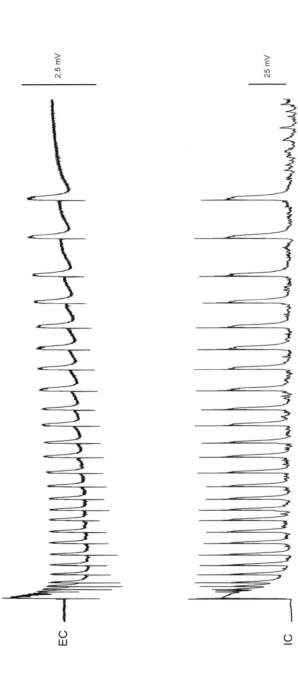

Figure 5.7
Sustained epileptiform events, resembling seizures, can occur in vitro. The experiment was performed in a ventral hippocampal slice from an adult rat, bathed in solution with $[K^+]_o = 5$ mM and with $GABA_A$ receptors blocked with biciculline. The epileptiform event was triggered by a shock to the perforant path. Intracellular (IC) recording below, extracellular (EC) above. The periods of primary, secondary, and tertiary bursts are shown. The $2°$ bursts ride on an intracellular depolarization; membrane potential returns to near resting values during the $3°$ bursts. All three types of burst are synchronized, as indicated by the extracellular recording. Note the increased membrane potential noise during and after the $3°$ bursts, presumably reflecting synaptic activity. (From Traub,

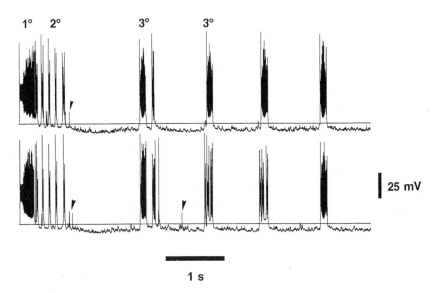

Figure 5.8
Simulation of primary, secondary, and tertiary bursts. The simulation shows potentials from the somata of 2 out of the 192 pyramidal cells in a network, interconnected by synapses with AMPA and NMDA receptors and with synaptic inhibition absent. NMDA receptor-mediated conductances desensitize to $1/10$ of their maximum value, with a time constant of 300 ms. Noise is present in this system in the form of random ectopic action potentials originating in axons, producing random EPSPs, as well as antidromic spikes that often block to reveal partial spikes (➤). Primary, secondary, and tertiary bursts are apparent. Cells in this simulation are not as depolarized during the 2° bursts as in the experiment shown in Figure 5.7, but model neurons' dendrites are depolarized. Note the synaptic noise between the 3° bursts. (From Traub, Borck, et al., 1996 with permission)

gree, and there are increasing numbers of EPSPs (Chamberlin et al. 1990) and/or unit activity (Ives and Jefferys 1990) just prior to a fully synchronized burst. This latter basic experimental observation—a build-up of activity prior to full synchrony—emerges in network models in a simple way: with a background random process for generating EPSPs or ectopic spikes and with the decline of the AHP, a few cells will eventually be stimulated to fire. The output of these few cells will be amplified by the divergence of the synaptic connections so that orthodromically activated firing occurs in some cells, and the

EPSPs so generated by the firing neurons add to those occurring spontaneously. This process becomes regenerative, and eventually cells start to burst, with propagation of bursting taking place as for the 1° burst. What is special about this process is that, in the initial stages, cells may be firing single spikes, rather than bursts, and furthermore, that no single neuron can be said to initiate the process.

An example of a simulation of a 4AP-induced population burst is shown in figure 5.9. The notation in this figure is as follows. The a indicates an antidromic spike, spontaneously occurring in an axon and propagating retrograde; the d, an antidromic spike that blocks at the soma, leaving a partial spike. This terminology goes back to the 1970s when such potentials were recognized and were attributed to dendritic spikes, as indeed some of them may be (Spencer and Kandel 1961). The o is an orthodromic spike. The background EPSPs are most apparent in the dendrite. In both high $[K^+]_o$ and in 4AP, the excitatory propagation of firing that is required for this type of synchronization requires AMPA receptors and does not require NMDA receptors (Chamberlin et al. 1990; Perreault and Avoli 1991; Traub, Colling, and Jefferys 1995).

Secondary Bursts, But Not Primary or Tertiary Bursts, in the Disinhibited Slice Require NMDA Receptors

A critical test of our hypothesis on epileptogenesis in the disinhibited hippocampal slice is that pharmacological blockade of NMDA receptors should abolish the 2° bursts, although not necessarily the initial burst. Dingledine et al. (1986) showed that NMDA receptor blockade would shorten somewhat the primary burst without abolishing it, and this observation has been confirmed by others (see below). Loss of 2° bursts with NMDA receptor blockade was shown by Lee and Hablitz (1990) and by Traub, Miles, and Jefferys (1993) and is confirmed by the experiment shown in figure 5.10. Note as

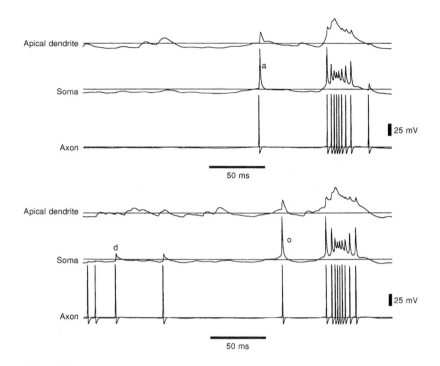

Figure 5.9
The 4AP model: simulation of synchronized bursting in the presence of enhanced EPSPs and spontaneous synaptic noise. The two sets of traces (apical dendrite, soma, and axon) are simultaneous. The network contains 128 pyramidal cells and 24 interneurons, including axo-axonic cells, basket cells, dendrite-contacting cells, and cells activating GABA$_B$ receptors. EPSC decay time constant was 3 ms, and noise was present in the form of ectopic axonal spikes occurring randomly at high frequency (mean interval 80 ms in each axon). Ectopic spikes can partially invade the soma to produce partial spikes or d-spikes (*d*) or to produce full antidromic spikes (*a*). In addition, orthodromic spikes (*o*) occur just prior to the synchronized burst. (From Traub, Colling, and Jefferys, 1995)

A)

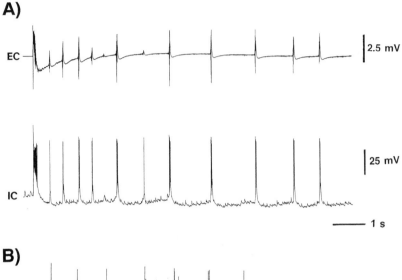

B)

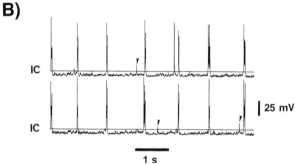

Figure 5.10
In disinhibition-induced epileptiform events, blocking NMDA conductance short-
ens the primary burst and removes secondary bursts, but tertiary bursts can persist.
(A): An epileptiform event in a ventral hippocampal slice, as in Figure 5.7, but with
the NMDA antagonist D-AP5 (50 μM) in the medium. Simultaneous extracellular
(EC, from s. pyramidale) and intracellular (IC) recordings. Both primary and tertiary
bursts are narrower than in Figures 5.7, and secondary bursts have disappeared.
Note the persistent membrane potential noise between the 3° bursts. (B): Simulated
epileptiform event, as in Figure 5.8, but with NMDA receptors blocked. Two pyramidal cell somatic potentials are shown. Again, primary and tertiary bursts are
narrowed, secondary bursts are gone, and membrane noise persists. Symbol ➤
shows partially blocked ectopic action potentials. (From Traub, Borck et al., 1996
with permission)

well the shortening of the initial burst during NMDA receptor blockade. What is interesting, and also predicted by the computer network model, is that tertiary bursts continue, although perhaps reduced in number, despite NMDA receptor blockade. This finding is consistent with a similarity (although not identity) in mechanism for the 1° and 3° bursts.

In Epilepsy Models Other Than Disinhibition, Sustained Depolarizations and Secondary Bursts Need Not Depend on NMDA Receptors

It will be shown in chapter 9 that tetanically induced gamma oscillations are associated with a large prolonged intracellular depolarization that drives the oscillation. This depolarization is only in small part produced by NMDA receptor activation. Evidently, the brain has a number of different means of inducing prolonged depolarizations of neurons.

An interesting means of producing such a depolarization in the 4AP epilepsy model involves the normally inhibitory transmitter GABA. It is believed that, at concentrations in the tens of μM, 4AP acts to block the D current postsynaptically (Storm 1988) and to enhance transmitter release (Buckle and Haas 1982). In addition, pools of interneurons are prone to burst in 4AP even without synaptic excitation from pyramidal cells (Müller and Misgeld 1991; Michelson and Wong 1991, 1994; chapter 6). Perhaps for these reasons, enough GABA is released in 4AP to spill over to (presumably) extrasynaptic depolarizing GABA receptors. Following synchronized bursts, prolonged depolarizing GABA-dependent potentials have been described in 4AP epileptogenesis (Avoli 1990; Perreault and Avoli 1992), and such depolarizations can even drive 2° bursts (figure 5.11). Unfortunately, the slow depolarization remaining after blockade of GABA and NMDA receptors in 4AP (figure 5.11) has not been further characterized.

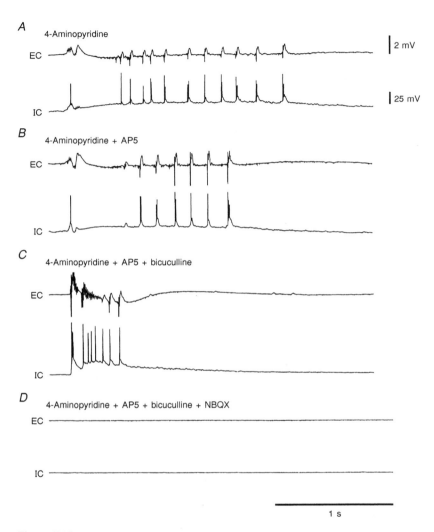

Figure 5.11
The slow depolarization in 4AP, giving rise to a series of synchronized bursts, has several components: NMDA, depolarizing GABA$_A$ and an unidentified element. There is no synchronized excitatory activity when AMPA receptors are blocked. (A): Spontaneous epileptiform event, lasting about 1 second, in 70 μM 4AP. EC, extracellular recording; IC, intracellular recording. (B): The event is slightly shortened by blockade of NMDA receptors with 20 μM D-AP5. (C): The event is further shortened by the additional blockade of GABA$_A$ receptors with 30 μM bicuculline methiodide. (D): No synchronized activity remains after the additional blockade of AMPA/kainate receptors with 20 μM NBQX. (From Traub, Colling, and Jefferys, 1995)

Population Oscillations Resembling Secondary Bursts That Occur in the Presence of Metabotropic Receptor Activation

Metabotropic receptors, both glutamate and muscarinic, contribute to the slow depolarization underlying tetanically evoked gamma oscillations in the CA1 region (chapter 9). It is therefore of interest to examine briefly the synchronized population oscillations induced by activation of these receptors in the CA3 region in vitro. Such oscillations provide a conceptual link between epileptogenesis and gamma oscillations.

Carbachol (tens of μM concentration) induces oscillations at theta frequency (4–12 Hz) in CA3 (in vitro) in the hands of some investigators (MacVicar and Tse 1989), while the nonspecific metabotropic glutamate receptor agonist, ACPD (> 60 μM), induces oscillations at 8–27 Hz (Taylor, Merlin, and Wong 1995) (figure 5.12). In both cases, pyramidal cells fire (usually) one or more action potentials on the crests of the voltage waves. The words "theta frequency" should not be taken to imply that such in vitro oscillations are mechanistically similar to in vivo theta rhythm, and indeed, the mechanisms appear to be quite different (see discussion in Traub, Miles, and Buzsáki 1992 and in Williams and Kauer 1997). In one study (MacVicar and Tse 1989), blockade of GABA$_A$ receptors had little effect on in vitro carbachol oscillations, while in another (Williams and Kauer 1997), such blockade led to synchronized population bursts that were poorly rhythmic. Blockade of GABA$_A$ receptors increases the amplitude and decreases the frequency of metabotropic glutamate receptor-induced oscillations (Taylor et al. 1995). This effect is analogous to what is seen with spontaneous partially synchronized synaptic potentials, in slices without ACPD, as synaptic inhibition is gradually reduced (Miles and Wong 1987a; Traub and Miles 1991). In neither case, that is, neither carbachol nor ACPD, do NMDA receptors contribute significantly. In both cases,

A

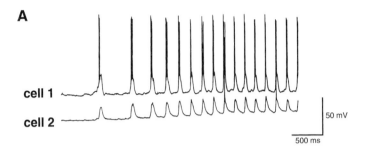

cell 1

cell 2

50 mV

500 ms

B

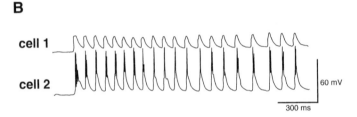

cell 1

cell 2

60 mV

300 ms

Figure 5.12
CA3 synchronized oscillations driven by metabotropic receptor activation. (A:) Dual intracellular recording in CA3 pyramidal neurons with carbachol in the bath. This type of activity was observed with carbachol concentrations of 10–60 μM. The lower cell does not fire as often as the upper one. (From MacVicar and Tse, 1989). (B) Similar activity in two CA3 neurons in the presence of the metabotropic glutamate receptor agonist, ACPD. Similar oscillations were observed with ACPD 100–200 μM in the bath or after focal application of ACPD, 200–350 μM. (From Taylor, Merlin, and Wong, 1995 with permission)

however, AMPA receptors are required for the oscillations to synchronize. Individual pyramidal cells in the presence of carbachol can continue to fire on their own when AMPA receptors are pharmacologically blocked (Williams and Kauer 1997), as would be expected if carbachol can induce a slow inward current.

Based on the data of MacVicar and Tse (1989), we proposed a model of the in vitro carbachol oscillations (figure 5.13; Traub, Miles, and Buzsáki 1992) that may apply to ACPD-induced oscillations as well. The underlying idea is that these oscillations are rather like the 2° bursts in disinhibition-induced epileptiform discharges, that is to say,

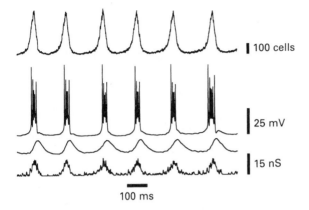

Figure 5.13
Simulation of carbachol-induced oscillation resembling in structure an epileptic afterdischarge. The network consisted of 1,000 pyramidal neurons (as in Traub et al., 1991) with the Ca^{2+}-dependent AHP conductance reduced, with tonic excitation of the pyramidal cells present and with synaptic coupling between pyramidal cells via AMPA receptors—all features consistent with the experimental situation. Upper trace is the number of neurons depolarized more than 20 mV from rest, the middle two traces are somatic potentials of two neurons (the lower one hyperpolarized by current injection), and the bottom trace shows the AMPA receptor-mediated conductance in a single neuron. (From Traub, Miles, and Buzsáki, 1992)

they result from dendritic depolarization evoking rhythmic Ca^{2+} spikes, with AMPA receptors serving to provide phase-locking between different cells. Yet, in the case of metabotropic receptor-induced CA3 oscillations, it is not NMDA receptors that provide the depolarization, but rather metabotropically activated inward currents (Benson et al. 1988; Guérineau et al. 1994), with metabotropic reduction of K currents also contributing (Cole and Nicoll 1984; Charpak et al. 1990). IPSPs, while present in carbachol or ACPD, are expected to be reduced in amplitude, owing to presynaptic inhibition of transmitter release (Valentino and Dingledine 1981; Poncer, Shinozaki, and Miles 1995). Our model explains the observation that progressive blockade of ionotropic glutamate receptors will reduce the amplitude of carbachol oscillations without much change in the frequency until finally the cells become uncoupled from each other

(Traub et al. 1992). We shall see later that some of the principles underlying beta (10–25 Hz) oscillations in CA1 in vitro resemble the principles at work in metabotropic oscillations in the in vitro CA3 region.

Recently, it has been shown that carbachol can also induce gamma oscillations in the CA3 region in vitro (Fisahn et al. 1998). These gamma oscillations depend on both AMPA and $GABA_A$ receptors. Further details of the mechanisms are being investigated.

In Summary

Some of the common principles of in vitro epileptogenesis are these:

1. Strong coupling between pyramidal cells is required for the first interictal burst, particularly if this first burst arises out of relative silence of the neuronal population. By strong coupling is meant the ability of firing in single neurons to induce firing in other neurons. Strong coupling is not required in situations where a stimulus is given simultaneously to sufficiently many cells (Traub and Miles 1991, figure 6.11).

2. Background excitation of one or more of the neurons is required to start the synchronization process. In the brain, this background process can be spontaneous synaptic noise and/or ectopic spikes.

3. There must be strong tonic depolarization of pyramidal cell dendrites if secondary bursts are to occur. Such depolarization can originate in a number of different ways, e.g., NMDA receptors, depolarizing $GABA_A$ receptors, or metabotropic receptor activation.

4. The background excitatory noise may need to be more intense after the primary burst than before, if tertiary bursts are to occur because pyramidal cell membranes will be shunted and hyperpolarized by K currents after the initial burst. Metabotropic receptors, either glutamate or muscarinic, could counteract some of this intrinsic inhibitory effect.

6

Networks of
Interneurons I:
Synchronized Bursts

We shall show in chapter 8 that networks of interneurons can generate synchronized gamma oscillations by virtue of mutual synaptic inhibition, mediated by hyperpolarizing $GABA_A$ receptors. In order to understand this important result, it is necessary to place the result in the context of other known behaviors of interneuron networks, behaviors that arise because of other sorts of interaction between interneurons. It is the purpose of this chapter to establish such a context. We shall review interneuron network bursts mediated, at least in part, by depolarizing $GABA_A$ receptors and bursts that are probably mediated through gap junctions.

Synchronized Interneuron Bursts Mediated by Depolarizing $GABA_A$ Receptors

These events have been studied in hippocampal slices from mature animals in the presence of 4-aminopyridine (4AP, at concentrations up to about 75 μM), together with drugs to block ionotropic glutamate receptors (i.e., AMPA and NMDA receptors) (Michelson and Wong 1991; Müller and Misgeld 1990). The relevant action of 4AP is perhaps to enhance GABA release in sufficient quantities to activate depolarizing $GABA_A$ receptors, as well as hyperpolarizing $GABA_A$ receptors. In these conditions, one observes, both spontaneously and in response to a stimulus, giant (sometimes 10 mV or more) triphasic potentials, predominantly hyperpolarizing, in principal neurons throughout the in vitro hippocampal formation (e.g., in dentate, CA1, and CA3). The first two components of the triphasic potential are, respectively, hyperpolarizing and depolarizing $GABA_A$ receptor-mediated events. The third, slower component is almost certainly a $GABA_B$ receptor-mediated IPSP.

Simultaneous intracellular recordings have been made of pyramidal neurons and interneurons in the dentate hilus in order to find interneurons that fire preferentially in phase with one or another component of the triphasic response (Michelson and Wong 1991, 1994; Forti and Michelson 1998). In this way, one could hope to correlate a) interneuron morphology, b) burst-generating mechanisms in the interneuron, and c) postsynaptic action of the interneuron. Some hilar interneurons near to the cell bodies of dentate granule cells had dendrites confined almost exclusively to the hilus and fired in phase with the earlier portions of the triphasic response, those portions mediated by $GABA_A$ receptors (Michelson and Wong 1994; Forti and Michelson 1998). Furthermore, the burst in such interneurons, Type 1, had a large depolarizing envelope, resembling the potential that occurs during a synchronized population burst in pyramidal cells, an epileptiform burst (chapter 5, figure 5.1). This potential in the interneuron is a synaptic potential: during strong hyperpolarization of the interneuron, the potential increases in amplitude even as action potentials are blocked (figure 6.1).

When, in addition to 4AP and blockers of ionotropic glutamate receptors, picrotoxin is added to the bath, blocking $GABA_A$ receptors, two findings are noted. First, not surprisingly, the initial two components of the triphasic response disappear. Second, remarkably, the depolarizing envelope in Type 1 interneurons also disappears. The large $GABA_B$ IPSP persists in pyramidal cells so that the triphasic response becomes monophasic, and some Type 1 interneurons may exhibit an uncovered slow IPSP (Michelson and Wong

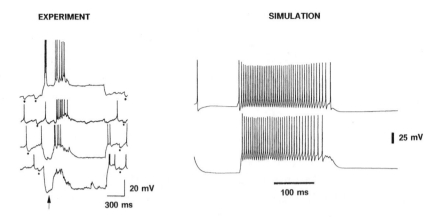

Figure 6.1
Synchronized burst mediated by depolarizing GABA$_A$ receptors. Experiment: intracellular recordings from a hilar interneuron (guinea-pig hippocampal slice) in medium containing 4AP (75 μM), the AMPA receptor blocker CNQX (10 μM), and the NMDA receptor blocker CPP (10 μM). The cell was held at different membrane potentials, while a shock was delivered nearby ($\uparrow$), revealing the large synaptic event underlying the burst. Such events are blocked by bicuculline and are presumed to be synchronized because of their temporal correlation with large IPSPs in pyramidal cells. Symbol ●, spontaneous hyperpolarizing IPSPs. Simulation: two cells (the lower one held hyperpolarized to reveal the depolarizing synaptic potential) out of 128 in a network of interneurons (as in Traub and Miles, 1995). Each interneuron is synaptically connected to 20 others, with unitary IPSC of 10 nS, 5 ms decay time constant and with reversal potential 35 mV depolarized to resting potential. Compare to Figure 5.1. (Experiment by H. Michelson and R. K. S. Wong; from Traub, Wong et al., 1997 with permission)

1991, 1994). It is further to be noted that, in normal media, puffing GABA onto certain interneurons in the dentate hilus can induce a mixture of hyperpolarizing and depolarizing potentials, or, depending on the position of the pipette, it can induce what appears to be a pure depolarizing response.

The most economical interpretation of these results is that, at least in 4AP (and also in 12 mM [K$^+$]$_o$), a subset of interneurons excite each other via depolarizing GABA$_A$ receptors. Consistent with this idea, bicarbonate ions must be available for the triphasic response to occur (Lamsa and Kaila 1997). With mutual GABA$_A$

receptor-dependent synaptic excitation, something resembling an epileptic chain reaction occurs among the interneurons (cf. chapter 5). We say resembling a chain reaction, because it is not yet known how this interneuron population event is initiated or whether firing can propagate from interneuron to postsynaptic interneuron solely via GABA$_A$ receptors. Certainly, however, it is clear that the depolarizing GABA$_A$ receptors play a major role in the synchronization process. Interestingly, giant IPSPs sometimes can precede epileptiform bursts induced by 4AP without blockers of ionotropic glutamate receptors (Avoli 1996), as if the interneuron burst were causally related to the ensuing synchronized pyramidal cell burst.

Giant Depolarizing Potentials in Hippocampal Slices from Immature Animals

The depolarizing GABA-dependent interneuron network bursts, expressed in 4AP, that we have been discussing, may be a holdover of a sort of activity expressed in neonatal cortical circuits and are believed to be important for the normal development of the brain. By way of background, three facts are pertinent. First, in the rat, GABAergic circuits, i.e., interneurons that are synaptically connected with each other and with pyramidal cells, are developed at birth. Second, in neonatal animals, the primary action of GABA is depolarizing due to a difference in transmembrane Cl$^-$ gradient from the more mature state (Cherubini, Gaiarsa, and Ben-Ari 1991). Only after a week or two do hyperpolarizing actions develop. Finally, AMPA receptor-mediated synaptic actions develop later than do NMDA receptor-mediated synaptic actions. It is thought that coincident firing of pre-and postsynaptic neurons with Ca^{2+} entry into the postsynaptic neuron is required for a Hebbian LTP-like mechanism to permit expression of functional AMPA receptors at synapses in the postsynaptic cell. This notion is similar to that by which NMDA receptor-mediated LTP leads to expression of AMPA receptors at previously silent synapses (Liao et al. 1995).

These three concepts are useful in interpreting the following experimental results. In CA3 slices from postnatal rats (e.g., age 2–5 days, never more than 12 days), spontaneous giant depolarizing potentials (GDPs) occur, synchronously, in pyramidal cells and in s. radiatum interneurons (Ben-Ari, Cherubini, et al. 1989; Khazipov, Leinekugel et al. 1997; figure 6.2). GDPs can be found in the isolated CA3 region. GDPs last a few hundred ms, are crowned with action potentials in both pyramidal cells and interneurons, and are associated with synaptic conductances in both cell types. In addition to synchrony between cell pairs, several other criteria for network behavior apply to GDPs, as they do to epileptiform bursts (Johnston and Brown 1981; Wong and Traub 1983). There is a long and variable latency to the GDP after a stimulus; the amplitude in a single cell, but not the frequency of GDPs is altered by manipulation of the membrane potential in that cell; and the events depend upon synaptic activity.

There are several lines of evidence that $GABA_A$ conductances participate. Bicuculline abolishes GDPs in pyramidal cells and in s. radiatum interneurons, and in both cell types, the reversal potential of the GDP in one neuron moves in a depolarizing direction, with Cl^- loading of that neuron in the same manner as happens to the voltage response evoked by GABA application (Khazipov, Leinekugel, et al. 1997).

NMDA receptors are also required, however, for GDPs to occur. NMDA blockers reduce the amplitude and duration of evoked GDPs, Ca^{2+} signals develop in neurons coincident with GDPs in pyramidal cells (Leinekugel, Medina et al. 1997), and a portion of the inward synaptic current in interneurons rectifies in a manner expected for an NMDA current. It should be noted that in CA3 pyramidal cells, NMDA conductances are slower in postnatal animals than in adult animals, although Mg^{2+} regulation of the channel

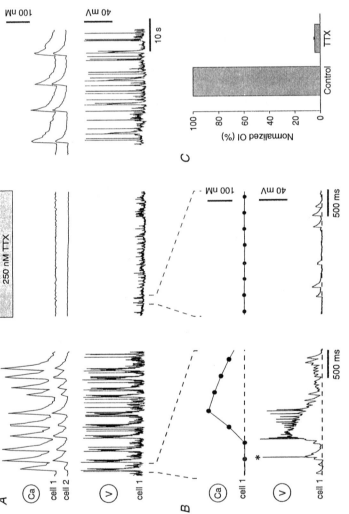

Figure 6.2

[Ca²⁺]ᵢ and membrane voltage correlates of giant depolarizing potentials in CA1 pyramidal cells, neonatal rat hippocampal slice (P1). (A) Spontaneous waves of activity are associated with synchronized intracellular Ca²⁺ signals and with membrane depolarizations with superimposed action potentials. Cell 1 was loaded with 150 μM fura-2, which led to loading of the nearby cell 2; cell 1 was also recorded from electrically in whole-cell current-clamp mode. The activity is reversibly blocked by tetrodotoxin (TTX), indicating that it is a network phenomenon. (B) Signals on expanded time scale. Single isolated action potentials (*) and spontaneous miniature synaptic potentials (lower middle trace) do not elicit Ca²⁺ signals. (C) Mean effect of TTX on optical signal in 18 cells in 7 slices. (From Garaschuk et al., 1998.).

is similar, a factor that may contribute to the long duration of the GDP (Khazipov, Ragozzino, and Bregestovski 1995). Finally, AMPA receptors are not required for GDPs to occur (Khazipov, Leinekugel, et al. 1997).

The relevant synaptic interactions in this CA3/interneuron network, then, are all excitatory and occur between pyramidal cells, between interneurons (as in the Michelson/Wong experiments), and between the respective cell populations. The effect of the GDP is to produce temporally coincident bursts in different cell pairs. As noted above, one interpretation of this effect is that it allows the development of AMPA receptor-mediated synaptic interactions (Ben-Ari et al. 1989; Hanse et al. 1997).

GDPs have also been found in CA1 in a similar preparation. These GDPs are temporally coincident between CA3 and CA1 (Garaschuk et al. 1998; figure 6.2) and are likewise associated with contemporaneous intracellular [Ca^{2+}] signals.

Interneuron Network Bursts Probably Synchronized by Gap Junctions

We shall now return to the work of Michelson and Wong (1994) on giant IPSPs in pyramidal cells, recorded in mature hippocampal slices, in media containing 4AP (e.g., 75 μM) and blockers of ionotropic glutamate receptors. It will be recalled that with blockade of GABA$_A$ receptors, after adding picrotoxin to the bath, the third component persists of the triphasic pyramidal cell potentials, the component that is presumed to be a large GABA$_B$ receptor-mediated potential. Additionally, it will be recalled that some interneurons (Type 2) in the hilus continue to generate bursts of action potentials, coincident with the residual pyramidal cell IPSP even with GABA$_A$ receptor blockade. Bursts in Type 2 interneurons (figure 6.3) either lack a depolarizing envelope or continue to persist when the cell is hyperpolarized. Action potentials may exhibit an abrupt onset, fail

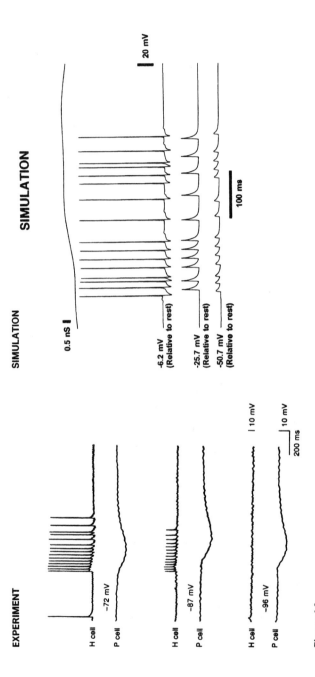

Figure 6.3

Interneuron network burst that is probably dependent upon nonsynaptic mechanisms. Experiment: Simultaneous recordings of a hilar inter-neuron (H cell) and a CA3 pyramidal cell. The medium contained 4AP and blockers of GABA$_A$ receptors and of ionotropic glutamate receptors. The large amplitude of the GABA$_B$ receptor-mediated IPSP in the pyramidal cell indicates that multiple interneurons are bursting synchro-nously. Progressive hyperpolarization of the hilar interneuron (middle traces) uncovers partial spikes, indicating that action potentials can be initiated remotely from the cell body under these conditions. Simulation: a network of interneurons was simulated, each having electrically active dendrites. The dendrites were interconnected by gap junctions in a random pattern with an average of 2 gap junctions per neuron. The coupling conductance allowed action potentials to propagate from one neuron to another and thus permitted reentrant activity in the population that could lead to sustained bursts. Under these conditions, hyperpolarization of a single neuron also uncovers partial spikes, which in this case are generated in dendrites. (From Traub, Wong et al., 1997; experiment originally from Michelson and Wong, 1994; simulation originally from Traub, 1995 with permission)

to be preceded by a depolarizing ramp, or begin from different levels of membrane potential—all characteristics of action potentials initiated at some site or sites remote from the soma. Furthermore, more extreme hyperpolarization of the membrane uncovers partial spikes of amplitude less than 10 mV, another characteristic of remote action potential initiation. Given that at least some of these interneurons are dye-coupled via dendrites to other, similar-appearing interneurons (Michelson and Wong 1994; figure 6.4), it seems likely that synchrony of bursting is mediated via gap junctions. The relevant gap junctions mediating synchrony are presumed to be dendro-dendritic, but axo-axonic gap junctions, as can occur in the retina (Vaney 1993), should also be considered (Draguhn et al. 1998).

This type of synchrony has been studied in network simulations by Traub (1995) (figure 6.3). In the conditions of these simulations (128 model interneurons), interconnected with nonrectifying, symmetric gap junctions, several criteria had to be met in order to obtain firing behaviors that agreed with experiment. These behaviors included synchrony, duration of the burst lasting many tens of ms, abrupt initiation of action potentials from baseline membrane potential, and partial spikes upon hyperpolarization of a single cell.

There were two criteria that had to be met. First, gap junction conductance had to be large enough and dendrites excitable enough that action potentials could propagate from one neuron to an electrotonically coupled neuron. In other words, strong coupling had to exist.

Second, gap junctions could neither be too sparse nor too plentiful. Of course, with too few gap junctions, isolated clusters of mutually coupled cells exist, rather than a connected syncytium, and there is no way for a large number of neurons to become synchronized. The reason why junctions could not be too plentiful is more subtle, and has to do with reentry. For a population burst to be sustained by gap junctions under the present conditions, with a series of action potentials occurring, there must be paths through the circuit, from the soma of each cell back to itself, so that reexcitation can occur.

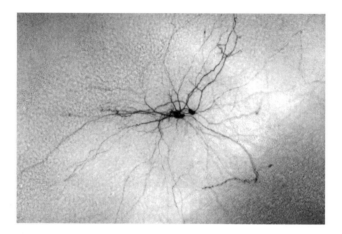

Figure 6.4
Oviform hilar interneurons, dye-coupled in the dendrites (Courtesy of H. Michelson)

(When there is an underlying slow synaptic depolarization, this criterion is unnecessary, but such a slow depolarization does not exist in the present situation.) Propagation of firing from the cell back to itself must also take long enough that the reentrant spike arrives when the neuron is no longer refractory: hence, the cycles can not be too short, on average, a matter well-known to those who study cardiac arrhythmias. When gap junctions are too plentiful, many short cycles occur, preventing the burst from sustaining itself.

There is ultrastructural evidence for the presence of gap junctions in the dendrites of interneurons in CA1, CA3, and the hilus (Kosaka 1983a,b; Katsumaru et al. 1988). What the Michelson-Wong experiments suggest is that these gap junctions can contribute directly to, or even be essential for, the generation of population behaviors, at least under certain conditions. For this reason, we must keep an open mind concerning the participation of gap junctions in other sorts of population behavior, including gamma oscillations, even if present data suggest that chemical synaptic interactions are the prime movers (so to speak) in gamma oscillations.

7   Gamma Oscillations in Vivo

In this chapter we shall review data on this set of questions: where in the brain do gamma oscillations occur and during what sorts of behavioral states? What might be the functional and physiological significance of gamma oscillations?

Gamma Oscillations in the Hippocampus in Vivo

In the hippocampus, gamma oscillations can be observed during at least four different conditions. First, they occur as a transient phenomenon, lasting a few hundred ms at most, following a physiological sharp wave (Buzsáki 1986; Traub, Whittington, Colling et al. 1996). Something like this phenomenon is also recorded in vitro following a synchronized burst induced by 4AP (see chapter 8). During a sharp wave, the firing rates of pyramidal neurons are increased (Ylinen et al. 1995a), but at least judging from extracellular unit activity, the pyramidal cells are largely silent after the sharp wave. The transient gamma following the sharp wave is, therefore, presumed to be generated by the interneuronal network, possibly as a consequence of the interneurons having become tonically depolarized from glutamate, released during the sharp wave, acting on NMDA and/or metabotropic receptors (see next chapter).

Second, during the theta state in the rat, gamma oscillations occur as a background rhythm superimposed on the theta waves. Gamma is observed superimposed on theta waves (4–12 Hz), both in rats anesthetized with ketamine/xylazine (Soltesz and Deschênes 1993; Sik et al. 1995; Ylinen et al. 1995b; Penttonen, Kamondi et al., 1998) and also in awake behaving rats (Bragin et al. 1995; figure 7.1). The amplitude of the gamma waves is modulated at theta frequency; and the firing of anatomically identified basket cells is time locked to both rhythms (chapter 3, figure 3.1; Sik et al. 1995; Penttonen et al., in 1998). Intracellular recordings of gamma activity have been obtained from the hippocampus of anesthetized rats by Penttonen et al.(1998): the gamma-frequency potentials occur in pyramidal cells (up to 2 mV in amplitude, in soma and in the apical dendrites) and also in basket cells. In the latter interneurons, subthreshold oscillatory potentials behave like $GABA_A$-receptor mediated IPSPs, so far as the reversal potentials are concerned. Firing rates of pyramidal cells are low in during the theta state (Buzsáki, Leung, and Vanderwolf 1983), but injection of a tonic current into the pyramidal cell—strong enough to induce repetitive firing—reveals that frequency accomodation is suppressed, as if there were some sort of metabotropic receptor influence present (Penttonen et al., 1998; cf. chapter 2 figure 2.9). Gamma oscillations also occur during spontaneous theta in the entorhinal cortex (layers II/III) of rats under ketamine/xylazine anesthesia (Chrobak and Buzsáki, 1998).

Not only is the mean firing rate of pyramidal neurons low during the theta state (and population spikes are never found during theta in normal conditions), but when pyramidal cells do fire, they tend to do so during the opposite phase of theta than when the interneurons usually fire (Buzsáki, Leung, and Vanderwolf 1983). At least, this pattern of firing is the case during anesthesia. Thus, there is evidence for participation of basket cells during hippocampal gamma during the in vivo theta state but not for the participation of pyramidal cells, at least not in a phasic manner. This observation suggests that gamma oscillations, which are superimposed on theta waves, might be generated by networks of interneurons that are tonically depolarized, as will be discussed in the next chapter.

Third, in vivo limbic seizures may end with a period of STO, seizure termination oscillation, at gamma frequency. The STO is apparently not generated by interneurons, as judged by extracellular unit recordings (Bragin et al. 1997). Hippocampal seizures in vitro in the high $[K^+]_0$ model are also sometimes initiated with a period of gamma-frequency population spikes (figure 5Ab of Jensen and Yaari 1997). Fourth, gamma oscillations may persist for minutes, following a limbic seizure via some completely unknown mechanism (Leung 1987).

Gamma Oscillations in Sensory, Motor, and Auditory Cortices

In awake cats, 35–45 Hz EEG activity occurs during focused attention, such as watching a mouse in another cage. This EEG activity was found only in certain regions of sensorimotor cortex (4γ, $6\alpha\beta$, 5a) but not in intervening cortical regions (Bouyer, Montaron et al. 1987). These authors pointed out that the cortical areas with 35–45 Hz EEG activity contain large pyramidal cells.

Murthy and Fetz (1992) described 25–35 Hz field potential activity and correlated unit activity in the sensorimotor cortex of awake, behaving monkeys. This gamma activity occurred in bursts lasting about 100 ms to a few hundred ms. Gamma bursts were most common when the monkey was performing a sensorimotor task that required attention, such as reaching for a raisin that it could not see, but bursts could also occur, albeit less often, spontaneously or during the performance of repetitive motor tasks. (Donoghue et al. [1998] found that gamma oscillations were most likely to occur just before a movement was made by an alert monkey.) Field potentials associated with gamma bursts reversed polarity at cortical depths of about 800 μm. Murthy and Fetz provided further significant in-

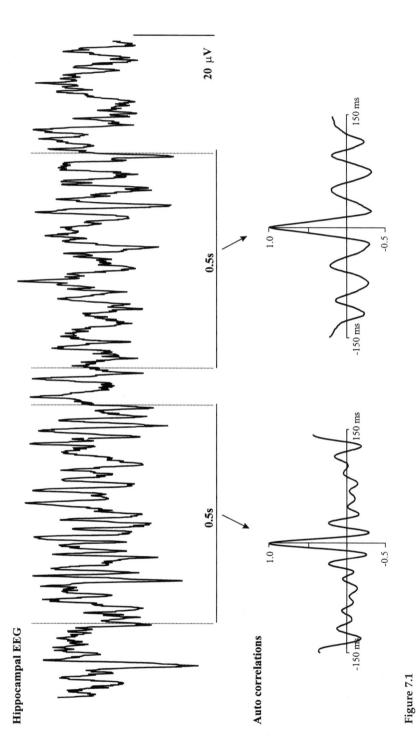

Figure 7.1
Hippocampal EEG from an awake behaving rat, showing first theta activity with superimposed gamma, then beta activity. The gamma frequency is 38 Hz and the beta frequency, 20 Hz. (H. Doheny and M. Whittington, unpublished data.)

formation in two subsequent papers (1996a,b): gamma oscillations can occur synchronously in sensorimotor cortex with near-zero phase lag at distances up to about 2 cm. Two-site synchronization can also occur across the corpus callosum, as it does in visual cortex (see below).

For several reasons, the functional significance of these gamma bursts is not clear. First, the incidence of gamma bursts is about the same with one-handed as with two-handed tasks. Second, two different units can become synchronized whether or not both participate in the ongoing task (participation being judged by an increase in firing rate during the task). Rather, during the oscillation, the firing rate of the neuron is clamped at its pre-oscillation rate. Murthy and Fetz offered this summary statement: "Widespread synchronization of LFP (local field potential) oscillations in the sensorimotor cortex appears to be too nonspecific and episodic to be directly involved in mediating motor control."

When synchronized gamma oscillations appear in the sensorimotor cortex of awake cats during a task, the oscillation frequency decreases during the reward phase that follows, and significant phase lags develop between previously synchronized areas (Roelfsema, Engel, König, and Singer 1997). Barth and MacDonald (1996) studied gamma oscillations in the auditory cortex of lightly anesthetized rats, using 8×8 arrays of electrodes placed onto the cortical surface, with inter-electrode spacing 500 μm. Then, 500 ms trains of current pulses were delivered to the posterior intralaminar nucleus (PIL, the nonspecific part of the auditory thalamus), and these trains evoked a burst of gamma oscillations in the auditory cortex (figure 7.2). The latency to onset of the evoked oscillations was hard to define precisely but was about 100–200 ms, with the oscillations outlasting the stimulus by about 100 ms. Spontaneous bursts of gamma waves, lasting more than 100 ms, also occurred, as is the case in sensorimotor cortex in awake monkeys (see above). Both evoked and spontaneous auditory cortical

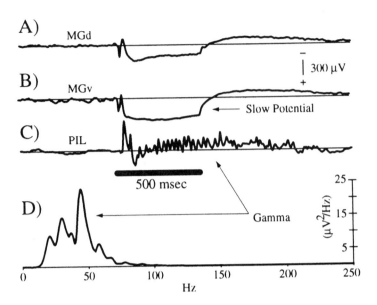

Figure 7.2
Gamma waves in auditory cortex evoked by stimulation of the acoustic thalamus.
Potentials were measured in the auditory cortex of rats (halothane anesthesia) during and after stimulation of different thalamic regions with 500 ms trains of 500 Hz
current pulses. (A, B) stimulation of dorsal medial geniculate (MGd) and of ventral
medial geniculate (MGv) evoke only slow potentials. (C) Stimulation of the posterior
intralaminar nucleus (PIL) evokes gamma oscillation that outlasts the stimulus
(power spectrum in D). Mapping studies showed this oscillation to occur in the
boundary region between primary and secondary auditory cortex. Spontaneous
gamma activity could occur in this region as well, even after lesions of PIL, suggesting that the cortex is able to generate gamma oscillations on its own, at least in
some conditions. (From Barth and MacDonald, 1996, with permission of *Nature*, ©
Macmillan Magazines Ltd.)

gamma oscillations were centered between the 1° and 2° regions
of auditory cortex. Following an electrolytic lesion of PIL, spontaneous gamma oscillations still had the same spatial distribution
as before the lesion. Stimulation of the medial geniculate nucleus,
either the ventral or dorsal parts, that is to say, stimulation of the
specific auditory thalamus, not only failed to elicit cortical gamma
oscillations, but it suppressed spontaneous gamma bursts in the
cortex. During both evoked and spontaneous bursts of gamma ac-

tivity, gamma waves in 2^0 auditory cortex lagged behind those in 1° auditory cortex by 2–4 ms.

Barth and MacDonald concluded that auditory cortex alone is sufficient to generate gamma oscillations, but that cortical gamma can be triggered by thalamic inputs as well. This group has subsequently shown that focal electrical stimulation of nucleus reticularis thalami could evoke gamma oscillations in cortex, either in auditory or somatosensory regions, depending on which part of nRT was excited (MacDonald et al. 1998).

In a subsequent study (Brett and Barth 1997), it was found that stimulation of the centrolateral nucleus (CL) of the thalamus or stimulation of nucleus basalis (basal forebrain) failed to elicit gamma oscillations in auditory cortex. Anatomical data were consistent with the physiology: HRP injections into regions of auditory cortex, where oscillations could be evoked, led to labeling of cells in PIL and the nearby acoustic thalamus but did not label CL or nucleus basalis.

Using rats, MacDonald, Brett, and Barth (1996) recorded spontaneous runs of gamma oscillations, lasting more than 100 ms and occurring independently in both auditory and somatosensory cortex. Oscillations were only found in these granular cortices and were not found in the intervening nongranular cortex (cf. the comparable results of Bouyer et al. 1987, cited above). There was an approximately 2 ms phase lag in oscillations from 1° to 2° somatosensory cortex. When oscillations occurred simultaneously between auditory and somatosensory cortex of one hemisphere or in auditory (respectively somatosensory) cortex of both hemispheres, the oscillations were not phase-locked; this observation stands in contrast to stimulus-evoked visual cortical oscillations, which do synchronize across corpus callosum and with which synchrony depends on the corpus callosum (see below). MacDonald et al. (1996) noted that callosal connections in the rat, running between auditory and between SS regions, do not interconnect precisely homotopic regions.

Instead, they tend to run from granular to dysgranular cortex; the latter type of cortex may be unable, or less able than the granular cortex, to express gamma oscillations in vivo. Jones and Barth (1997) also described gamma oscillations produced in somatosensory cortex by stimulation of the mystacial pad and of contralateral vibrissae. These oscillations were confined to primary and secondary somatosensory cortex.

In the Galambos classification of gamma oscillations (see chapter 1), the oscillations so far discussed in this chapter are spontaneous and induced (occurring after a stimulus, but not time locked to the stimulus). Time-locked evoked oscillations in auditory cortex have also been recorded, including in humans (Galambos, Makeig, and Talmachoff 1981; Joliot, Ribary, and Llinás 1994). Steady-state gamma oscillations during periodic stimulation occur as well.

Sniff-evoked Oscillations in Olfactory Bulb

Physiological stimulation of the olfactory bulb with odors leads to the appearance of runs of 40–80 Hz EEG waves (Adrian 1942, 1950). These oscillations are generated within the olfactory bulb itself, as the olfactory nerve does not show evidence of oscillatory activity, and are associated with increased firing of mitral cells. In a remarkable series of experiments, Freeman and colleagues showed that olfactory-induced oscillations in the bulb are spatially distributed, at near constant frequency, but with the oscillation amplitude being modulated by position in the bulb. Furthermore, this spatial modulation carries information about the identity of the odor and of the behavioral relevance of the odor, so that the same odor can evoke different spatial patterns over the bulb, in different experiments (Freeman 1978; Bressler and Freeman 1980; Freeman and Schneider 1982; Viana di Prisco and Freeman 1985). Interestingly, in the locust olfactory system, temporal modulation of firing patterns also carries information about odor identity (see below). In the olfactory system, therefore, it appears likely that gamma oscillations have behavioral relevance.

The cellular mechanism of gamma oscillation that has been proposed for olfactory bulb (Freeman 1974; Gray and Skinner 1988) involves recurrent excitation of granule (inhibitory) cells by the mitral (excitatory) cells, followed by inhibition by the granule cells. This scheme predicts that mitral cells should exhibit a phase advance with respect to the field IPSPs of about ¼ cycle, or about 4.2 ms at 60 Hz; unit recordings were consistent with the existence of such a phase advance. This finding is in contrast to tetanically induced gamma oscillations in the hippocampal slice: in this latter case, pyramidal neurons and inhibitory neurons fire nearly in phase. This firing pattern is a consequence of interneurons in the hippocampus inhibiting each other, as well as pyramidal cells, and both pyramidal cells and inhibitory neurons being tonically depolarized after a tetanic stimulus (chapter 4; see also chapter 9).

Stimulus-Evoked Oscillations in the Visual Cortex

Visual cortical gamma oscillations can be either time locked to a stimulus, or of delayed onset and not time locked to the stimulus. In humans, relatively short-latency (tens of ms) oscillations are time locked; these oscillations are also rather fast, more than 100 Hz (Lopez and Sannita 1997). In contrast, in cat visual cortex (Eckhorn et al. 1988; Gray and Singer 1989; Gray, Engel, König, and Singer 1990), oscillations evoked by sensory stimulation are not time locked to the stimulus. Much of the interest in gamma oscillations and their relevance to cognition has been motivated by studies of the non-time-locked events, as these latter appear capable of encoding certain global features of the inducing visual stimulus.

Properties of Visual Cortical Oscillations at a Single Recording Site

We present here some of the important details from the three papers just cited. Gamma-frequency oscillations in voltage occur in field potential and in unit recordings (figures 7.3 and 7.4); this presence implies that local populations of neurons develop correlations in their mutual firing times, as well as oscillating individually. The optimal visual stimulus for evoking the oscillations is moving rather than stationary, and the movement velocity should not be either too fast or too slow. Synchronization lasts for 100 to 900 ms, and there are "multiple epochs of correlated oscillations" over about 1 second after a moving bar stimulus (Gray, Engel, König, and Singer 1992). Individual cells with oscillatory properties, evoked by visual stimulation, are to be found in cortical layers 2/3 through layer 6, but not all cells with the appropriate receptive field and orientation preference oscillate: oscillations were found in 7 out of 60 simple cells and in 30 out of 54 standard complex cells (Gray, Engel, König, and Singer 1990). Besides receptive field and orientation preference, which have strong effects, what additional underlying factors distinguish oscillating from non-oscillating cells are not clear. In addition, in squirrel monkey visual cortex, action potentials in deep layer 3 lead action potentials in layer 2/3 by about 3 ms on average (Livingstone 1996).

Visual evoked oscillations are most apparent with binocular stimulation or with stimulation of the dominant eye for those cells with clear ocular dominance (see also Eckhorn and Obermüller 1993). A change in orientation of the stimulus from the optimal orientation attenuates the degree of modulation in the oscillation in spike-time histograms (note that these are extracellularly recorded data), or the change in orientation may abolish the oscillation altogether. Simultaneous visual stimulation with an optimally oriented bar and with

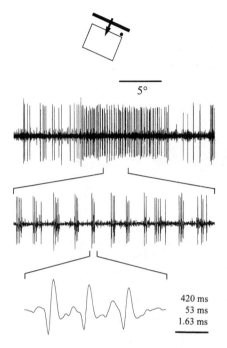

5°

420 ms
53 ms
1.63 ms

Figure 7.3
Gamma oscillation evoked in visual cortex (area 17) by visual stimulation in awake cat. The oscillation (shown in field potential recordings on three different time scales) was evoked by visual stimulation with a moving bar, as shown in the inset above (●, fixation point; □, receptive field). Brief bursts occur at about 40 Hz. The fine structure of this unit activity (bottom trace) suggests that the cell is chattering (see appendix 1 of this chapter.) (From Gray, 1994 with permission)

an orthogonally oriented bar interferes with the oscillation. Visual evoked oscillations are also to be found in awake cats and monkeys (figures 7.3 and 7.4; Eckhorn, Frien, et al. 1993; Frien, Eckhorn, et al. 1994; Gray and Viana Di Prisco 1997), and thus they are not an artefact of the anesthesia. Visually induced oscillations can be found in area V2 of the monkey, as well as area V1 (Frien, Eckhorn, et al. 1994).

The firing patterns of visual cortical units that oscillate at gamma frequency suggest that the cells are bursting on each

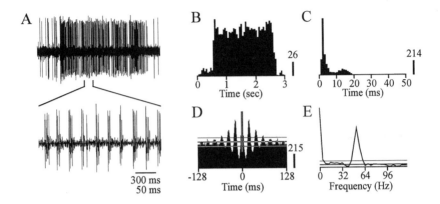

Figure 7.4
Gamma oscillations evoked by visual stimulation, in visual cortex of awake monkey.
(A) Unit activity of a cortical neuron responding to visual stimulation, shown on
two time scales. As in Figure figure 7.3, the unit chatters. (B) Firing rate as a function
of time. (C) Spike interval histogram shows two peaks, corresponding to the high
intra-burst frequency and to the gamma frequency of bursting. (D) Autocorrelation
of unit activity reveals rhythmicity of the bursting discharge. (E) Power spectrum
of autocorrelation shows gamma-frequency peak. (Courtesy of C. M. Gray)

gamma wave at high intra-burst frequencies (several hundred Hz)
(figures 7.3 and 7.4; see also Gray and Singer 1989). This notion
has been confirmed with intracellular recordings, the high-
frequency bursting sometimes being called chattering (Gray and
McCormick 1996). Chattering is discussed further in an appendix
to this chapter. Intracellular recordings in visual cortex also suggest the occurrence of gamma-frequency synaptic potentials
(probably a mixture of EPSPs and IPSPs) during a visual stimulus
(Jagadeesh et al. 1992).

In humans, visually evoked gamma oscillations can appear after
a latency as long as 280 ms (Tallon-Baudry et al. 1997), and the
gamma activity can be followed by beta waves (Pantev 1995). This
latter finding is of particular interest, as beta oscillations follow
gamma oscillations in vitro in slices that have been strongly stimulated (see chapter 10).

Properties of Visual Cortical Oscillations Recorded at Two Sites

Visual cortical oscillations can be synchronized over long distances—at least 7 mm in the cat—when the evoking visual stimulus has an appropriate structure, i.e., with respect to receptive field, orientation, and spatial continuity of the object (Gray, König, Engel, and Singer 1989). With regard to the distance over which oscillations can synchronize, it should be noted that neocortical pyramidal cell collateral axons are estimated to conduct at 0.15 to 0.55 m/s (Murakoshi et al. 1993). An axon conducting at 0.55 m/s would take 12.7 ms to propagate a signal for 7 mm. As gamma oscillations can be synchronized (on average) with phase lags of 1 or 2 ms, it becomes an intriguing physical problem (and a problem on which in vitro studies shed light—chapter 9) how such tight synchrony can be achieved despite such long conduction delays. It seems unlikely that synchronization over such distances, which is specific for features of an object, is generated entirely within the thalmus and then projected to discrete cortical areas, as feature recognition itself is generated intracortically. In addition to long-range synchrony within primary visual areas of the cat, synchronization can occur as well between areas V1 and V2 of the monkey (Frien, Eckhorn, et al. 1994), between striate and extrastriate cortex of the cat (Engel, Kreiter, König, and Singer 1991), and across the corpus callosum in the cat (Engel, König, Kreiter, and Singer 1991). In the latter case, anatomical integrity of the corpus callosum is required for synchronization: cortical-cortical connections must be preserved.

The most commonly used paradigm for studying long-range synchrony in the visual system is to use a long bar as a test stimulus, followed by variations of this test, the long bar with its middle third removed, and the proximal and distal thirds of the bar moving in opposite directions. For within-hemisphere synchrony, the cross-correlations between oscillating cortical sites are strongest when both sites are stimulated by the same (collinear) object, for example a single long moving bar (Gray, König, Engel, and Singer 1989). Synchronization is less optimal when the middle portion of the bar is removed, and synchronization may not occur at all if the two sites are stimulated by bars moving in opposite directions. In contrast, and somewhat mysteriously, when oscillations are synchronized across the corpus callosum, neither receptive field nor orientation preference must overlap in order for two separated regions to oscillate synchronously (Engel, König, Kreiter, and Singer 1991).

It is possible for some neurons at site 1 to oscillate synchronously with some neurons at site 2 (several mm away), while being phase-advanced up to 4.5 ms with respect to other neurons at site 1 (König, Engel, Roelfsema, and Singer 1995). It was hypothesized that the phase-delayed neurons were driven less than optimally, perhaps due to differences in orientation selectivity; a network model, based on studies of gamma oscillations in the hippocampal slice, is consistent with this idea (Traub, Whittington, and Jefferys 1997).

Amblyopia Studies in Cats: Evidence That Gamma Oscillations Are Important in Perception

Roelfsema, König, Siretano, and Singer (1994) induced esotropia (inward deviation of one eye) in cats surgically. They demonstrated behavioral confirmation of amblyopia (reduced visual perception through a structurally normal eye) by failure of the esotropic cat to respond correctly to gratings presented to the amblyopic eye, in contrast to a correct response on presentation of the grating to the normal eye. Recordings were made in area 17, using multiunit recording electrodes, with the electrodes up to 2 mm apart. With interelectrode separations this small, oscillation-synchronization between 2 sites does not depend on the relative orientation preference of the 2 sites (in contrast, say, to 7 mm separation). Visual stimulation of either eye with a grating produced a comparable increase in firing rates in neuronal units responding to the respective eye; such responsive units were found with about equal frequency when the stimulation of the two eyes was compared. In response to bars, however, synchronization was nearly absent between two sites when site 1 was driven by the normal eye and site 2 by the amblyopic eye. In addition, if both sites were driven by the amblyopic eye, synchrony was decreased in response to a high-spatial-frequency grating when compared to the case where both sites were driven by the normal eye.

The authors argued that perceptual deficits could arise from abnormal timings, both across amblyopic stimuli and with simultaneous normal/amblyopic stimuli. This conclusion is interesting, especially as individual neurons seemed to respond normally to single-site stimulation. As we will show later, loss of long-range synchronization could have a number of different cellular mechanisms. One example of a means for two oscillating sites (at gamma frequency) to become incapable of mutual synchronization is depression of the pyramidal cell synaptic connections from one site to interneurons at the other site (chapters 9 and 10).

On the Uncertain Uses of Distributed Synchronization for Cerebral Representation of an Object That Is Spatially Distributed in the Visual Field

Brosch, Bauer, and Eckhorn (1995) found synchrony of visually driven oscillations in cat visual cortex, areas 17 and 18, only when the respective receptive fields overlapped or were adjacent. If this observation is valid in general, it implies that for synchrony to be used in the representation of a large object, then the object must be topologically connected. In other words the object in visual space can be covered with a set of overlapping or touching visual field patches in such a way that a path exists from any patch to any other patch via intermediate patches. This notion is perhaps consistent with experimental data (Engel, Kreiter, König, and Singer 1991) that synchrony elicited by two separated collinear bars is at least slightly less robust than synchrony elicited by a single long bar. On the other hand, it is not yet precisely worked out which conditions evoke long-range synchrony, and which conditions do not:

1. As mentioned above, synchrony across the corpus callosum does not depend on orientation preference or receptive field (Engel, König, Kreiter, and Singer 1991).

2. Engel, Kreiter et al. (1991) recorded from sites in striate and extrastriate cortex, respectively, with nonoverlapping receptive fields and similar orientation preference. They found clear synchrony between the two sites when both were activated by a single moving bar or by two separated bars moving coherently in the same direction. However, they found no synchrony when the stimulus consisted of two bars moving in opposite directions. Yet, when this experiment was repeated in the squirrel monkey for sites 5 mm apart, there *was* synchrony between the two sites using two bars moving in opposite directions, albeit not as strong as the synchrony induced by a single bar (figure 15 of Livingstone 1996).

3. Stimuli moving at right angles to each other tend not to evoke synchronized oscillations, or to reduce the modulation amplitude in the oscillation evoked by a single optimal stimulus (Gray, Engel, König, and Singer 1990). How then are objects with corners represented?

Thalamocortical Gamma Oscillations: Human Studies with Magnetoencephalography (MEG)

Ribary et al. (1991) performed MEG measurements with a 14–channel system, having 1 ms temporal resolution and 2–5 mm spatial resolution in the cortex but with less spatial resolution in deep structures. They made recordings in 5 normal young adults, 5 normal elderly subjects, and 5 demented elderly patients. Recordings were made during continuous auditory stimulation at 40 Hz. Ribary et al. observed a roughly 40 Hz signal that was widespread across the cortical mantle, as well as being present in or near diencephalic structures. There was a progressive phase shift from the the front of the head to the back, the front leading, with the maximum phase shift across the brain of 4–6 ms. In the demented patients, the ratio of cortical-signal amplitude to thalamic-signal amplitude was reduced, relative to age-matched normal subjects.

Llinás and Ribary (1993) reported further measurements using a 37–channel MEG apparatus. They found that 40 Hz activity occurred spontaneously in spindlelike events lasting hundreds of ms. This duration of 40 Hz transient oscillations is comparable to the observations of Murthy and Fetz (1992, 1996a, b) in the monkey.

The 40 Hz events in humans occurred during wakefulness, REM (rapid eye movement) sleep, and slow-wave sleep, with significantly greater amplitude during wakefulness and REM sleep. The rostral-caudal phase shift, found during evoked 40 Hz, was also found during spontaneous 40 Hz events, both in wakefulness and REM sleep; the phase shift was most apparent during REM sleep.

Joliot et al. (1994) recorded MEG signals from awake human subjects during and after the presentation of auditory clicks. When two clicks were presented within 12–15 ms, only one gamma-wave was evoked, and the subject reported hearing a single click. In contrast, when the clicks were presented at longer intervals, two gamma-waves were evoked, and the subject heard two separable clicks. The authors, noting that 12–15 ms is one-half of a gamma cycle (about), thus had discovered a clear correlation between evoked—time-locked—gamma activity in the brain, and perception.

Thalamocortical Gamma Oscillations: Animal Studies

Thalamocortical gamma oscillations occur spontaneously and can be potentiated by stimulation of cholinergic nuclei in the mesopontine reticular formation. Spontaneous oscillations are synchronized between areas of thalamus and cortex that are reciprocally interconnected, with phase delays up to 5–6 ms (Steriade, Contreras, Amzica, and Timofeev 1996); oscillations appear in both principal thalamic nuclei and in nucleus reticularis thalami (nRT). Spontaneous gamma oscillations occur during the intracellular depolarizing phase (recorded in neocortical cells) of the slow rhythm (< 1 Hz), a rhythm that is seen during slow-wave sleep in chronically implanted cats and during ketamine/xylazine anesthesia in cats. Gamma oscillations, however, do not occur during the hyperpolarizing phase of the slow rhythm (Steriade, Amzica, and Contreras 1995; Steriade and Amzica 1996; figure 7.5). (It is also the case that in vitro gamma oscillations are associated with slow cellular depolarizations.) Gamma waves may follow a sleep spindle, a phenomenon reminiscent of gamma waves following hippocampal sharp waves. In contrast to Murthy and Fetz (1992), Steriade and colleagues did not find a phase reversal of gamma oscillations recorded through the depths of the cortex (Steriade, Amzica, and Contreras 1995). Interestingly, intrinsic 40 Hz oscillatory properties are found in some cells of intralaminar nuclei (CL region) and of the VA/VL thalamic nuclei (Steriade, Curró Dossi, Paré, and Oakson 1991), with this rhythmicity potentiated by mesopontine stimulation, which likewise potentiates gamma oscillations in neuronal populations. The facilitation of thalamic gamma (which can be recorded in cortical field potentials as well) is mediated by muscarinic receptors, either in cortex and/or thalamus, and is not dependent on a pathway running through basal forebrain nuclei (Steriade, Curró Dossi, Paré, and Oakson 1991).

The spatial extent of synchronization of cortical gamma appears to be limited during slow-wave sleep, although this observation has not been fully quantitated. Gamma, activated by stimulation of the pedunculopontine tegmentum (see below), is synchronized across all cortical layers within a column but is not synchronized between cortical areas 5 and 6 in ketamine/xylazine anesthesia (Steriade, Amzica, and Contreras 1995). Similar results were found for spontaneous gamma oscillations in the awake animal, comparing potentials in a single column or in nearby columns (< 1 mm away), using paired extracellular recordings from cortical areas 3 and 4. One may speculate that wide-spread (but still patchy) synchrony of gamma oscillations is what counts for cognition, not the localized oscillations themselves.

The long phase delays that can occur between thalamic and cortical gamma oscillations are unlike the tighter synchronization seen intracortically with gamma oscillations evoked by visual stimulation or occurring in sensorimotor cortex of awake monkeys, but this difference may be related to the anesthesia. The mechanisms of thalamocortical oscillations are nevertheless critical to understand, given the dense interconnections of the participating neuronal structures and given the human MEG data.

Facilitation of Gamma Oscillations by Brainstem Stimulation

Steriade and Amzica (1996) stimulated the pedunculopontine nucleus (PPT, a cholinergic nucleus) at 300 Hz in adult cats anesthetized with ketamine/xylazine. This stimulation evoked gamma oscillations in field potential recordings in neocortical area 5 and synchronously in the CL nucleus of the thalamus (a region reciprocally connected with area 5). The evoked oscillations occurred after a latency of approximately 150–200 ms, lasted some hundreds of ms, and outlasted the stimulus. In intracellular recordings from neocortical regular-spiking neurons, the evoked response consisted of a slow EPSP with superimposed gamma oscillations, not time locked to the stimulus, the gamma having latency of about 200 ms (figure 7.6; see also Steriade, Amzica. and Contreras 1995). The slow depolarization observed in these experiments—having a superimposed oscillation that appears with latencies of 100–200 ms—bears

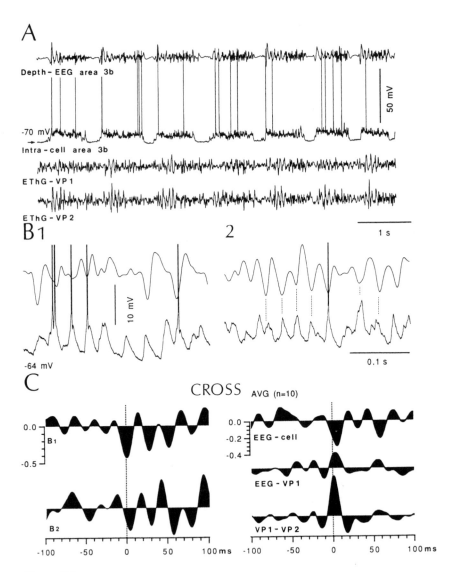

Figure 7.5
Thalamocortical gamma during the slow (< 1 Hz) oscillation. Cat under ketamine/
xylazine anesthesia. (A) Simultaneous recordings of EEG in cortical area 3b, intracellular recording of an area 3b neuron, and EEG signals (electrothalamograms,
EThG) from two sites in ventral posterior nucleus (VP) of the thalamus. (EEG signals
filtered between 10 and 100 Hz.) Note the slow (about 1 Hz) oscillation, with waves

a striking resemblance to gamma activity evoked in vitro by tetanic stimulation (chapters 9 and 10). There is a suggestion of some common underlying mechanism.

Munk, Roelfsema, et al. (1996) further developed the idea of brainstem-potentiated cortical gamma oscillations, using anesthetized cats (N_2O plus halothane, with pancuronium paralysis) to investigate how brainstem stimulation would interact with visual stimulation. Visual stimulation with one or two moving bars was used, both before and after stimulation of the mesencephalic reticular formation, while recording multiple unit activity in visual cortex. Mesencephalic reticular formation (MRF) stimulation did not increase the mean number of spikes occurring in response to visual stimulation, but it did 1) enhance the appearance of frequencies above 14 Hz, both in spontaneous activity and in response to stimulation, and 2) enhance the synchronization of responses between the two hemispheres, at sites close to the vertical meridian. On the other hand, MRF stimulation did not lead to synchronization of oscillatory responses to two light bars moving in opposite directions; this control observation implies that activation of synchrony is not nonspecific, given that, under normal conditions, there is little 2-site response synchronization to light bars moving in opposite directions. The cellular basis of this MRF-oscillation-facilitating effect is not known, but it could also depend on muscarinic receptor activation of thalamic and cortical neurons.

of depolarization in the neuron and in the cortical EEG, a few spindle-frequency waves followed by higher frequency oscillations. (B) Two epochs on expanded time scale of gamma activity in cortical neuron (below) and nearby EEG (above). (C, left) Cross-correlations between field recording and cell potential for epochs shown in B1 and B2, revealing ˜40 Hz rhythmicity; phase lag is near 0 for B1 and about 5 ms for B2. (Right) average of 10 cross-correlations between cortical EEG and cortical intracellular recording, between cortex and thalamus, and between two thalamic sites. Correlation is strongest within thalamic VP for these signals. (From Steriade, Contreras, Amzica, and Timofeev, 1996 with permission)

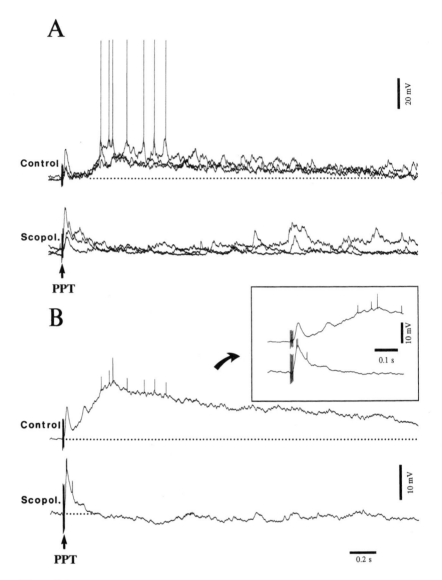

Figure 7.6
Muscarinic activation of the cortex. Cat under ketamine/xylazine anesthesia. (A) Intracellular recordings from a regular-spiking neuron in cortical area 5, depth 0.8 mm. Superimposed traces showing response to stimulation of the cholinergic pedunculopontine tegmental nucleus (PPT, 5 stimuli at 300 Hz) under control conditions and in the presence of the muscarinic blocker scopolamine (administered systemically). (B) Average of 15 traces before and after scopolamine administration. PPT stimulation leads to an early EPSP and then to a delayed, slow depolarization, with latency 150–200 ms, lasting for 2–2.5 seconds. Action potentials can be superimposed on this slow depolarization. (From Steriade and Amzica, 1996 with permission of the National Academy of Sciences, U.S.A.)

Gamma Oscillations Originating in the Deep Cerebellar Nuclei

Under certain conditions at least, thalamic (VL nucleus) and motor-cortical gamma appear to originate in the deep cerebellar nuclei (Timofeev and Steriade 1997): gamma-frequency EPSPs and fast prepotentials, appearing spontaneously in VL neurons, depend on the integrity of the brachium conjunctivum (the superior cerebellar peduncle, interconnecting the deep cerebellar nuclei with the VL region of the thalamus) and can in addition be evoked by stimulation of the brachium conjunctivum. VL gamma rhythms evoked in this way project on to motor cortex, with phase lags of 1.7–2.8 ms for durations of hundreds of ms. Spontaneous gamma oscillations in VL and motor cortex can also drift apart in frequency over time (Timofeev and Steriade 1997). If deep cerebellar nuclear gamma turns out to be widely synchronized within these nuclei, then one can speculate about a role of gamma oscillations in the timing functions of the cerebellum. The deep cerebellar nuclei/VL gamma projection may also be analogous to the fast oscillations observed by Neuenschwander and Singer (1996) that are visually induced and are coherent between retina and lateral geniculate nucleus.

Further Anatomical and Cellular Aspects of Thalamocortical Gamma

Thalamocortical Circuits

Many projection neurons in thalamic nuclei receive extrathalamic afferents coding for sensory information (e.g., retinal and spinothalamic projections). These connections are well ordered and involve mainly privileged primary target nuclei (Macchi et al. 1986). This segregation of inputs has the effect of restricting specific thalamic nuclei to particular functional modalities. For example, ventral thalamic nuclei are almost exclusively involved in motor function, with further subdivisions for discrete primary receptive fields. In the ventral posterior nucleus, the lateral area receives afferents coding for somatosensory information from the body, and the medial area receives similar afferents from the face. Remarkable somatotopic organization has been seen within portions of some thalamic nuclei. In the rat ventrobasal thalamic nucleus, projection neurons are arranged in laminar patterns which correspond to the barrels seen in somatosensory cortex (Land et al. 1995). These barreloids represent a detailed somatotopic map of the sensory field lying at an angle of $180°$ to the corresponding cortical map due to rotation of thalamocortical afferents within bundles in the internal capsule (Bernardo and Woolsey 1987). A similar, highly specific topographical interaction is seen between the primary visual cortex and the lateral geniculate nucleus (Reid and Alonso 1995).

Projection neurons in most thalamic nuclei send well-ordered efferents to the corresponding cortical area or areas (e.g., the primary visual cortex for the lateral geniculate nucleus), with reciprocal corticothalamic projections again precisely arranged to provide a thalamo-cortico-thalamic loop, allowing reinvasion of the projection site (Colwell 1975). Such an anatomical arrangement is presumably what underlies the occurrence and synchronization of gamma oscillations in reciprocally connected regions of thalamus and cortex. This excitatory loop can be highly specific and can take the form of a monosynaptic feedback loop (Hersch and White 1981; Reid and Alonso 1995). This loop is mainly located ipsilaterally, but projections of thalamic neurons to the contralateral cortex have been seen (Preuss and Goldman Rakic 1987). The precise projection site within the laminae of the neocortex is variable, depending both on the origin of the thalamic projection neuron and the target area (Robertson and Kaitz 1981; Craig et al. 1982). Strong thalamocortical projections terminate in the deeper layer of the cortex, although possible connections are seen in layers I and III. In general, the only cortical layer not seen to be a target for thalamocortical neurons was layer II (but see Livingstone and Hubel 1982).

The corticothalamic half of the loop usually involves axon collaterals from layer V and VI projection neurons, with some projections from layer IV (Jacobson and Trojanowski 1975). Some corticothalamic neurons target the thalamus specifically, with no axon collateralization within the cortex and subcortical white matter (Bernardo and Woolsey 1987). A large proportion of both thalamic and cortical afferents send out collaterals within the thalamic reticular nucleus and associated areas (ventral lateral geniculate nucleus, zona incerta) on their way to more medial thalamic nuclei. The thalamic reticular nucleus and associated areas also have some degree of somatotopic organization (Pollin and Rokyta 1982). This strong innervation of the mainly inhibitory reticular neurons (Houser et al. 1980) by collaterals of both thalamic efferents and afferents has led to the suggestion that the thalamic reticular nucleus may act as a gate controlling the activity of the thalamocortical loop.

Relevant Local Circuits

Within the deeper thalamic nuclei, the large projection neurons constitute the majority of cells seen, with only a paucity of smaller cells. These smaller cells stain positively for glutamic acid decarboxylase (GAD), suggesting that they are inhibitory interneurons (Houser et al. 1980; Kultas Ilinsky et al. 1985). The smaller cells also show extensive arborization within specific thalamic nuclei and possess serial and symmetrical synapses. This arborization suggests that these smaller neurons constitute local circuit interneurons providing blanket inhibition after activation by thalamic projection neurons. A far greater number of GAD-positive synaptic structures are present on thalamic projection neurons than would be expected from the small number of local circuit interneurons (Houser et al. 1980). Many of these inhibitory synapses on projection neurons come from axon

collaterals of reticular cells (Ohara et al. 1980). As well as the connections into deeper thalamic nuclei, reticular neurons, of which
there are two main types (Mulle et al. 1986; Contreras et al. 1992),
show strong axon collateralization for long distances with the thalamic reticular nucleus itself, possibly providing a substrate for recurrent inhibitory interactions.

Cortical local circuits, of relevance to thalamocortical interactions,
are numerous, but are in many cases poorly characterized. In its simplest form, the cortical component of the thalamocortical loop is a
monosynaptic interaction between thalamic and cortical projection
neurons (Hersch and White 1981). Within the deeper layers (IV–VI),
the proportion of synapses of thalamocortical origin on cortical projection neurons appears to depend on the major projection site of the
cortical principal cell (White and Hersch 1982). Cells with defined
thalamic projections were seen to have up to 20% of their synaptic input derived from thalamic projection neurons. In contrast, cells with
cortical or striatal projections had very few synapses from thalamic
cells (< 7% and < 1%, respectively). These observations suggested
that the thalamocortical loop was a specific substructure in the CNS
involving specific subsets of cortical neurons. Labelling experiments
have also shown that, even with monosynaptic connections, thalamocortical afferents send collaterals to synapse onto local inhibitory
interneurons within the deeper cortical layers (Keller and White
1989). These interneurons also receive input from axon collaterals of
cortical projection neurons. This reception suggests an arrangement
of both feed-forward and feedback inhibition within the cortical section of the loop, analogous to that seen in the hippocampus.

The fate of thalamocortical projections to layers III and I is less
clear. Layer V cortical pyramids send their major dendrite up
through layer III to arborize extensively within layers II and I. The
projections to layers III and I may, therefore, again represent monosynaptic connectivity with thalamocortical projection neurons, albeit with less influence on neuronal activity due to the distance of

the synapses in question from the soma. Alternatively, there are associational pyramidal neurons with their soma and dendritic arborizations within layer III, whose axons are seen to arborize extensively in the horizontal plane (Manzoni et al. 1979) and which provide inhibitory input to layer III cortical neurons via basket cell activation. These layer III neurons also innervate both deeper and more superficial cortical layers (Mitani et al. 1985). They may form part of a polysynaptic reflex pathway for thalamocortical information entering the cortex, or they may provide a mechanism for the lateral spread of this activity away from the precise somatotopic thalamocortical areas.

Sites of Generation of Fast Oscillations: the Cortex

Fast oscillations have been observed in cortical cells and populations of cells both in vivo (as reviewed above) and in cortical slices in vitro (next chapters). In the cat, about 20% of corticothalamic and corticocortical neurons exhibited intrinsic 40 Hz oscillations on depolarization (Nuñez et al. 1992a). In the visual cortex, as noted above, these fast oscillations have been seen to be generated in populations of neurons by visual stimuli, such as a bar of light, but in many of these experiments, no oscillation was seen in the corresponding thalamic region (Gray and Singer 1989; Gray et al. 1992). As well as fast oscillations in excitatory cells, intrinsic fast oscillations have been recorded in layer IV sparsely spiny neurons that are presumed to be inhibitory (Llinás et al. 1991).

In the isolated cortical slice, application of the metabotropic glutamate receptor agonist ACPD generated fast inhibitory oscillations in layer II cortical neurons (chapter 8; Whittington et al. 1995b). Similar experiments generated fast inhibitory oscillations in presumed layer III pyramidal cells, a major target for the layer IV interneurons mentioned above. The ability of rhythmic inhibitory input to entrain principal cell firing appears to be strong (Whittington et al. 1995b; Cobb et al. 1995). Such a mechanism—of oscillations being generated in networks of interneurons—permits the super-imposition of fast rhythms on many cortical principal cells due to the marked axon collateralization of layer II and layer IV basket cells. As we shall show later, however, when sufficiently many py-ramidal cells participate in the oscillation, new features of the os-cillation, related to the ability to synchronize over long distance, emerge.

Sites of Generation of Fast Oscillations: Thalamic Nuclei

Thalamic projection neurons display two distinct modes of activity (Jahnsen and Llinás 1984; Steriade and Deschênes 1984). A 4–8 Hz os-cillatory mode is well documented, consisting of rhythmic burst fir-ing generated by reciprocal activation of low-threshold calcium currents and potassium currents (intrinsic and GABA-activated), as well as the H-current (Sawyer et al. 1994). These cells also display a membrane potential-dependent transfer mode, which allows spike-for-spike following of primary afferent input, with fast oscillations of 40–70 Hz often seen. Fast spiking in projection neurons appears to be facilitated by the development of fast prepotentials of presumably dendritic origin (Deschênes 1981). In thalamic intralaminar nuclei, with diffuse projections to the cortex, depolarization of single cells generated 20–80 Hz activity that was clearly separate from spindle activity (Steriade et al. 1991; Steriade et al. 1993). Similar fast oscilla-tions were seen spontaneously during wakefulness and REM sleep.

Sites of Generation of Fast Oscillations: Thalamic Reticular Nuclei

The majority of research on the fast component of thalamocortical oscillations has implicated the thalamic reticular nucleus and re-lated structures in the generation of fast rhythms within the thalamocortical circuit as a whole. The cellular organization of the reticular nucleus itself has a number of properties relevant to the generation of fast oscillations.

Two types of reticular thalamic neurons have been reported (Contreras et al. 1992). Approximately one-quarter of reticular cells showed no bursting activity. Instead, slight depolarization led to the generation of a stable 40 Hz firing without a subthreshold oscillation. This type of oscillation can be generated by networks of inhibitory neurons reciprocally interconnected by synapses using $GABA_A$ receptors, provided the neurons are all depolarized by about the same amount (chapter 8; Whittington et al. 1995b; Traub et al. 1996). The evidence for this type of mutually inhibitory synaptic connectivity within the reticular nucleus is strong, with the majority of axon collaterals being present within the nucleus (Scheibel and Scheibel 1966) and with all identified cells being GABAergic inhibitory neurons (Houser et al. 1980). Circumstantial evidence for the dependence of this fast rhythm on mutual $GABA_A$ receptor-mediated inhibition was seen in experiments where metabotropic excitation of cell populations generated 40 Hz oscillations that were sensitive to bicuculline in a manner similar to the well-characterized 40 Hz oscillation in the hippocampus, occurring during blockade of ionotropic glutamate receptors (Pinault and Deschênes 1992a; Traub et al. 1996). Despite clear evidence, however, for fast population oscillations within the thalamic reticular nucleus, simultaneous recordings of pairs of reticular neurons showed little synchrony (Pinault and Deschênes 1992a). This lack suggested a limited involvement, perhaps highly restricted spatially, of reticular neurons in the population oscillation, possibly fitting with the topographic features of the nucleus. Synchronization within the reticular nucleus can also occur during periods of spindle oscillation (Steriade et al. 1993).

In order to understand the functional significance of oscillatory behavior of neurons, it is necessary to consider the impact of such activity on relevant CNS regions. The thalamocortical circuit involves the interaction between deep thalamic nuclei, the reticular thalamic nucleus, and cortical projection sites, with gamma oscillations present in each site. Despite clear evidence for intrinsic fast-oscillation generators within the neocortex (see above), no fast oscillations were seen in deep layer projection neurons in isolated neocortical slices during metabotropic activation and blockade of ionotropic glutamate receptors (Whittington et al. 1995b). We have, however, been able to induce gamma oscillations in the neocortical slice in layer IV neurons, using tetanic stimulation (see chapter 9). Clear evidence for fast oscillations in deep layer projection neurons was seen in vivo with thalamocortical connections intact, suggesting a role for corticothalamic linkages in generation and/or synchronization, at least under certain conditions (Nuñez et al. 1992). Still, the precise nature of the interactions responsible for cortical fast oscillations is not yet clear, either in vitro or in vivo.

Within the diencephalon itself, generation of fast oscillations may represent the synaptic interaction between principal neurons and the reticular nucleus, in a manner analogous to what has been proposed for spindle generation in ferret diencephalic slices (Bal, von Krosigk, and McCormick 1995a, 1995b). It has been shown that thalamic projection neurons can fire for long periods of time at 40–70 Hz, but during this transfer mode, a range of frequencies is often seen. In contrast, the reticular thalamic nucleus displays population activity at frequencies close to 40 Hz. There is a strong inhibitory influence of reticular neurons on thalamic projection neurons, as well as on each other, both influences mediated mainly by $GABA_A$ receptors, but with participation of $GABA_B$ receptors when enough reticular neurons are firing (see above; Sanchez-Vives and McCormick 1997; Sanchez-Vives, Bal, and McCormick 1997). In addition, there is excitatory activation of reticular neurons by both thalamocortical afferents and efferents. Oscillatory interactions between thalamic nuclei and the inhibitory reticular neurons have been demonstrated (Warren et al.

1994), and it has been suggested that fast inhibitory oscillations in the lateral geniculate nucleus act to drive the output of thalamocortical cells (Williams et al. 1996). In anterior thalamic nuclei, a group devoid of input from the thalamic reticular nucleus, no spindles or fast spike rhythms were seen (Paré et al. 1987). Having an inhibitory cell network, capable of oscillating autonomously but also driven by excitatory synaptic potentials, provides an oscillatory system that can be modulated in interesting ways. We shall discuss later some remarkable emergent phenomena that appear when excitatory cells join in to the oscillation in the hippocampal slice.

Modulation of Thalamocortical Oscillations by Extrinsic Influences

The occurrence of fast oscillations within the thalamocortical loop can be controlled by a number of external regions providing input to the major components (thalamus, reticular nucleus, and cortex): there are serotoninergic, adrenergic, dopaminergic, cholinergic and GABAergic synaptic interactions. As discussed above, cholinergic inputs from the pedunculopontine tegmental nucleus and from nucleus basalis potentiate fast oscillations in cortical EEGs (Metherate et al. 1992; Steriade et al. 1993) and provide strong cholinergic input to the reticular thalamic nucleus (Hallanger and Wainer 1988). Opposite effects to cholinergic ones are seen in both cortical and reticular thalamic areas when noradrenergic-activating regions are activated: fast oscillations were inhibited or abolished by noradrenergic locus coeruleus input or by direct activation of reticular $\alpha 1$ adrenergic receptors (Pinault and Deschênes 1992b; Steriade et al. 1993).

Concerning muscarinic actions in diencephalon, it is interesting that LGN interneurons do not depolarize in response to immediate metabotropic glutamate or muscarinic activation (Pape and McCormick 1995). In addition, muscarinic receptors hyperpolarize nRT cells as an initial effect, while a cholinergic activation of these cells is via nicotinic receptors (Lee and McCormick 1995). On the other hand, there is a delayed muscarinic depolarization, which presumably is the relevant effect. Concerning metabotropic receptor-mediated activation of the cortex, CL is part of the intralaminar complex; these nuclei project to the corpus striatum and layer I of various cortical areas, including area 5. Because the projection is to layer I, it is not likely to induce metabotropic glutamate receptor activation, as iontophoretically applied ACPD induces excitatory effects mainly in layer V (Cahusac 1994). If CL does induce a metabotropic excitation of the cortex, it may therefore be via muscarinic receptors.

GABAergic and cholinergic inputs from areas such as the mesopontine reticular system, the entopeduncular nucleus, and the substantia nigra also appear to influence ventral thalamic nuclei (Kultas Ilinsky et al. 1985). The neighboring dopaminergic ventral tegmental projection area as well appears to have strong control over the generation of fast oscillations within the thalamocortical loop (Montaron et al. 1984). Lesions of the ventral tegmental area abolished spontaneous fast oscillations, a process that could be partially reversed by the administration of apomorphine. The thalamic reticular nucleus contains a large number of D1 dopamine receptors (Huang et al. 1992). In cats, some A10 cells (ventral tegmental dopaminergic neurons, projecting to frontal cortex) appear to act as gating neurons controlling the generation of beta rhythms in the thalamocortical system (Galey et al. 1977).

Appendix 1: Chattering Cells

A critical physiological question asks is there a specific cell type that generates neocortical gamma or whose participation is at least necessary? In this appendix, we shall review data that suggest that chattering cells make a unique contribution to neocortical gamma oscillations, although it is not yet clear whether chattering cells correspond to a morphological cell type. We have already noted above that extracellular recordings in the visual cortex suggest that units fire high-frequency bursts that repeat at gamma frequencies (figures 7.3 and 7.4). Intracellular recordings have since demonstrated that visual stimulation does indeed produce gamma-frequency bursting in individual neurons (figure 7.7); in fact, of those cells that oscillate in response to visual stimulation, chattering cells are the most common type (Gray and McCormick 1996). Progress has been made in understanding some of the intrinsic cell properties that contribute to this pattern of bursting.

Based on the firing responses to depolarizing injected current, Gray and McCormick (1996) classified neocortical cells (in vivo) into IB (intrinsic bursting), RS (rhythmic spiking), FS (fast spiking), and chattering cells (bursting at gamma frequency, with many hundreds of Hz intraburst firing rate). The IB, RS, and FS cell types are well known (Connors, Gutnick, and Prince 1982; McCormick, Connors, et al. 1985). In chattering cells, extra spikes arise from spike depolarizing afterpotentials to produce doublets and bursts. The entire sequence of events is able to repeat at gamma frequency (figure 7.7). Gamma-frequency bursts of this sort, in response to strong injected current, have also been described by Steriade, Amzica, and Contreras (1995, their figure 7.10), in cat neocortical cells at depths of 0.5 and 0.8 mm (see also Steriade et al. 1998). The current required to elicit gamma-frequency chattering is large, about 1 nA (figure 7.7).

What might be the cellular mechanism of intrinsic (current-driven) chattering? One can imagine intrinsic mechanisms that involve either Ca spikes or bursts dependent upon a persistent g_{Na} (see chapter 2). McCormick and Nowak (1996) showed that the bursts in chattering cells are not solely dependent on Ca^{2+} currents, although the bursts do become irregular when extracellular Ca^{2+} concentration is reduced and Mg^{2+} concentration raised. The absence of subthreshold oscillations in chattering cells makes one

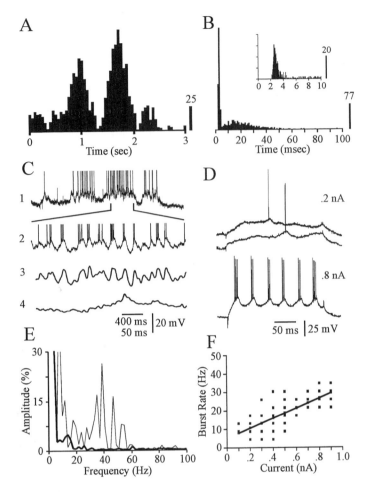

Figure 7.7
Intracellular recordings showing that chattering can be evoked in cortical neurons by visual stimulation, as well as by injection of tonic current. Cat under ketamine/ xylazine anesthesia. This striate-cortical cell had a simple receptive field and was orientation-selective but not direction-selective. (A) Peristimulus-time histogram, 20 presentations of an optimally oriented bar to the opposite eye. (B) Interspike interval histogram during the visual response showing two peaks, the slower one corresponding to gamma frequency (c.f. Figure 7.4, C). Inset: intervals at < 10 ms, with peak at about 2.5 ms (400 Hz). (C) Cellular response, at two time scales to visual stimulation (action potentials truncated), showing chattering (trace 2). In traces 3 and 4, action potentials have been removed, and trace 4 is spontaneous activity (no oscillations). (D) Response to steady current injections; the larger current evokes ˜30 Hz chattering. (E) Power spectrum of traces 3 (thin line) and 4 (thick line) from (C), showing gamma activity only in response to visual stimulation but not spontaneously. (F) Burst (chattering) rate as a function of injected current. (From Gray & McCormick, 1996 with permission of the American Association for the Advancement of Science)

wonder if persistent g_{Na} really could play a role in chattering. It is worth considering, however, the modeling work of X-J Wang (1993, 1998): an intrinsic 40 Hz oscillation, in response to steady depolarization, could arise from an interaction between $g_{Na(P)}$ and $g_{K(S)}$. The latter conductance is a K^+ conductance with $\tau_m = 5$ to 10 ms and with two phases of inactivation, both of which are slow ($\tau > 200$ ms) (Huguenard and Prince 1991) The intrinsic frequency of such a cellular oscillation is signficantly influenced by the activation time constant of $g_{K(S)}$ and by the membrane time constant as well. Slow inactivation of $g_{K(S)}$ can lead to intermittent runs of firing, rather than subthreshold oscillation. But this type of model (Wang 1993) when embodied in a single compartment by itself does not chatter. A 2-compartment model (soma + dendrite) *can* chatter, however, by an interaction between a 40 Hz wave generator as above in the dendrite and a system (with fast g_{Na} at the soma) capable of high-frequency firing. This mechanism is analogous to our model of repetitive bursting in CA3 cells, although operating at much higher frequencies. The common principle is localize $g_{Na(P)}$ and $g_{K(S)}$ to the dendrites (before it was g_{Ca} and $g_{K(C)}$) and couple the dendrites to a spike generator with fast kinetics at the soma/initial segment (Wang 1998; Traub et al. 1991 and 1994). It is perhaps relevant that persistent g_{Na} does actually occur in dendrites of neocortical cells (Mittman et al. 1997). It is also of interest that visual cortical neurons can chatter in response to muscarinic or metabotropic glutamate receptor activation (McCormick and Nowak 1996), just the type of receptors that seem critical for gamma oscillations in vitro.

For comparison with these findings, other sorts of chattering-like bursts have been described:

1. rostral intralaminar (IL) thalamic cells also can fire in the chattering mode (Steriade, Curró Dossi, and Contreras 1993). Extracellular recordings were obtained during the waking state in vivo, and also intracellular recordings in vivo from anesthetized animals. In-

traburst frequencies approached 1000 Hz. Doublets develop as an intrinsic property in these cells as well. Low-threshold Ca^{2+} spikes (LTS) are present in IL cells, but the kinetics are fast enough that IL cells can burst on almost every wave in a spindle, in contrast to principal TCR cells, which typically miss waves.

2. Chattering has been observed in neocortical neurons that were morphologically identified as aspiny, and hence that were probably interneurons (Steriade et al. 1998).

3. chattering-like behavior (40–80 Hz bursts, 2–6 spikes/burst) has been observed in pyramidal cells of the electrosensory line lobe of weakly electric fish (Turner, Maler et al. 1994). Again, the data suggest an interaction between somatic and dendritic Na^+ currents.

Neocortical chattering cells in vivo have been filled and reconstructed. In one study, such cells were spiny and occurred in layers II and III; they exhibited multiple intracortical collaterals to different layers and possibly a branch to the deep white matter (Gray and McCormick 1996; figure 7.8). Steriade et al. (1998) have reported also that at least some cells, capable of fast rhythmic bursting, can be antidromically activated by thalamic stimulation. Steriade and colleagues, working in cats in vivo found fast rhythmic bursting (FRB) cells in deep cortical layers (V and VI) as well as superficial layers. EPSPs were recorded in runs at 300–400 Hz in FRB cells themselves, suggesting that the FRB cells interconnected with each other. Remarkably, as noted above, at least some of the FRB neurons in the study of Steriade et al. were sparsely spiny local circuit neurons. The visual responsiveness of these cells was not studied.

Several important questions about chattering remain outstanding:

1. What is the functional significance of chattering? To answer this question, one would like a dual intracellular recording, in which the

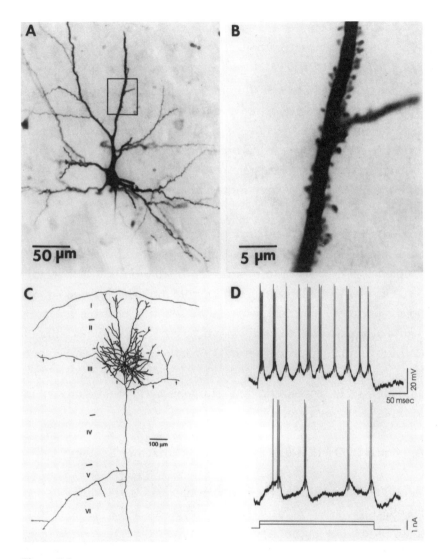

Figure 7.8
Morphology of a layer 3 spiny, striate-cortical neuron that chatters in response to current injection. (A) The biocytin-filled cell resembles a superficial pyramidal cell. (B) Higher-power view of the rectangular region in (A), showing high density of spines. (C) Camera lucida reconstruction of the cell, soma/dendrites thick lines, axon thin lines (small arrow, axon collaterals); the cell also projected into the white matter. (D) Response to tonic current injections. Smaller currents (below) do not reveal subthreshold oscillations, but the cell chatters in response to injection of a larger current (above). (From Gray and McCormick, 1996 with permission of the American Association for the Advancement of Science)

presynaptic cell chatters. Perhaps chattering induces striking synaptic depression or facilitation.

2. As it takes a rather large depolarizing current to elicit chattering, can one conclude that the physiological stimulus that evokes gamma includes a strong inward current as one of its components? If this possibility is the case, it would provide an important link between in vivo gamma oscillations, evoked by visual stimuli, and tetanically evoked gamma oscillations in vitro, as the latter are correlated with large intracellular depolarizations (chapter 9).

3. How can intrinsic oscillatory properties in neurons, such as the tendency to chatter and to develop subthreshold oscillations, be coupled together, so as to produce an oscillation that is synchronized throughout a large neuronal population? This is a deep question, especially given that, as we shall see, it is possible for large neuronal populations to produce synchronized oscillations without intrinsic oscillatory properties in the component neurons. Yet, one feels strongly, the widespread ability of single neurons to oscillate on their own in response to tonic stimulation can not be present in the brain without a reason.

Appendix 2: Oscillations in the Locust Olfactory System

Gilles Laurent and colleagues have published a series of papers on the olfactory system of locusts and honeybees that is of great interest to the student of gamma oscillations in the mammalian brain (e.g., MacLeod and Laurent 1996; Wehr and Laurent 1996.) In this appendix, we shall briefly review some of the data. As background, we note that the cell types in the locust olfactory system include the following:

1. In the antennal bulb, there are projection neurons (PNs) that are spiking and non-spiking local neurons. Local neurons produce

monosynaptic IPSPs in PNs via GABA$_A$ receptors, and a single local neuron can suppress firing in a PN that is tonically depolarized (compare Miles et al. 1996), although each PN still receives multiple GABA$_A$ inputs.

2. In the mushroom body, there are so-called Kenyon cells.

Puffing an odor over an antenna of a locust leads to an oscillation at about 20–30 Hz in the antennnal bulb and mushroom body. The oscillation can be recorded as field potentials and in intracellular recordings of bulb PNs and local neurons. Field potential oscillations are time locked to the stimulus and can be averaged. About 10% of PNs fire in response to a given odor. Individual PCs fire only during selected subintervals of the total time over which the oscillation lasts, and in fact, one can recognize cycle-by-cycle changes in firing probability that are specific for neuron/odor pairs. Phase differences between pairs of PNs do not appear to be odor-specific, but the overall temporal pattern of active subintervals is specific for the odor and for the cell. One wonders if this behavior reflects the existence of an underlying attractor network (Amit 1989; Griniasty, Tsodyks, and Amit 1993). The physiological mechanisms by which these selected subintervals are generated are not yet clear.

Application of picrotoxin to the bulb, blocking GABA$_A$ receptors, abolishes the local oscillation, as might be expected. Remarkably, however, there is persistence of the overall temporal pattern, the pattern of which subintervals during which any particular neuron fires. Of course, the cycle-by-cycle structure no longer exists after picrotoxin application. Picrotoxin in the bath abolishes oscillations in the bulb, but population spikes—at about 30 Hz—persist in the mushroom body.

Can one conclude from the picrotoxin data that oscillations are unnecessary for olfactory information processing in the locust? Probably not. Even though GABA$_A$ receptor blockade leaves intact an overall temporal pattern of odor-evoked firing, nevertheless one might guess that the oscillations are still somehow important for olfactory network function. To show this Laurent and colleagues (Stopfer et al. 1997) first demonstrated that the physiological properties of the honeybee olfactory system are similar to the locust. The honeybee has the advantage, however, that it exhibits an observable behavior (proboscis extension) that can be conditioned by smells. In the honeybee preparation, the oscillation-blocking drug picrotoxin interferes with the discrimination between similar odors, although the animal can still discriminate between dissimilar odors.

One possible conclusion from these data is that a $GABA_A$ receptor-gated oscillation provides a fine temporal structure that is not required for the slower temporal pattern of active subintervals. The latter may be what encodes odor specificity, at least in part. Why then have the 30 Hz oscillation at all? Our data on synaptic plasticity induced by gamma oscillations (reviewed in chapter 10) suggest the hypothesis that the oscillation might be important for laying down memories of odors.

8

Networks of
Interneurons II: Gamma
Oscillations in Vitro

Steriade et al. (1987) reported that the surgically deafferented nucleus reticularis thalami (nRT), in acute experiments in vivo, could autonomously generate synchronized spindle oscillations. This observation is a most interesting finding, for nRT consists of GABAergic inhibitory neurons, although nucleus reticularis thalami in vitro appear to require phasic AMPA receptor-mediated inputs from principal thalamic nuclei in order to oscillate (Bal, von Krosigk, and McCormick 1995a,b). When nRT neurons are held at appropriate membrane potentials, they are able to act as intrinsic oscillators, in a manner largely defined by the properties of T-type Ca^{2+} channels and a Ca^{2+}-gated AHP conductance (Bal and McCormick 1993). Destexhe and Babloyantz (1992) reported that interneuron networks could generate synchronized oscillations, and Wang and Rinzel (1993) analyzed conditions under which inhibitory neurons could entrain each other, so as to produce—counterintuitively, it would seem—a synchronized oscillation. Wang and Rinzel found that such entrainment was possible if, first, the IPSPs were hyperpolarizing, and if, second, the IPSPs had a longer time course than the intrinsic oscillatory period. Both the hyperpolarizing action and the long time course of the IPSPs were necessary for them to exert an entraining effect. (See also Destexhe et al. 1994).

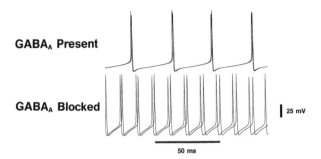

Figure 8.1
GABA$_A$ receptor-mediated IPSPs can produce zero-phase-lag synchronization, in principle. Simulation was of a fully interconnected network of 96 interneurons producing GABA$_A$ receptor-mediated synaptic actions. Potentials of two cells are shown superimposed. The cells were depolarized by slightly different driving currents to simulate the effects of metabotropic glutamate receptor-mediated excitation. When the GABA$_A$ receptors are functional (above), there is synchronized gamma-frequency oscillation. Blocking the receptors (below) shows that the intrinsic frequencies of the tonically excited, but synaptically uncoupled, cells are faster than the frequency of the network oscillation. The trace also shows that the cells become unsynchronized. The physical principles here are similar to those described by Wang and Rinzel (1993).

Such findings suggested the possibility that hippocampal and cortical interneurons, which do contact each other synaptically (chapter 4), might also generate synchronized oscillations gated by mutually induced hyperpolarizing GABA$_A$ receptor-mediated IPSPs. If such oscillations were to occur, they would be expected to have a frequency in the gamma range, given that the time constant of GABA$_A$ receptor-mediated IPSCs is approximately 10 ms (chapter 4; figure 4.1). These questions began to be approached experimentally in 1994 by Jefferys and Whittington (then both at St. Mary's Hospital Medical School, Imperial College, London) and in simulations by Traub (then at the IBM T. J. Watson Research Center), first separately and then collaboratively (Whittington et al. 1995b).

The Generation of Gamma-Frequency Oscillations by
Networks of Interneurons (Interneuron Network Gamma)

Gamma-frequency oscillations can be induced in hippocampal and neocortical brain slices under conditions when pyramidal cells are not firing or when ionotropic glutamate receptors are blocked. Although it is not clear if slices of nRT in isolation can generate synchronized oscillations, populations of interneurons in the CA1 region in vitro can do so. Such oscillations can be induced in a number of different ways. One means, shown in figure 8.2, is to apply a short conditioning tetanus to the slice in drug-free medium, followed by a single shock. This sort of simulation will activate ionotropic receptors, but it is also expected to liberate neuroactive substances, including glutamate and perhaps acetylcholine, which could act on metabotropic receptors. Recording from pyramidal neurons, one observes trains of bicuculline-sensitive (hence $GABA_A$ receptor-dependent) synaptic potentials at gamma frequency (33.4 Hz in the example shown in figure 8.2b). The synaptic potentials have the appearance of reversed (i.e., depolarizing, as can occur after afferent stimulation) IPSPs. The trains last some hundreds of ms and even longer when $GABA_B$ receptors are pharmacologically blocked (Whittington et al. 1995b). Trains of synaptic potentials are produced by stimuli that do not cause the pyramidal cells to fire, suggesting that the firing of one or more interneurons is responsible for generating the potentials.

In order to confirm that gamma-frequency trains of IPSPs are not somehow gated by oscillatory firing of pyramidal cells, experiments were performed in which ionotropic glutamate receptors, that is, AMPA/kainate and NMDA receptors, were pharmacologically blocked. Under these conditions, gamma oscillations, as recorded in CA1 pyramidal cells or in s.pyramidale/oriens interneurons, could still be evoked when metabotropic glutamate receptors were

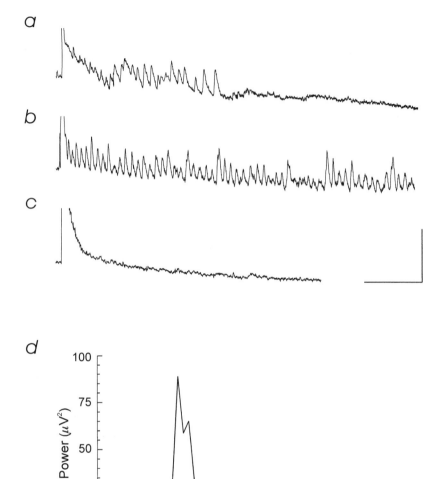

Figure 8.2
A train of gamma-frequency IPSPs can be induced by a single afferent shock after a weak conditioning train in a drugfree medium. (a) Intracellular recording of a CA1 pyramidal cell, showing rhythmic potentials induced by a shock 2 seconds after a weak conditioning train (amplitude = one-half threshold for action-potential

activated (Whittington et al. 1995b; Traub, Whittington, Colling et al. 1996). The activation of mGluRs could be achieved by puffing on glutamate itself, puffing on the metabotropic agonist ACPD, or by applying a single electrical pulse when ACPD was present in the bath. Furthermore, metabotropic glutamate receptor activation could induce trains of IPSCs in neocortical slices, as well as hippocampal slices, of greater amplitude and regularity in neocortical layer II than in the deeper layers. Interestingly, in vivo, neocortical gamma in awake monkeys, performing a visual/motor task such as seeking a raisin, seems to be generated in superficial layers (Murthy and Fetz 1996a). On the other hand, however, Brosch, Bauer, and Eckhorn (1995) found that two oscillatory sites in cat visual cortex areas 17 and 18 were most likely to be synchronized when the recording electrodes were in the deeper layers.

Examples of metabotropically induced oscillations appear in later figures in this chapter. We note that, as expected, pharmacological blockade of metabotropic receptors prevents the generation of oscillations under the experimental in vitro conditions described above.

As metabotropic glutamate receptor-elicited EPSPs are relatively slow, with time courses of hundreds of ms at least (Bianchi and Wong 1995; Pozzo Miller et al. 1995), these data suggested an hypothesis: tonic activation of mutually inhibitory interneurons was sufficient under certain experimental conditions to elicit gamma oscillations, perhaps by a mechanism similar in its basic physics to what is believed to occur in nRT in vivo. It remained to answer many significant questions: how are the oscillations organized, and

generation, 100 Hz, 1 s). (b) The rhythmic potentials last considerably longer after $GABA_B$ receptors are blocked with 2-OH-saclofen (0.2 mM). (c) Bicuculline (10 μM) blocks the rhythmic potentials, indicating that they are depolarizing IPSPs mediated by $GABA_A$ receptors. Pyramidal cells themselves do not fire under these conditions. (d) Power spectrum of the last 1.8 s of the signal in (b), showing a peak at about 33 Hz. (From Whittington et al., 1995b with permission of *Nature*, © Macmillan Magazines Ltd.)

what determines the frequency? And what determines the degree of synchrony and the spatial scales over which synchronization is possible? Some of these questions are considered in this chapter, but the issue of spatial scale is deferred to the next chapter, as it appears that pyramidal cell firing is critically involved in allowing synchronization to exist over scales that are large with respect to the axonal extent of most interneurons (about 1 mm).

Are the Oscillations Generated by a Single Interneuron or by a Network of Interneurons?

Before one asks how a network generates an oscillation, one should check that a network is truly involved, rather than a single oscillating cell or a group of cells oscillating independently. The fact that bicuculline blocks the oscillations, illustrated in figure 8.2, does not prove that $GABA_A$ receptors on interneurons are necessary in any way because the recording is from a pyramidal cell, and the drug will block $GABA_A$ receptors on the pyramidal neuron membrane as well, preventing observation of the oscillation, however it is generated. (Indeed, a means of selectively blocking $GABA_A$ receptors on interneurons, but not on pyramidal cells, and vice versa, would be most useful for the study of gamma oscillations.) Gamma oscillations do not occur in the presence of tetrodotoxin (TTX) (Whittington et al. 1995b), but this absence could, in principle, simply reflect the requirement for some interneuron to fire repetitively in order for oscillations to be generated.

There are several pieces of indirect evidence that interneuron-generated gamma oscillations must be a network phenomenon, no single one of these pieces being definitive:

1. Synchronized IPSPs occur in pyramidal cells 1 mm apart (see below), but single interneurons can have an axon spanning this distance.

2. Synchronized IPSCs in pyramidal neurons can reach 2 nA, large for induction by a single presynaptic interneuron. In a cell held at -40 mV, or about 35 mV positive to the $GABA_A$ reversal potential, 2 nA corresponds to a synaptic conductance greater than 50 nS, while Buhl, Cobb et al. (1995) estimated the unitary basket cell $\rightarrow$CA1 pyramidal cell synaptic conductance to be about 1 nS.

3. IPSCs in pyramidal cells can be inflected in their rising phase, suggesting induction by presynaptic interneurons firing slightly out of phase, but possibly explicable by a single interneuron firing a spike doublet.

Short of the technically demanding feat of recording gamma oscillations simultaneously in pairs of interneurons, is there a way to be sure that the oscillations are generated by a network? The answer is yes. Suppose one applies a drug at concentrations which have no effect, or negligible effects, on the intrinsic properties of interneurons; suppose further that this drug alters some property of unitary $GABA_A$ IPSCs, either conductance or time course, or both; and suppose, finally, that this drug alters the frequency of the oscillations. How could the frequency be altered? There are only three possibilities: a) the mechanism is by an action on pyramidal cell $GABA_A$ receptors; b) the mechanism is by an action on interneuron $GABA_A$ receptors; or c) both. We can eliminate possibilities a and c because, when ionotropic glutamate receptors are pharmacologically blocked and the pyramidal cells are not firing, the pyramidal cells are acting solely as measuring devices, through which one observes the gamma oscillation, but which have no effect on the oscillation. Greater or lesser hyperpolarization of the pyramidal cells can not influence the oscillation frequency. Hence, the mechanism is by an action on interneuron $GABA_A$ receptors. It follows, therefore, that the oscillations are generated by an interneuron network. Of course, in theory, a single interneuron with autapses (Tamás et al. 1997) could constitute a network!

One further argument remains. If a single interneuron were generating the IPSPs and projecting to pyramidal cells via synaptic connections with multiple release sites (hence low or negligible transmission failure rates), then IPSPs induced in different pyramidal cells should be virtually superimposable. This, however, is not so (see figure 8.10 below).

The above arguments are not just logical abstractions. Whittington et al. (1995b) showed that pentobarbital in concentrations less than 2 μM would slow oscillation frequency (see also below). We, therefore, designate the phenomenon interneuron network gamma. The scientific task is then to investigate if the concept of an interneuron network with mutual GABA$_A$ receptor-mediated synaptic inhibition can be used to generate specific and testable predictions concerning gamma-frequency oscillations. One step in pursuing this task is to develop a computer model. The value of modeling gamma oscillations was shown in Whittington et al. (1995b), who argued that network frequency was expected to decrease with slower $\tau_{GABA(A)}$. A similar conclusion had been reached by Wilson and Bower (1992), based on their pyriform cortex model.

Network Modeling Considerations

Given that it is appropriate to approach gamma oscillations using interneuron network models as a tool, how should one go about it? There are several main issues, including how to model the individual interneuron, network connectivity (how many cells, what sort of wiring patterns, etc.), and synaptic actions. The authors of this book have used a multicompartment interneuron model, as described in chapter 3, which allows inclusion of interesting details, such as the dendritic sites of certain synaptic receptors and gap junctions (Whittington et al. 1995b; Traub, Whittington, Colling, et al. 1996; Traub, Jefferys, and Whittington 1997). On the other hand, the basic physical principles of interneuron network gamma can be captured using a single-compartment interneuron model (Wang and Buzsáki 1996).

Regarding connectivity, there are several considerations. Most importantly, a single interneuron with autapses would work for studying the effects on frequency of manipulating $GABA_A$ conductance and time course, but such a model would not be appropriate for studying other important issues, such as the effects of stimulating different cells with different current amplitudes or how oscillations lose synchrony as they slow down. Assuming, then, that multiple interneurons are to be used, how many should one employ? There is no definite answer to this question, but we have used models with 16, 96, 120, and 384 interneurons. Larger numbers of interneurons are required if one hopes to capture something of the actual connectivity in the slice.

With respect to patterns of connectivity, there are four approaches that have been used: a) all-to-all (conceptually the simplest), b) globally random, c) spatially localized but structured, and d) spatially localized but random within the spatial field. Patterns *a* and *b* have the advantage of providing physical intuition about the system that is independent of spatial effects. The problem with these patterns is that they do not correspond precisely to actual experimental paradigms: if oscillations are evoked, for example, by local application of a drug or an electrical stimulus, then there will be boundary effects, with interneurons on the border of the stimulus "feeling" different degrees of activation (and of inhibition by neighboring cells) than do interneurons in the center of the stimulated region. On the other hand, bath application of drugs will activate spatially distributed networks of interneurons, whose connectivity is not globally random. As we shall see in the next chapter, such spatially distributed interneuron networks tend not to oscillate synchronously, so that new physical principles are introduced that are not apparent in globally connected networks. In approaching this modeling issue, what has worked historically is to analyze physical principles first in all-all or randomly connected networks (Traub, Whittington, Colling et al. 1996; Wang and Buzsáki 1996) and, afterwards, to try to incorporate more realistic topologies. What should be the quantitative extent of the connectivity? In the first model of CA1 gamma oscillations (Whittington et al. 1995b), a random connectivity of about 16% was used. The signals generated by this model appear—qualitatively—noisier than the actual experimental data, although basic features of the oscillation could still be reproduced. Wang and Buzsáki (1996) analyzed the effects of connectivity in large networks of randomly connected interneurons and found that synchronization was possible when each interneuron had more than a certain fixed number of presynaptic inputs—in the range of 40 to 50—and this fixed number was the important variable, rather than the percentage connectivity. We have found that in networks with locally random connections, synchrony is possible with smaller numbers of inputs per neuron: 20 is an adequate number (Traub, Whittington, et al., 1999).

With regard to synaptic actions, many (but not all) of the experiments have been performed in the presence of $GABA_B$ receptor blockade, so that these receptors are generally not modeled explicitly. As 4AP is not present in the medium in most of the experiments and as the interneurons do not generate high-frequency bursts, depolarizing $GABA_A$ receptors are assumed not to play a primary role. $GABA_A Cl^-$-dependent hyperpolarizing IPSCs have rapid onset, and their decay can be approximated by a single exponential. It is true that $\tau_{GABA(A)}$ in principal neurons increases with depolarization (Segal and Barker 1984; Otis and Mody 1992), but this effect is assumed not to be significant for understanding the structure of the gamma oscillation. The role, if any, of gap junctions in contributing to interneuronal synchrony during gamma oscillations remains to be investigated further. In many of the simulations, pyramidal cells are not simulated at all, or if simulated, then their synaptic outputs are assumed to be blocked, so that they act as measuring devices. In other simulations, however, pyramidal cells do excite the interneurons synaptically, as this excitation leads to new phenomena and represents a situation closer to what happens in vivo and in certain experiments, such as where gamma activity is evoked by strong tetanic stimulation (next chapter).

A final issue in model construction is especially knotty: should all the model interneurons have the same intrinsic properties and/ or types of input and output synaptic connections? This issue is difficult because the types of interneurons participating, or failing to participate, in network gamma have not yet been determined morphologically. We do know experimentally that s. pyramidale and s. oriens interneurons participate in gamma oscillations most reliably and that such interneurons are mostly, but not entirely, parvalbumin-positive basket and axo-axonic cells. In addition, as axo-axonic cells do not contact other interneurons, they most likely do not participate actively in generation of interneuron network gamma. Thus, it is reasonable—and conceptually simplest as well— to begin by modeling a single functional type of interneuron, the s. pyramidale basket cell, and to assume that the connectivity of each cell is uniform, at least in a statistical sense. Even if this approach needs to be modified in future as more data become available, the approach is a sensible starting point for grasping the physical ideas underlying gamma oscillations. We shall now show that network models of interneurons provide insight into a number of experimental features of interneuron network gamma in vitro.

Interneuron Network Gamma Frequency Depends on Driving Currents or Conductances to the Inhibitory Neurons

Individual interneurons fire faster as they are progressively depolarized. One expects that a network of mutually inhibitory interneurons, firing synchronously, would also fire at higher frequency if all of the cells are depolarized more, at least provided that the amount of depolarization is about the same in all of the cells. A simple way to visualize this situation is to picture a single interneuron that synaptically inhibits itself; this is an adequate representation of a system in which the connectivity is uniform, the different synapses have identical properties, the cells are depolarized identically, and noise is negligible. In such an autaptic single-neuron network, the GABA IPSP follows immediately upon each action potential, as a form of self-inhibition, to produce an interneuron to which one additional outward current has been added. Such a cell will fire faster as it is depolarized. Consistent with this idea, network models of interneurons with mutual $GABA_A$ receptor-mediated IPSPs and with sufficiently high connectivity produce an almost linear relationship between mean driving currents and output frequency (figure 8.3; see also figure 12 of Wang and Buzsáki 1996).

The experimental manipulation of driving currents in a population of cells is not straightforward. One approach is to puff on glutamate for different time intervals, regulating the total dose of drug delivered to a small area and hence the local concentration. Puffing on more glutamate does increase the frequency, over the range 20 to about 50 Hz (consistent with model prediction), but further increases in drug delivery slow the oscillation frequency (figure 8.3). There are at least two possible interpretations of the frequency-decrease:

1. Higher concentrations of glutamate engage a second population of metabotropic receptors (Poncer et al. 1995), other than the ones that depolarize basket cells (see also next chapter). This relationship is not straightforward: presynaptic metabotropic receptors should diminish transmitter release, which would be expected to increase oscillation frequency, not decrease it (see below). On the other hand, at higher glutamate concentrations, another population of interneurons could become excited, perhaps cells whose postsynaptic

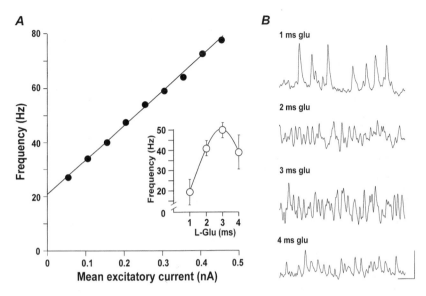

Figure 8.3
Interneuron network gamma: oscillation frequency depends on the driving current
or conductance to the interneurons. (A) In an all-all connected model with 96 interneurons, the dependence of frequency on mean driving current is linear. In experiments in which gamma activity is induced by puffs of L-glutamate, the frequency
first rises with the duration of the puff, then begins to decline (inset). In these experiments, ionotropic glutamate receptors and GABA$_B$ receptors were pharmacologically blocked. (B) Sample experimental records in voltage-clamp mode
recording from pyramidal cells held at −40 mV. Scale bars 80 ms, 200 pA. (From
Traub, Whittington, Colling et al., 1996).

GABA$_A$ receptor-mediated effects have a longer time constant
(Pearce 1993); activation of such interneurons could, in principle,
slow the oscillation.

2. As more glutamate is puffed on, it will diffuse away from the
application site, to activate more interneurons, in effect changing
the connectivity of the activated network. Synchronized GABA$_A$
conductances will become larger, reflecting the larger number of
oscillating interneurons, and this increase should slow the oscillation.

Interneuron Network Gamma Frequency Depends on $\tau_{GABA(A)}$, the Decay Time Constant of Hyperpolarizing $GABA_A$ Receptor-Mediated Conductances

The close agreement between model (●, 96 interneurons with all-all connectivity) and experiment (o, $\tau_{GABA(A)}$ prolonged with increasing concentrations of thiopental) is shown in figure 8.4. Two specific features of this figure require further comment.

First, the relation between $\tau_{GABA(A)}$ and frequency is not linear. This result is to be expected. Imagine the simplest possible model, of a single autaptic neuron having no membrane capacitance, so that voltage is instantaneously determined by membrane conductance, which we shall assume is dominated by the GABA synaptic conductance. After an action potential, the membrane conductance G will then be $G_0 \exp(-t/\tau)$, where G_0 is the initial GABA conductance and τ is the $GABA_A$ receptor decay time constant. The cell will fire again when membrane potential reaches some particular value, that is, when membrane conductance reaches some particular value, say G_1. This event will occur when $t = \tau \log(G_0/G_1)$, so that the frequency will be proportional to $1/\{\tau \log(G_0/G_1)\}$, i.e., the frequency is proportional to the inverse of the $GABA_A$ relaxation time constant.

Second, the experimental system is capable of oscillating at lower frequencies than is the model. In the model, as $\tau_{GABA(A)}$ becomes sufficiently prolonged, the oscillation begins to lose synchrony, so that the period becomes impossible to define. This outcome is actually expected because with long GABA relaxation times and with different driving currents to different neurons, the temporal dispersion—in times at which various cells fire after a given synchronized action potential—will increase: a consequence of heterogeneity in the system (White et al. 1998). The exact frequency at which synchrony disappears is hard to predict, as it will depend on the extent

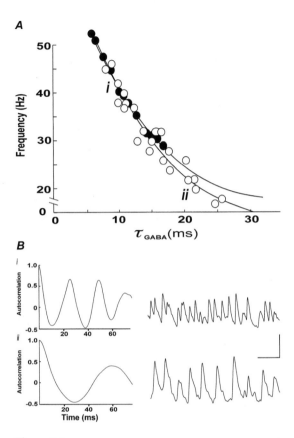

Figure 8.4
Interneuron network gamma: oscillation frequency slows as $\tau_{GABA(A)}$ is prolonged. (A) Network frequency as a function of $\tau_{GABA(A)}$ for the model (●, simulations in a 96-interneuron all-all connected network) and experiment (○). The experimental recordings were obtained (in voltage-clamp, holding at -40 mV) from interneurons in s. pyramidale and s. oriens, as it is interneuron $\tau_{GABA(A)}$ that is expected to regulate network frequency. Drugs were present to block ionotropic glutamate and $GABA_B$ receptors. $GABA_A$ decay time constant was prolonged by wash-in of thiopental, 2–20 μM. (B) Sample experimental records and current autocorrelations from the points i and ii in (A). Note that high concentrations of barbiturates can induce an increase in $GABA_A$ receptor-mediated conductance as well as time constant and can eventually induce a bicuculline-blockable GABA-dependent leak current (Rho, Donevan, and Rogawski, 1996; Whittington, Jefferys, and Traub, 1996). This mechanism is the most likely explanation for why the experimental system can oscillate at lower frequencies than can the model. Calibration 100 ms, 200 pA. (From Traub, Whittington, Colling et al., 1996)

of heterogeneity and on connectivity, as well as on the amount of noise in the system. In the experiments, at large enough concentrations of barbiturate, GABA conductance is increased, as well as time constant, and this increase tends to compensate for the heterogeneity. With still higher concentrations of thiopental (thiopentone) (> 50 μM), the experimental network can even oscillate at frequencies below 10 Hz. At such concentrations, still another effect comes into play, the induction of a $GABA_A$ receptor-mediated leak conductance (Whittington, Jefferys, and Traub 1996).

Interneuron Network Gamma Frequency Depends on the Amplitude of Unitary $GABA_A$ Receptor-Mediated Conductances

Again (see figure 8.5), the agreement between model prediction (●) and experiment (o) is good. Some of the experimental points occur at lower frequencies than is the case for the model. This result may be a consequence of the slight increase (about 14%) in $\tau_{GABA(A)}$ that occurs with higher concentrations of diazepam.

Interneuron Network Gamma Oscillations Cannot Be Generated at Arbitrarily Low Frequencies

We have mentioned above that the consequences of heterogeneity require a network for their study, and we have described how heterogeneity leads to a breakup in the simulated oscillation as $\tau_{GABA(A)}$ becomes sufficiently prolonged. A similar breakup in the oscillation occurs during the slowdown associated with a driving current that declines over time, an effect also seen experimentally at about the same frequency (15–20 Hz) in figure 8.6.

This figure illustrates two other important features of interneuron network gamma. First, the generating mechanism is stable enough to allow for frequency modulation and for the oscillation to synchronize quickly after a current pulse, perhaps corresponding to

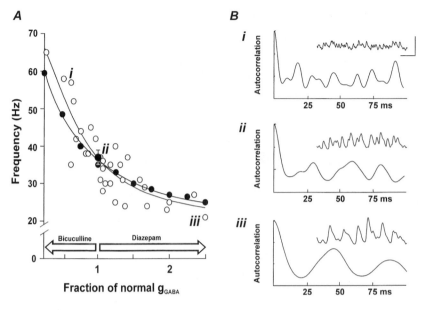

Figure 8.5
Interneuron network gamma: oscillation frequency is inversely related to $g_{GABA(A)}$.
(A) Network frequency as a function of $g_{GABA(A)}$ (relative to a fixed value) for the
model (●, simulations in a 96-interneuron all-all connected network, with τ_{GABA} 13
ms) and experiment (○). The experimental recordings were obtained (in voltage-
clamp, holding at −40 mV) from s. pyramidale interneurons with oscillations
evoked as in Figure 8.4, and ionotropic glutamate and $GABA_B$ receptors blocked as
in Figure 8.4. The $g_{GABA(A)}$ was decreased by bath application of bicuculline (0.5–5.0
μM) and increased by bath application of diazepam (0.05–0.5 μM). (B) Sample raw
voltage-clamp data from interneurons and autocorrelations from the points i, ii, and
iii in (A). Point ii is control, and the error bars around this point in (A) are the S.E.M.
of the frequency (n = 6 observations). Calibration 50 ms, 200 pA. (From Traub,
Whittington, Colling et al., 1996)

evoked gamma oscillations in vivo (chapter 1). Second, when a mi-
nority of the pyramidal cells are firing during interneuron network
gamma, the pyramidal cells fire in phase with the interneurons,
unlike the model of Freeman discussed in the previous chapter. The
physical reason for the in-phase firing in the present sorts of experiments is that the pyramidal cells and interneurons are both being
clocked by the interneurons. Additionally, the interneurons are ton-

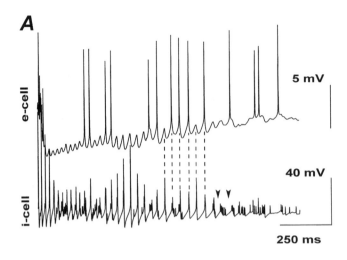

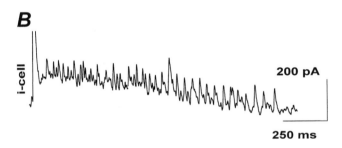

Figure 8.6
Interneuron network gamma: when $g_{GABA(A)}$ and $\tau_{GABA(A)}$ are fixed, there is a minimum network frequency; when pyramidal cells are depolarized enough to fire, they fire in phase with the interneurons. (A) Simulation of 96 interneurons (basket cells and axo-axonic cells, i-cells) with all-all connectivity and of a pool of pyramidal cells (e-cells) that are inhibited by the interneurons but whose excitatory synaptic output is blocked. One of the pyramidal cells receives a constant excitatory input that causes it to fire; the interneurons receive an exponentially decaying current ($\tau = 350$ to 375 ms) that is different in each cell. The figure shows the average somatic potential of 8 pyramidal cells and 16 basket cells. The interneuron network produces a synchronized oscillation of gradually diminishing frequency until synchrony is lost (arrowheads). The last interval is 22 Hz. The interneuron network output produces synchronized IPSPs in the pyramidal cells, entraining the firing to occur in phase with the firing of the interneurons (see also Figure 8.9). (B) Experimental oscillations. A single shock was given in the presence of the metabotropic glutamate receptor agonist ACPD, as well as drugs to block ionotropic glutamate and $GABA_B$ receptors, while recording in voltage-clamp from an interneuron. The initial oscillation frequency was 46 Hz, but it progressively slowed to 17 Hz. (From Traub, Whittington, Colling et al., 1996)

ically excited by metabotropic receptors, rather than being phasi-cally triggered to fire by action potentials in the pyramidal cells, this latter mechanism leading, in the Freeman model, to the time lag from pyramidal cell-to-interneuron firing.

Interestingly, during theta rhythm in vivo, firing rates of pyramidal cells tend to be low, even though basket cells fire at high frequency during the intracellular-depolarizing phases of the theta waves (Sik et al. 1995). Possibly, basket cells are being driven to fire by a slowly time-varying input, rather than by discrete AMPA receptor-mediated EPSPs. Furthermore, pyramidal cells and interneurons in vivo tend to fire on the same phase of gamma waves (Bragin et al. 1995; Penttonen et al. 1998). This issue is illustrated further below.

Synchrony of Interneuron Network Gamma Oscillations Is Disrupted, at Least in Principle, by Small Degrees of Nonuniformity in the Driving Currents or Conductances

In the simulations illustrated in figures 8.4–8.6, the heterogeneity in driving currents was deliberately kept small ($< 10\%$) in order to improve the stability of the oscillation. The quantitative effects of heterogeneity in driving currents to the interneurons were examined by Wang and Buzsáki (1996) (figure 8.7). These authors studied an ensemble of normally distributed driving currents ($S.D. = I_o$) in a randomly connected network of 100 interneurons, examining the effects on their measure of synchrony, the coherence index κ, which was defined as follows. First, fix the length of a time window, δt. Consider the spike trains of two neurons, i and j, over K time windows, the spike trains being called $X(l)$ and $Y(l)$ and taking on the values of 0 or 1. Define the coherence of these two neurons as

$$\kappa_{ij} = \{\Sigma_l = {}_{1\ldots K} X(l)\, Y(l)\} / \{[\Sigma_1 = {}_{1\ldots K} X(l)] \times [\Sigma_l = {}_{1\ldots K} Y(l)]\}^{1/2}.$$

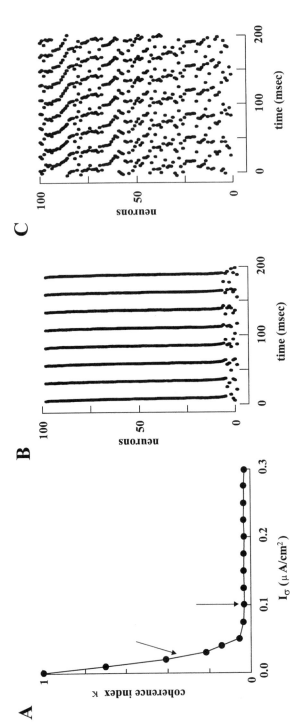

Figure 8.7
Interneuron network gamma: effects in simulations of heterogeneity in driving currents. Simulations were performed in a fully interconnected network of 100 mutually inhibitory neurons. The coherence index $\kappa(\Delta t)$ is defined in the text ($\Delta t = 1$ ms in this figure). κ is a measure of the coherence of the population and I_σ is the standard deviation of the distribution of currents applied to the different interneurons and is a measure of heterogeneity. (A) Coherence (κ) drops steeply as heterogeneity increases. (B) Firing times of the 100 different neurons (arranged along the vertical axis) over 200 ms when $I_\sigma = 0.03$ (first ↑ in A). (C) Firing times of the 100 different neurons when $I_\sigma = 0.1$ (second ↓ in A). Note the disorganization of the population. (From Wang and Buzsáki, 1996 with permission)

The coherence κ of the entire population is the average of κ_{ij} over all pairs i,j.

Wang and Buzsáki (1996) found that coherence disappeared rapidly as I_σ increased from 0 to 0.03, with mean driving current 1.0 (in units of $\mu A/cm^2$). In other words, synchrony is possible only when the intrinsic properties/driving currents of the constituent neurons are relatively homogeneous, although of course, these properties need not be identical. This finding has important implications for the generation of synchronized network gamma oscillations in vivo under conditions where pyramidal cells are silent, at least relatively so. If the interneurons are to oscillate together, the driving inputs must be correlated between the different interneurons, so that intercellular differences in input remain small. Furthermore, interneuron oscillations seem to work most readily when temporal fluctuations in input are limited as well (although a 5 Hz input signal can certainly be tolerated: Traub, Whittington, Colling, et al. 1996).

Short Runs of Interneuron Network Gamma Can Follow Synchronized Pyramidal Cell Bursts

A serious question that arises in the study of any network activity in a model system is, does something like the same activity occur in vivo? We have been discussing experiments in which oscillations are evoked by afferent shocks or by stimulation of metabotropic glutamate receptors with applied chemicals. It would be useful to know if interneuron network activity can arise spontaneously as a result of neuronal activity.

One suggestion that this activity might occur arose fortuitously. Simulations of epileptic activity induced by 4AP were being run and compared with experimental recordings (Traub, Colling, and Jefferys 1995). 4AP has the property that it enhances synaptic conductances, including inhibitory conductances, rather than blocking inhibition as in the more commonly studied disinhibition epilepsy model (in which interneuron network gamma would also be suppressed, given the blockade of $GABA_A$ receptors). The network being simulated contained synaptic interactions between pyramidal cells, between interneurons, and between the two respective cell populations, including excitation of interneurons by recurrent connections activating both AMPA and NMDA receptors. The latter sort of synaptic interaction was modeled with a slow conductance that relaxed with a time constant of 60 ms.

It was noted in the simulations that, following a synchronized burst, there was a transient interneuron network oscillation at gamma frequency that evoked a series of rippling IPSPs in pyramidal cells (figure 8.8). This oscillation resulted because the synchronized pyramidal cell discharge produced a large slow EPSP in the interneurons from the NMDA receptors. The interneurons then synchronized because of the mutual IPSPs (as discussed above). Similar-appearing rippling synaptic potentials were observed following experimental 4AP-induced synchronized bursts (figure 8.9), although with different pharmacology than in the model. In the experiment, the tail of gamma oscillation was dependent upon activation of metabotropic glutamate receptors (presumably in the interneurons), rather than upon NMDA receptors. Nevertheless, the suggestion was that synchronized bursting in pyramidal cells might induce slow EPSPs—by whatever means—in populations of interneurons, which could secondarily synchronize.

Review of in vivo recordings from the laboratory of G. Buzsáki showed that gamma oscillations could follow hippocampal sharp waves, most prominently in animals that had been subjected to entorhinal cortex lesions (see figure 9 of Traub, Whittington, Colling et al. 1996). A possibly related phenomenon is the in vivo neocortical gamma that occurs during the intracellular-depolarizing phases of the slow sleep-related rhythm (see previous chapter). It would be interesting to determine if other physiological sorts of synchronized

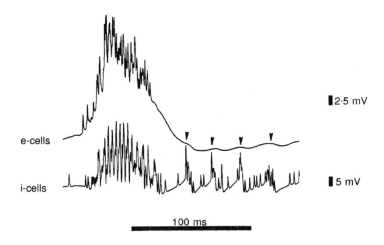

Figure 8.8
Interneuron network gamma: a tail of gamma oscillation can follow a synchronized burst induced by 4AP (simulation). The network contained 1,024 pyramidal cells (e-cells) and 256 inhibitory cells (i-cells), including axo-axonic cells, basket cells, dendrite-contacting cells, and cells eliciting GABA$_B$ IPSPs. Pyramidal cells activate both AMPA and NMDA receptors on other pyramidal cells and on interneurons. Noise was present in the form of spontaneous ectopic action potentials, which originated in axons. The action of 4AP was simulated by increasing the amplitude and duration of AMPA receptor-mediated conductances (compare with Figure 5.9). The synchronized burst induces slow EPSPs in the interneurons, which by virtue of mutual synaptic inhibition, produce a brief epoch of interneuron network gamma (40–46 Hz). This latter, in turn, induces a series of IPSPs in the pyramidal cells (➤). (From Traub, Whittington, Colling et al., 1996).

activity, such as vertex waves and PGO (ponto-geniculo-occipital) waves, are followed by transient gamma oscillations, detectable in local field potentials.

Entraining Effects of Interneuron Network Gamma on the Firing of Pyramidal Neurons

The synchronized output of an oscillating interneuron network can entrain and synchronize the firing of groups of pyramidal neurons. We have mentioned that experimental interneuron network gamma

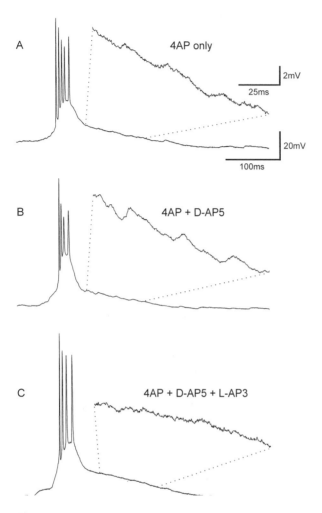

Figure 8.9
Interneuron network gamma: a tail of gamma oscillation can follow a synchronized burst induced by 4AP (experiment). The tail probably results from metabotropic glutamate receptor-mediated excitation of the interneurons. Intracellular recordings were taken from CA3 pyramidal cells (rat) during synchronized bursts induced by 4AP (70 μM). (A) Under these conditions, bursts are followed by small rhythmic potentials at about 40 Hz, resembling the IPSPs in simulations (Figure 8.8). (B) The gamma-frequency potentials are not blocked by the NMDA receptor-blocker D-AP5 (50 μM). (C) The gamma-frequency potentials were suppressed by the nonspecific metabotropic glutamate receptor-blocker. L-AP3 (0.2 mM). These data suggest that a slow, metabotropic glutamate receptor-mediated excitation of interneurons is driving the gamma tail. (From Traub, Whittington, Colling et al., 1996)

appears in multiple pyramidal cells as synchronized IPSPs, which of course, is not surprising. A direct experimental demonstration of this observation is shown in figure 8.10. The fact that the IPSPs in the two pyramidal cells do not have identical time courses favors, in our opinion, the network generation of the rhythm. This figure also demonstrates experimentally that, as predicted by Lytton and Sejnowski (1991), sufficiently large synchronized IPSPs are capable of mutually entraining pyramidal cells that are excited enough to fire, this being possible when the cells are not so excited that the IPSPs become irrelevant. Hence, interneuron network gamma is, in principle at least, functionally useful—this assuming that synchronization of pyramidal cells is useful!

Finally, figure 8.10 introduces another idea of great biological significance. The same chemical (glutamate) that triggers the network oscillation by acting on interneuron metabotropic receptors also primes the pyramidal cells to participate in the oscillation. One of the metabotropic actions on pyramidal cells is to block accomodation. This theme will be further explored in the next chapter when we examine gamma oscillations involving large populations of interneurons and pyramidal cells together.

The Synchronized Output of an Oscillating Interneuron Network Allows for Phase coding of Pyramidal Cell Firing with Respect to the Gamma Rhythm

O'Keefe and Recce (1993) described how in behaving rats the phase of firing of hippocampal place cells—relative to the ongoing theta rhythm—carried information about where the rat was in the respective place field. Hopfield (1995) discussed more generally how information can be encoded in the phase of firing of principal cells relative to an ongoing population oscillation.

An interesting physical principle allows such phase coding to be possible in gamma-oscillating networks of interneurons and pyram-

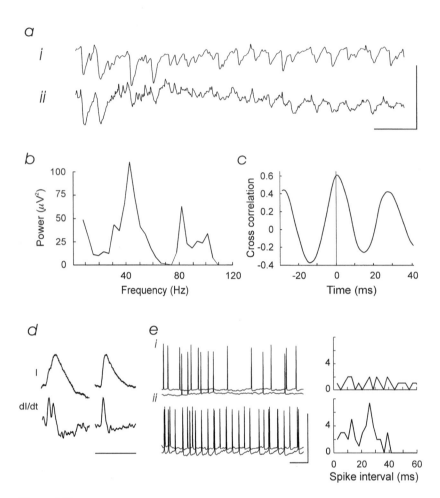

Figure 8.10
Interneuron network gamma: synchronized IPSPs appear in pairs of pyramidal cells
and can entrain their firing. Experiments were performed in the CA1 region of rat
hippocampal slices, with drugs in the medium to block ionotropic glutamate and
$GABA_B$ receptors. Gamma oscillations were evoked by pressure ejection of glutamate. (a) Synchronized synaptic potentials in 2 pyramidal cells, 1 mm apart, held
at −40 mV by current injection. Calibrations: 10 mV, 60 ms. (b) Power spectrum of
a signal from a recording similar to a, revealing a peak at 42 Hz. (c) Cross-correlation
of the signals in (a); the frequency is 37 Hz and the phase delay 1.5 ms. (d) Voltage-
clamp recordings of IPSCs in pyramidal cells under these conditions were
sometimes notched or inflected (as on the left), suggesting that multiple interneurons were participating. Calibration: 30 ms. (e) Top traces are superimposed recordings from 2 pyramidal cells during injection of 0.6 nA current into each: firing is not

idal cells under conditions where the pyramidal cells provide a uniform slow excitation to the interneuron population. We have discussed how isolated networks of mutually inhibitory neurons do not oscillate in phase when there is much heterogeneity in the driving currents. Nevertheless, provided the interneuron population is homogeneously excited, there can be considerable heterogeneity in the driving currents to the pyramidal cells, at least over a factor of two. The gamma oscillation persists, gated by the interneuron population, while the heterogeneity amongst the pyramidal cells expresses itself by a) a cell not firing at all, b) firing only on some of the gamma waves, c) firing on most or all of the gamma waves but with phase advance occurring in the most depolarized pyramidal cells. An example of this process is illustrated in figure 8.11 (simulation) and in figure 8.12 (experiment). We have found in simulations, however, that this distribution of phases relative to the gamma oscillation is easily disrupted by recurrent AMPA receptor-mediated excitation between pyramidal cells (Traub, Jefferys, and Whittington 1997), so that it is not clear if so-called phase coding would work in vivo in, say, neocortical circuits, wherein recurrent excitation between pyramidal cells is so prominent.

Possible Biological Relevance of Interneuron Network Gamma: Gamma-Frequency Rhythms Concurrent with the Theta Rhythm

In the previous chapter, we have described how in vivo gamma and theta oscillations appear together in the hippocampal and ento-

correlated, and there is frequency adaptation. The spike interval histogram, combined for the two cells, is flat (right). Bottom traces: when the same pyramidal cells are depolarized during an oscillation induced by glutamate ejection, there is much less frequency adaptation, and the firing times become correlated, as shown by the peak in the combined spike interval histogram (right). Calibrations: 100 mV, 100 ms. (From Whittington, Traub, and Jefferys, 1995b with permission of *Nature*, © Macmillan Magazines Ltd.)

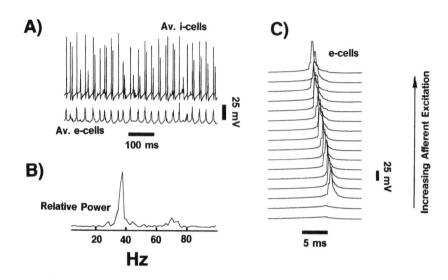

Figure 8.11
Interneuron network gamma: the synchronized IPSPs allow phase coding in which different pyramidal cells phase shift their firing relative to the gamma waves (simulation). The network contained 16 pyramidal cells and 16 basket cells with all-all connectivity but without pyramidal/pyramidal connections. Pyramidal cells excite interneurons via AMPA and NMDA receptors. The pyramidal cells are tonically excited by different currents: cell number L is driven somatically by $1.0 + 0.36 \ln (L)$ nA. (A) The average signals, representing the sum of interneuron and of pyramidal cell potentials, indicate a synchronized oscillation. (B) The frequency of the oscillation is near 40 Hz. (C) On a fine temporal scale, there is structure, however, in the firing times of each pyramidal cell, relative to the rest of the population. The most excited pyramidal cells fire first. (From Traub, Jefferys, and Whittington, 1997 with permission).

rhinal-cortical EEGs of rats. It is also the case that pyramidal cells fire, on average, infrequently during the theta/gamma state; and that in awake rats, but not in anesthetized rats, pyramidal cells and interneurons tend to fire during the same phase of theta (Buzsáki, Leung, and Vanderwolf 1983; G. Buzsáki, personal communication). It is possible to replicate the co-occurrence of theta and gamma oscillations (figure 8.13) in a manner that serves to highlight some of the principles that we have been discussing: the ability of interneuron network gamma to synchronize quickly (within a few cycles),

A

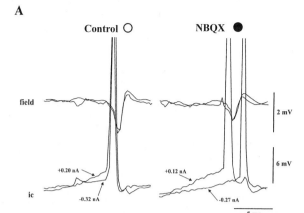

B

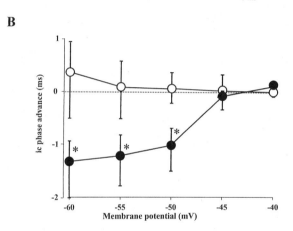

Figure 8.12
Interneuron network gamma: the synchronized IPSPs allow phase coding in which
different pyramidal cells phase shift their firing relative to the gamma waves, provided AMPA receptors are blocked (experiment). Experiments were done in the CA1
region of rat hippocampal slices, with NMDA receptors blocked by R-CPP (50 μM);
gamma oscillations were induced by pressure ejection of L-glutamate (1–10 mM).
Steady currents, either depolarizing or hyperpolarizing, were injected into a single
pyramidal cell (the monitor cell), and its firing phase was compared with the phase
of the population mean (as measured by the local field potential). (A) When AMPA
receptors are blocked with NBQX (50 μM), the phase of the monitor cell, relative to
the population, can be altered by tonic current injection. This outcome is not the
case under control conditions, even though recurrent pyramidal/pyramidal connectivity within the CA1 region is thought to be limited (however, see chapter 10).
(B) Averaged data showing relative phase of the monitor cell with respect to population gamma activity as a function of its membrane potential. Symbol ○, control
conditions (AMPA receptors unblocked, 147 events); ●, AMPA receptors blocked
with NBQX (129 events). (From T. R. Burchell H. J. Faulkner, and M. A. Whittington,
unpublished data.)

Number of pyramidal cells firing

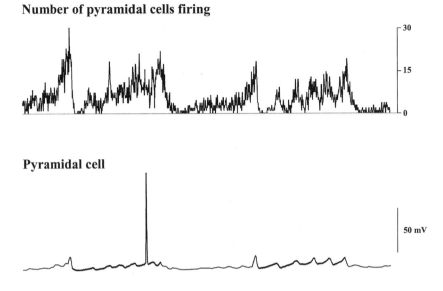

Pyramidal cell

Basket cell

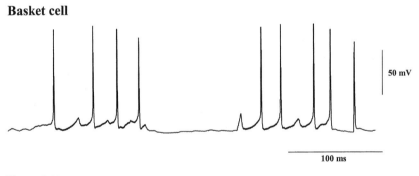

Figure 8.13
Simulation of simultaneously occurring theta and gamma rhythms. The network contained 3,072 pyramidal cells and 384 interneurons, including axo-axonic cells, basket cells and two types of dendrite-contacting cells. Mutual connections also exist between the interneurons, except for axo-axonic cells. Pyramidal cells were excited by stochastic trains of EPSPs to the distal apical dendrites with probability turning on and off at 100 ms intervals, and interneurons were depolarized by steady currents that also turn on and off at 100 ms intervals. The network then generates gamma oscillations that are superimposed on the imposed theta signal. Pyramidal cells fire rarely (provided the EPSPs are not too large), while basket cells are entrained to both theta and gamma rhythms. Compare with figure 3.1 (R. D. Traub, unpublished data)

its ability to entrain pyramidal cell firing, and the requirement to drive the interneurons homogeneously in order to induce synchronous oscillations.

The simulation of figure 8.13 was run on the most detailed hippocampal CA1 network model that we have. This model contains 3,072 pyramidal cells (with spatially random synaptic connections to each other at low density and to interneurons at higher density) and 384 interneurons, including 96 basket cells, 96 axo-axonic cells, 96 cells that contact distal apical dendrites, and 96 cells contacting basilar and mid-apical dendrites. The interneurons inhibit each other and the pyramidal cells, with localized random connectivity, producing IPSCs with decay time constant of 10 ms for the basket cells and axo-axonic cells and 50 ms for the dendrite-contacting interneurons. These time constants are for IPSCs produced in both pyramidal cells and in other interneurons. Further details are contained in (Traub, Whittington, et al., 1999).

The cells were excited as follows. First pyramidal cells were subjected to stochastic trains of EPSPs to the apical dendrites, the trains being turned on for 100 ms, then off for 100 ms. The amplitude and frequency of the EPSPs were adjusted so that no more than 40 pyramidal cells fired simultaneously, out of the 3,072 principal neurons. Second the interneurons were excited by depolarizing conductances, narrowly dispersed throughout the population (2% variation) and also turned on and off alternately at 100 ms intervals.

In this way, theta and gamma waves occur together, with entraining of both cell types at the two respective frequencies. The theta frequency is imposed by the external inputs (Kamondi et al. 1998), while the gamma frequency rhythm arises within the hippocampal network, as is believed to occur in vivo (Buzsáki et al. 1987; Bragin et al. 1995). The basket cell potentials closely resemble those recorded in vivo (Sik et al. 1995; figure 3.1). Interestingly, the gamma oscillation would not organize when the interneurons were driven by stochastic, rather than smoothly varying, synaptic excitatory inputs.

9 Gamma Oscillations in Networks of Interneurons and Pyramidal Cells in Vitro I: Mechanisms of Synchronization

In the previous chapter, we have considered gamma-frequency oscillations generated by networks of interneurons—presumably basket cells—under conditions in which pyramidal cells do not contribute to the shaping of the oscillation: the pyramidal cells either not firing very much or having their ionotropic glutamate-receptor outputs pharmacologically suppressed. We suggested that this so-called interneuron network gamma might serve as a model for two sorts of in vivo gamma-frequency EEG activity: (a) that which can transiently follow a physiological sharp wave in the hippocampus and (b) that which is recorded concurrently with the theta rhythm, also in the hippocampus. Interneuron network gamma is favored by blockade of $GABA_B$ receptors, can have its frequency regulated by the amplitude of driving currents, and can serve mutually to entrain the firing times of population cells.

On the other hand, synchrony is stable only when the population of interneurons is driven rather uniformly—a feature that forces one to question if interneuron network gamma by itself can be biologically useful. In addition, as we shall discuss below, if the axons of the interneurons all possess a limited spatial spread, then interneuron network gamma does *not* allow for synchrony across spatial scales that are large relative to the axonal spread. Thus, if the axons of an oscillating population of interneurons all run, let us say, at most 2 mm, then the population can not maintain synchrony across distances of, say, 4 mm. Hence, interneuron network gamma appears unlikely to explain, at least by itself, synchronization over the 7 mm or more that can exist in the neocortex in vivo.

In the present chapter, we shall examine in vitro gamma oscillations in which pyramidal cells contribute significantly to shaping the event by virtue of the fact that most of the pyramidal cells fire on most of the gamma waves and because the pyramidal cells synaptically excite the interneurons and, at times, each other. New technical experimental issues are involved in the ways such oscillations are elicited, and new physical principles appear. The most remarkable of the latter is that pyramidal cell oscillations can synchronize over long distances (up to 4.5 mm in vitro), even when the pyramidal cells excite each other weakly, or not at all, and despite the presence of significant axon conduction delays. The in vitro data will provide, therefore, a model for how long-range synchrony might arise intracortically without the requirement for participation by the thalamus or of any other central clock. Our simulation model is able to explain the effect of morphine and other μ-receptor agonists (including endogenous ones) on in vitro gamma oscillations: a disruption of long-range synchrony, which in turn suggests how opiate drugs might lead to mental confusion. Finally, we shall examine an experimental model in which gamma oscillations are projected from one cortical brain region to another: from CA1 to subiculum. We conclude with an experimental demonstration that gamma oscillations with pyramidal cell participation can be induced in neocortical slices.

Technical Considerations and Terminology

Most of the experiments described in this chapter were performed in transverse hippocampal slices, which contain subiculum and other parts of limbic cortex (Lorente de Nó 1933), or in longitudinal hippocampal slices, stimulating and recording in CA1 and/or sub-iculum. CA1 extends about 1.5 mm in a dorsal transverse slice from a rat, but up to 4 mm if the slice is cut obliquely. Longitudinal slices extend over 5 mm. Gamma oscillations, involving pyramidal cells and interneurons (s. pyramidale and oriens) can be evoked by te-tanic (repetitive) electrical stimulation at sites including s. radiatum, pyramidale, and oriens. Stimulation paradigms include 15–20 pulses of 50 μs width at 80–100 Hz. The amplitude of the pulses was adjusted so that gamma oscillations (recorded as field poten-tials near to the stimulation site) would be elicited by about half the stimulations, which are called threshold stimuli (1 × T for short) and which are the stimuli used in the figures in this chapter. In further experiments (described in the next chapter), twice threshold (2 × T) stimuli were also used. Gamma oscillations elicited by te-tanic stimulation in CA1 extend approximately 400 μm from the stimulating electrode (figure 9.15), less than the spread of most in-terneuron axons and significantly less than the spread of pyramidal cell axons (chapter 4).

In order to study synchronization on spatial scales > 1 mm, two stimulating electrodes are used up to 4.5 mm apart in longi-tudinal slices and 1.2 to 4 mm apart in transverse or oblique slices. It was found that for synchronization to occur over such distances, the amplitude of the two stimuli needed to be similar. In order to achieve this similarity, antidromic population spike amplitudes, elicited by single pulses, were compared at the two sites, and the relative intensity of the stimuli was adjusted to match the population spike amplitudes. When stimuli were not matched, it often occurred that oscillations were evoked at both sites that were phase locked (at nonzero phase) with each other (Whittington, Stanford, et al. 1997).

Figure 9.1 provides a cartoon of the synaptic interactions that can participate, in principle, in shaping oscillations at a single site and in providing for synchronization (or phase locking) between the two

Site 1   Site 2

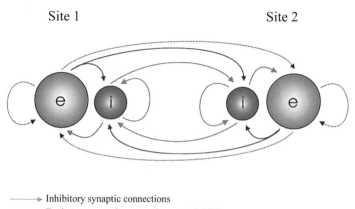

  ———→ Inhibitory synaptic connections
  ——▶ Excitatory synaptic connections onto inhibitory neurons
  ········▶ Excitatory synaptic connections onto excitatory neurons

Figure 9.1
Schematic illustrating synaptic interactions in tissue where oscillations are evoked
at two separated sites, 1 mm or more apart. The actual circuitry, both in real tissue
and in most simulation models, is distributed, rather than consisting of two discrete
sites. In addition, pyramidal cell and interneuron axons extend over different spatial
scales and have different connection densities. (From Whittington, Traub, Faulkner
et al., 1997 with permission of the National Academy of Sciences, U.S.A.)

sites. We emphasize that this figure is only a cartoon and not a
precisely accurate representation of the geometrical arrangement of
the circuitry. Most importantly, interneuron axons are unlikely to
run the entire distance between the two sites, which can be ≥2 mm
apart in the experiments. Either long-range synchrony is mediated
solely by pyramidal cell axons (contacting either other pyramidal
cells and/or interneurons), or else the intervening circuitry is important. We favor the view that both long-range axonal connections
and intervening circuitry matter, at least for studies of CA1 and for
this reason the computer models provide for distributed circuitry,
either with cell groups linked in a chain (cf. figure 1 of Traub et al.
1996) or with a long array of cells in which interneuron axons are
spatially localized (Whittington, Traub, et al. 1998; Traub, Whittington, et al., 1999). With this proviso, the diagram of figure 9.1 is

useful for keeping track of the different structural features of the system.

Basic Features of Tetanically Elicited Gamma Oscillations in CA1

Figure 9.2 illustrates a number of important facts which will require further analysis:

1. The oscillation takes the form of population spikes whose amplitude can reach 5 m V or more. This latter implies tight local synchronization of action potentials in pyramidal cells.

2. There is a latent period between the end of the stimulus artifact and the onset of the oscillation, which can be up to 150 ms and which can average 120–130 ms in rat CA1. (The latent period may be shorter in subiculum and in species other than the rat.) The latent period is reminiscent of that seen in neocortical neurons after stimulation of the PPT brainstem nucleus (chapter 7, figure 7.6).

3. The duration of the oscillation is hundreds of ms, sometimes up to 1.5 seconds. This range of durations is the same as for in vivo gamma oscillations that are evoked by visual stimulation or that occur spontaneously in monkey sensorimotor cortex or in human MEGs (chapter 7).

4. The oscillations have a frequency in the gamma range. Oscillations evoked by 2-site stimulation have a somewhat lower frequency than oscillations evoked by 1-site stimulation.

5. Oscillations evoked by 2-site stimulation can be synchronized with each other, with phase lags less than 1 or 2 ms.

6. S. pyramidale and oriens interneurons often fire doublets at gamma frequency during the oscillation evoked by 2-site stimulation, but they fire only singlets at gamma frequency during the oscillations evoked by 1-site stimulation. Doublets have also been

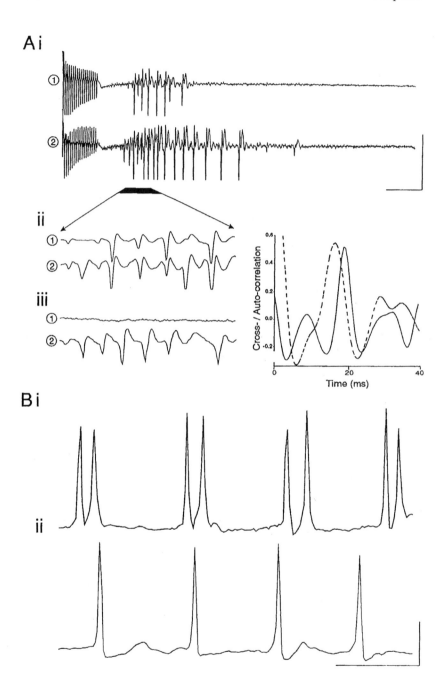

observed in vivo in a fast-spiking cell (a presumed interneuron with 0.8 ms-wide action potentials) during gamma activity (figure 8 of Steriade, Amzica, and Contreras 1995).

In the following sections, we will explore the physiological basis of these observations. One of the tools useful in this analysis is the computer model, which predicted many of these properties before they were known experimentally, including long-range synchrony, the existence of interneuron doublets, and the slowing of oscillation frequency with 2-site stimulation. The interaction between model and experiment promotes a better understanding of both physical and biological principles.

Simulations Replicate the Basic Features of 2-Site Synchrony

While the existence of interneuron doublets was predicted in the chain model of 5 cell groups, having synaptic connections within a group and to neighboring groups, a more geometrically accurate model gives a correspondingly more accurate picture of the physi-

Figure 9.2
Basic features of gamma oscillations elicited by tetanic stimulation of the CA1 region in vitro, either at one or two sites: the oscillations consist of population spikes that follow the tetanus after a latent interval. (A*i*) Tetanic stimuli were applied to two sites in the CA1 region (rat hippocampal slice, sites 4 mm apart); stimuli were 20 pulses, 100 Hz, sufficient to induce half-maximal population spike. After a latent period, rhythmic population spikes appear at both sites. The latent period varied from 50 to 150 ms. (Calibration 200 ms, 10 mV). (A*ii*) 2-site stimulation (above) leads to synchronized population spikes; results of stimulation of site 2 alone are shown below. (A*iii*) cross-correlation of signals evoked by 2-site stimulation (solid line) and autocorrelation of signal evoked by 1-site stimulation (dashed line). Two-site-evoked oscillations are synchronized between the two sites; the 2-site-evoked oscillations have a lower frequency (52 Hz) than do 1-site-evoked oscillations (62 Hz). (B) Electrophysiologically, s. pyramidale interneurons sometimes fire spike doublets during the 2-site-evoked oscillations (Bi), but never after 1-site-evoked oscillations (Bii). (Calibration 20 ms, 40 mV.) (From Traub, Whittington, Stanford, and Jefferys, 1996, with permission of *Nature*, © Macmillan Magazines Ltd.)

ology. The most accurate model that we have used is the one employed to generate the theta/gamma simulation of chapter 8, figure 8.13. To reiterate some of the structural features of that model (Traub, Whittington, et al., 1999), it contains 3,072 pyramidal cells in an array 1.92 mm long, together with 96 each of the following sorts of interneurons: basket cells, axo-axonic cells, bistratified cells, and oriens/lacunosum-moleculare (o/lm) cells that contact distal apical dendrites. Each pyramidal cell has synaptic input from 30 pyramidal cells, distributed randomly in space and making contacts onto basal dendrites, and 20 each of the 4 interneuron types. Also, critically (and as exists in the actual CA1 slice), inhibitory inputs are constrained to come from cells within 0.5 mm of the postsynaptic pyramidal cell. Each interneuron receives inputs from 150 pyramidal cells, distributed randomly in space—an important point, as will be seen below, and from 20 basket cells, no axo-axonic cells, 20 bistratified cells, and 20 o/lm cells. Only AMPA and GABA$_A$ receptors are simulated: it is known that gamma oscillations can persist when NMDA and/or GABA$_B$ receptors are blocked (chapter 8 and further on). Additionally, $\tau_{GABA(A)}$ is 10 ms for basket cells and axo-axonic cells and is 50 ms for dendrite-contacting interneurons. Pyramidal cell axon conduction velocity was 0.5 m/s (Colling et al., 1998), and interneuron axon conduction velocity was 0.2 m/s (Salin and Prince 1996); the shortest time it takes a signal to propagate from one end of the array to the other is 3.84 ms. Pyramidal cells and interneurons are simulated as multicompartment model neurons, as described in chapters 2 and 3 (Traub, Miles et al. 1994; Traub and Miles 1995). Simulated oscillations are studied in the steady state during the presence of large tonic excitatory conductances in both pyramidal cells and interneurons; the experimental justification for this assumption is described below. The excitation of the pyramidal cells is large enough to force them into a repetitive firing mode. In some simulations, the maximal $g_{K(AHP)}$ conductance is reduced, as is expected to occur during activation of metabotropic glutamate receptors. One-site stimulation is modeled by applying excitatory conductances to cells in the "left half" of the array only.

Figure 9.3 illustrates simulations of 1-site and 2-site stimulus-induced gamma oscillations, generated with this large network model. Let us compare the simulation with experiment point by point, referring to figure 9.2 as well:

1. Tight local synchrony exists in the simulations, although it is not shown in figure 9.3. Examples of local-average signals in simulations are to be found in figure 8A of Whittington, Stanford, et al. (1997) and in the conductance plots, which reflect average presynaptic activity, in the control panel of figure 9.11c.

2. Neither the latent period to oscillation onset nor the oscillation duration will be captured in a simulation of the steady-state oscillatory behavior, which figure 9.3 illustrates.

3. The simulated oscillation is at gamma frequency, as pyramidal cell and interneuron firing continue to be gated by IPSPs with $\tau_{GABA(A)}$ of about 10 ms. Oscillations evoked by 2-site stimulation have a lower frequency than those evoked by 1-site stimulation, as in the experiment.

4. In the simulations, 2-site evoked oscillations exhibit synchrony across the array.

5. In the simulations of 2-site evoked oscillations, interneurons often fire in spike doublets.

Where do the Interneuron Doublets Come From?

Our model interneurons do not generate spike doublets as an intrinsic property. On the other hand, in simulations of local networks producing gamma oscillations during sustained tonic driving currents, two features of the oscillation were noted. First, pyramidal

2-site stimulation   # 1-site stimulation

A

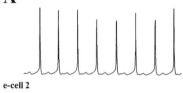

e-cell 2

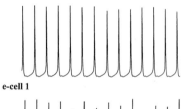

e-cell 2

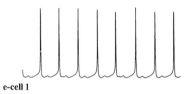

e-cell 1

e-cell 1

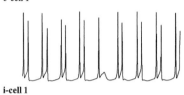

i-cell 1

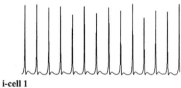

i-cell 1

50 mV

100 ms

B

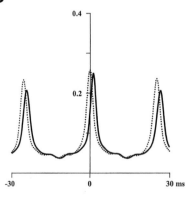

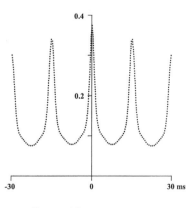

0.4

0.2

-30   0   30 ms

0.4

0.2

-30   0   30 ms

·············· Autocorrelation   ——— Cross correlation

cells and interneurons, on average, fired nearly in phase. Second, if the AMPA receptor-mediated pyramidal → interneuron synapse is powerful enough, synchronized pyramidal cell EPSCs, impinging on nearby interneurons within a few ms, can overcome the large interneuron spike AHP and induce a second interneuron spike, several ms after the first interneuron spike (Traub, Jefferys, and Whittington 1997). Note also that interneuron AHPs will be reduced by metabotropic glutamate receptors (see below; Miles and Poncer 1993). When these AMPA conductances are not quite strong enough, the interneuron spike is followed by an EPSP (as occurs also experimentally—see the interneuron during 2-site stimulation in figure 9.5b). In short, we predict that the second spike in the interneuron doublet is triggered by AMPA receptor-mediated conductances. Interneuron recordings taken during the course of our morphine work provide evidence for this concept (see later on). Doublet intervals in one set of distributed network simulations averaged 6 ms, compared to 5.2 ms experimentally (Whittington, Stanford, et al. 1997).

Oscillation intervals, at the start of which most interneurons fired doublets, were found in simulations to be longer than intervals in which most interneurons fire singlets—a straightforward conse-

Figure 9.3
Gamma oscillations in a distributed network model exhibit the same basic properties as do experimental oscillations (c.f. Figure 9.2). The same network model was used as in Figure 8.13, but tonic driving conductances were delivered to pyramidal cells and to interneurons (not identical in all cells), either across the whole array (2-site stimulation, left), or in one-half of the array only (1-site stimulation, right). e-cells (pyramidal cells) 1 and 2 are at opposite ends of the array. (A) Both pyramidal cells and interneurons oscillate. The oscillation is locally synchronized and would produce a field potential (although the figure does not show this). During 2-site stimulation (left), interneurons (i-cells) often fire doublets, but not after 1-site stimulation (right). (B) Autocorrelations of local average e-cell potentials and cross-correlation of local average e-cell potentials (near e-cells 1 and 2 for 2-site stimulation). The phase lag between sites 1 and 2 for dual stimulation is 1 ms. As in experiments, 2-site stimulation leads to an oscillation at lower frequency (41 Hz) than does 1-site stimulation (62.5 Hz). (From Traub, Whittington et al., 1999, with permission)

quence of the prolonged time course of the compound, doublet-elicited IPSP. This observation explains why 2-site stimulation-induced oscillations, which are associated with interneuron doublets, exhibit lower frequencies than 1-site stimulation-induced oscillations, which are not so associated.

Why do interneuron doublets occur after 2-site stimulation but not after 1-site stimulation? Given that pyramidal cell axons run long distances (several mm) so that interneurons are contacted by distant pyramidal cells, as well as nearby ones, 2-site stimulation will lead to greater AMPA receptor-mediated EPSPs in interneurons, than will 1-site stimulation. Hence, there is a higher probability of doublets after 2-site stimulation. For this notion to be applicable, two criteria must be met:

1. The pyramidal cell $\rightarrow$ interneuron AMPA conductance can not be too small or too large. If the conductance is too small, even 2-site stimulation will fail to cause interneuron doublets; while if the conductance is too large, then 1-site stimulation will cause interneuron doublets, something we have never seen experimentally. Unfortunately, it is difficult to measure experimentally some of the relevant parameters, such as the probability of connection between pyramidal cells and interneurons several mm away and the AMPA conductance required to force the occurrence of the second spike in an interneuron doublet. In models that have a network topology consisting of a chain of cell-groups, without long-range connections (e.g., Traub et al. 1996; Traub, Whittington, Colling et al. 1997), interneurons can not tell if the whole array is being excited or not, i.e., whether there is 1-site or 2-site stimulation: they only receive input from relatively nearby cells. In this case, depending on parameter choices, the interneurons either fire doublets or they don't, both during local and global stimulation. This is an important argument as to why a model with distributed connectivity is most appropriate, even though the chain model has proven most useful for other principles.

2. The two sites must, of course, oscillate synchronously. This process does indeed happen, but it seems—or ought to seem—mysterious, given that conduction times across the array are 3.5 ms at least; in simulations, synchrony can occur even when total conduction times are 20 ms or more. How can such synchrony occur and be stable even in the presence of noise and heterogeneity of driving currents/conductances to the pyramidal cells? Are interneuron doublets relevant to long-range synchrony, or are they just an epiphenomenon?

Before returning to these questions, we shall first address two sets of issues. First, can tetanically induced oscillations possibly be of physiological relevance given the occurrence of population spikes? Second, are the assumptions incorporated into the model experimentally justified and does the model make testable predictions?

Is Tetanically Evoked Gamma Activity Pathological?

We illustrated in the preface (see figure P. 1) that strong enough tetanic stimulation could induce a sequence of activities: gamma oscillations, beta oscillations (discussed in the next chapter), and then epileptiform bursts (chapter 5), which ride on intracellular depolarizations. Indeed, spreading depression can occur as well, following one or more epileptiform bursts. Figure 9.4 provides another illustration of the gamma → beta → epileptiform burst sequence, this time in the subiculum in vitro: these phenomena are not confined to CA1 and may represent common properties of all cortical structures (see also figure 9.21).

While few would question the resemblance of in vitro epileptiform bursts to interictal spikes in human patients (the latter tending, however, to be less perfectly synchronized than in vitro [Wyler et al. 1982]), what is the physiological significance of the in vitro gamma oscillation? We shall list arguments that a) favor this form

stimulation

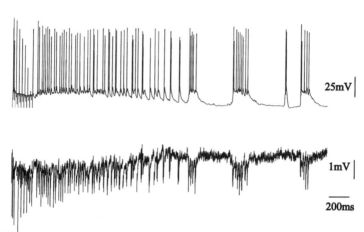

Figure 9.4
When tetanic stimulation is intense enough, the gamma oscillation is followed by lower-frequency population spikes (at beta frequency, 10–25 Hz) and sometimes by epileptiform synchronized bursts. Experiment in subicular region of rat, transverse slice. Note the tetanic stimulation artifact at the beginning of the traces (intracellular above, extracellular below). The late epileptiform bursts ride on intracellular depolarizations and have a distinct morphology from the gamma-frequency and beta-frequency population spikes. Compare with Figure P.2. Beta oscillations are considered further in Chapter 10. (I. M. Stanford and J. G. R. Jefferys, unpublished data.)

of gamma not being pathological, b) that favor its being pathological, and c) that favor the notion that in vitro gamma is worth studying even if it does prove pathological.

With respect to *a*, in vitro tetanically evoked gamma never becomes self-sustaining so as to persist longer than 1 or 2 seconds. The oscillation is shaped by the highly organized firing of interneurons in precise temporal patterns—something that is not a recognized feature of any cortical epilepsy, as far as we are aware. Precisely synchronized firing of populations of pyramidal neurons at gamma frequencies occurs in many cortical structures (reviewed in chapter 7) under what are believed to be physiological conditions. The difference in vitro in CA1 is in the size of the associated field potentials, a consequence of the fact that all (or nearly all) pyramidal cells in the local population participate in the oscillation. Also, the simpler lamination of CA1 and subiculum, compared with neocortex, amplifies the size of the field potentials.

With respect to b, gamma-frequency population spikes have not, so far as we are aware, been recognized in vivo in the hippocampus as a spontaneously occurring event (as opposed to following repetitive electrical stimulation or drug application (Dichter and Spencer 1969; Paré et al. 1992). Of course, it is conceivable that the correct behavioral context and sensory inputs remain to be found, which might be capable of eliciting hippocampal gamma with population spikes in, say, an awake behaving rat.

With respect to c, there are examples of pathological events in vitro that have shed considerable light on normal physiological events. One example is the interictal spike (i.e., synchronized burst), study of which has provided insight into physiological sharp waves, that is, partially synchronized bursts. Recurrent excitatory collaterals in CA3 are essential for interictal spikes and, therefore, may play a key role in physiological sharp waves. By analogy, the strongly synchronized gamma-frequency events in vitro may share common mechanisms with partially synchronized, less tightly organized, events in vivo. If this is the case (and we suspect that it is), then one needs to understand in vitro gamma mechanisms thoroughly enough that one can anticipate how the oscillation might be modified in vivo. Factors expected to come into play in vivo are modulators released by neurons whose cell bodies lie in subcortical structures, barrages of afferent inputs, and the likely absence of glutamate bathing large neuronal populations.

Metabotropic Glutamate Receptor-Induced Effects on Neurons That Are Elicited by Strong Tetanic Stimulation of CA1 and Their Implications for Network Modeling

Figure 9.5a shows that repetitive electrical stimulation at intensities adequate to induce gamma oscillations with pyramidal cell firing cause depolarizations (up to 20 mV) in both interneurons and pyramidal cells. The slow depolarization lasts for hundreds of ms in most cases. (Interestingly, the long bursts studied in CA3 by Bianchi and Wong (1995) last for more than 5 seconds. These events are blocked by MCPG, have an underlying synaptic conductance with reversal at-15 mV, and are presumably mediated by metabotropic glutamate receptors. The 4AP in the medium may have contributed to the long duration.)

Figure 9.5 also shows the latent period that is usually observed from the end of the stimulus to the onset of action potentials, despite the earlier onset of significant depolarization. The cause of this latent period is not known but may be related to the release of GABA induced by the stimulus and consequent membrane shunting. In addition, metabotropic EPSPs take 15–30 ms to reach 90% of their peak amplitude (Pozzo Miller et al. 1995). The latent period is variable from trial to trial, implying that no temporal feature of the subsequent oscillation can be time locked to the stimulus.

One implication arises out of the data shown in figure 9.5a. It is sensible to model the effects of the stimulus as a tonic excitatory conductance present in both pyramidal cells and interneurons.

The pharmacology of the slow depolarization in pyramidal cells was further investigated (bottom of figure 9.5). These data indicate that most of the depolarization is caused by metabotropic glutamate receptors, as most of the depolarization was eliminated by the nonspecific metabotropic glutamate blocker MCPG. (Boddeke et al. [1997] were additionally able to evoke population oscillations in CA1 with ACPD or quisqualate at about 20 Hz.) NMDA receptors made some contribution, as their blockade produced some short-ening of the duration of the induced oscillation, but this shorten-ing could be compensated simply by increasing the intensity of the stimulus. NMDA receptors, therefore, appear not to play a cru-cial role in the induction of gamma oscillations by tetanic stimuli. M1 muscarinic receptors make some additional contribution to the depolarization (Ncara is nitrocaramiphen, an M1 receptor-blocker; 4—DAMP is an M3 receptor-blocker; and had little, if any, effect).

The reader will note some residual depolarization, induced by the tetanus and resistant to the drug combination MCPG + 4—DAMP + Nitrocaramiphen. Possible factors in this residual depo-larization are a) activation of kainate receptors (Castillo et al. 1997; Vignes and Collingridge 1997), b) activation of depolarizing $GABA_A$ receptors, and c) elevation of $[K^+]_o$. Concerning the latter, we found that $[K^+]_o$ rose to an average of 8.2 mM, 200 μm from the tetanic stimulating electrode. Of crucial importance, however: in two cases, $[K^+]_o$ rose from 3 mM to just 4.1 or 5.5 mM, respectively, yet gamma oscillations continued to occur (Whittington, Stanford, et al. 1997). Hence, extravagant rises in $[K^+]_o$ are not a sine qua non for in vitro gamma oscillations.

Figure 9.5b serves to emphasize the difference in firing patterns between cells that are strongly depolarized individually and cells that are depolarized during a tetanically induced oscillation. De-polarization of pyramidal cells most often causes frequency-adapting trains of spikes, and depolarization of interneurons can easily cause firing at frequencies over 100 Hz. These are not the frequencies or patterns observed during the oscillation (lower two sets of panels in figure 9.5b). These data are a result of both meta-botropic suppression of the K conductances that lead to adaptation and, of IPSPs that limit the firing frequency of the interneurons, as well as shaping the oscillatory event in both cell types. Note again the interneuron doublets after 2-site stimulation but not after 1-site

Intracellular correlates of gamma oscillations

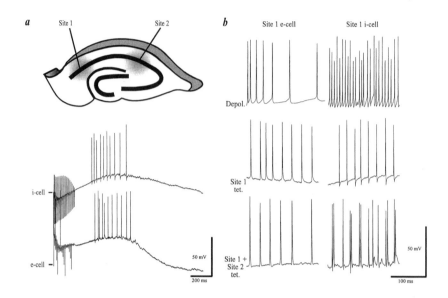

Origin of the post-tetanic depolarisation

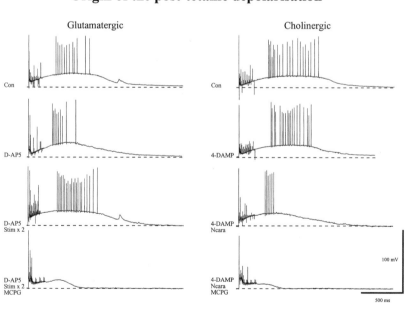

stimulation. It is interesting (as we have noted previously, but wish to emphasize again) that metabotropic receptors both induce the oscillation by exciting the neurons and permit the pyramidal cells to participate by blocking adaptation.

In network simulations, either of 1-site or 2-site stimulation, pyramidal cells and interneurons fire in phase to within a few ms. When interneuron doublets occur, it is the first spike in the doublet that is in phase with the spike in nearby pyramidal cells (figure 9.3, quantitated in one case in figure 9.6). Such an outcome occurs provided that the interneurons are depolarized enough to fire spontaneously on their own, as appears to be true experimentally (figure 9.5). (A phase difference between pyramidal cells and interneurons

Figure 9.5
Further experimental features of tetanically evoked gamma oscillations. (a) Schematic of the rat hippocampal slice, showing the locations of sites 1 and 2 within the CA1 region. Below are intracellular recordings from an interneuron (i-cell), and from a pyramidal cell (e-cell, not simultaneous) as they respond to a typical tetanic stimulus that evokes population oscillations. After the stimulus artifact (20 pulses at 100 Hz), a slow depolarization develops, followed in pyramidal cells by an AHP. After a latent period that averages about 125 ms, rhythmical action potentials begin. That this latter reflects population activity is shown in Figures 9.4 and 9.7. (b) Contrast between depolarization-induced firing in single neurons and the activity generated by the population. In response to depolarizing current, single pyramidal cells fire accomodating trains of action potentials, and interneurons fire rapid trains (upper traces). After tetanizing a single site (middle traces), both cell types fire rhythmically (40 and 46 Hz, respectively, in these examples). Tetanization of both sites (lower traces) leads to slower oscillation, and the interneuron fires many doublets. Singlet spikes in the interneuron are often followed by EPSPs. The lower part of the figure illustrates in pyramidal cell intracellular recordings some of the pharmacology of the slow depolarization induced by the tetanic stimulation. Upper traces are control conditions after the tetanus (different cells). Blockade of NMDA receptors with D-AP5 (50 μM) shortens the duration of the depolarization, but this shortening can be compensated by doubling stimulus intensity. Further addition of MCPG (0.2 mM), blocking metabotropic glutamate receptors, significantly reduces the depolarization, and prevents action potential generation. The M_3 muscarinic antagonist 4-DAMP has little effect on the depolarization, but the M_1 antagonist Nitrocaramiphen (*Ncara*) reduces the half-width by about 50%. [K^+]$_o$ elevations induced by the tetanic stimulus probably also contribute somewhat to the depolarization (not shown in this figure). (From Whittington, Stanford, Colling et al., 1997)

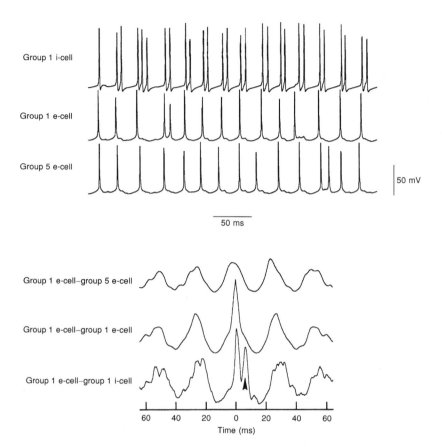

Figure 9.6
The network model predicts that, during synchronized gamma oscillations in a distributed network, pyramidal cell spikes are approximately in phase with the first spike of interneuron doublets. Simulations were done in the chain model, consisting of 5 cell groups in a chain, each group having 8 pyramidal cells (*e-cells*) and 8 interneurons (*i-cells*), with all/all connectivity within a group and with connections between each group and its neighboring group(s) in the chain. Tonic driving currents were applied to both pyramidal cells and to interneurons, not identical for each cell. (Above) The pyramidal cells fire mostly rhythmic spike singlets, the interneurons mostly spike doublets. (Below) Autocorrelations and cross-correlations of some of the different signals (obtained by averaging potentials of a given cell-type within a given group). The mean oscillation frequency was about 37 Hz, and the mean phase lag between opposite ends of the chain (groups 1 and 5) was 1.9 ms. The cross-correlation between pyramidal cells and nearby interneurons (lowest trace) shows that the pyramidal cell action potential is nearly in phase with the first spike of the interneuron doublet, and the mean doublet interval was 6.0 ms (➤). (From Whittington, Stanford et al., 1997)

can appear if the interneurons are held hyperpolarized enough so that only AMPA inputs cause them to fire, but this is not the situation after tetanic stimulation.) Some phase difference can be elicited as well by depolarizing the pyramidal cells enough, also increasing the oscillation frequency of the whole network, both pyramidal cells and interneurons (Whittington, Stanford, et al. 1997).

The prediction of small phase differences between pyramidal cells and interneurons was tested experimentally (figure 9.7) by simultaneously recording pyramidal cells (respectively, interneurons) intracellularly and population spikes nearby. Both pyramidal cell action potentials and the first action potential of the interneuron doublet are in phase with the local population spike, hence, with each other. Figure 9.7 (*Ad* and *Bd*) illustrates another point: synchrony of the population spikes between the two sites is not perfect, but it can, at times, jitter back and forth.

Why Might Interneuron Doublets Contribute, in Principle, to Long-range Synchrony?

König and Schillen (1991) considered the question of how synchronized oscillations might arise in a distributed system with conduction delays. They constructed a lattice, at each node of which was an excitatory neuron and an inhibitory neuron. Connections existed between neurons within a node and between neighboring nodes. Conduction delays between cells within a node were matched to delays between cells on neighboring nodes. Under these conditions, a synchronized oscillation could exist stably throughout the system. This model provides an existence proof that long-range synchrony is possible in the presence of significant conduction delays. The structure of this model, however, is wrong: measurements have been made of conduction times between nearby cells (chapter 4), and these times are short.

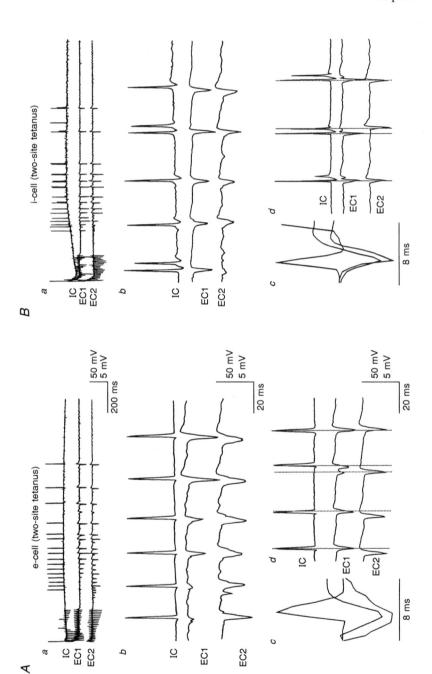

The notion that interneuron doublets served to match two time constants (the doublet interval and the delay time) was suggested (Traub et al. 1996), but this proposal is probably not the most fruitful way to view the physics of this system. Rather, as Ermentrout and Kopell (1998) have shown, the interneuron doublet interval serves to encode the difference in firing times between the two sites and to exert a corrective effect that brings the two sites back into register. Ermentrout and Kopell constructed a 2-site model, with an e-cell and i-cell at each site, mutually coupled with negligible delay and with $e \rightarrow i$ connections between sites that do have delays. Remarkably, this simple model replicates the basic behaviors of our more complex models and of the experiments: the two sites can synchronize, stably, and interneuron doublets occur and are necessary for the synchrony.

The Ermentrout/Kopell model is analytically solvable, but the following example, in words, gives some idea about the mechanism.

Figure 9.7
In experiments, during 2-site-tetanically-induced oscillations, pyramidal cells fire in phase with the local population spike, as does the first spike of the interneuron doublet; hence, pyramidal cells fire in phase with the first spike of the doublet. Gamma oscillations were induced by simultaneous 2-site tetanic stimulation in the CA1 region (see Figure 9.5). Intracellular (*IC*) recordings were obtained at site 1, with simultaneous extracellular recordings (EC) at each site. (Aa, Ab) Two different oscillatory epochs, on different time scales. The traces in a show the stimulus artifacts. These recordings demonstrate the tight correlation between action potentials in the single pyramidal cell and the nearby field potential, as well as correlations between field potentials at the two sites, confirming that the oscillation is a population phenomenon. (Ac) Further expanded time scale, showing tight synchrony between the different signals. (Ad) Sometimes a phase delay can exist between the two sites, which then switches to synchrony. (B) Corresponding phenomenology for interneurons. It is always the first spike of interneuron doublets that is best correlated with the nearby population spikes (*EC1*), even when, as in (Bd), there is jitter between sites 1 and 2. Because pyramidal cell action potentials are also in phase with the nearby population spikes, it follows that pyramidal cell action potentials and nearby interneuron action potentials (or the first spike of the interneuron doublet, if there is one) are in phase with each other. (From Whittington, Stanford et al., 1997)

Suppose, on a given cycle, that site 1 leads site 2. Then the inter-neuron doublet interval at site 1, will be prolonged because of the relatively delayed excitation from site 2, while the interneuron doublet interval at site 2 will be short because interneuron-2 will receive excitation from the two sites nearly simultaneously—or perhaps interneuron-2 will not fire a doublet at all. If the site-1 interneuron doublet interval is long, it will delay the next site-1 pyramidal cell spike. If the site-2 interneuron doublet interval is short (or there is a singlet), then the next site-2 pyramidal cell interval will be shortened. The result of this process is that on the next cycle, site 1 and 2 pyramidal cells will be more closely synchronized. In other words, the timing of the interneuron doublet intervals generates a feedback signal, which corrects for timing jitter between the two sites. Note that when interneurons only fire singlets, this feedback signal can not exist. The timing of the singlet spike in the interneuron is primarily determined by the balance between the tonic excitation and the relaxation of the compound $GABA_A$ IPSPs. The singlet spike timing does not contain information about the relative spike timing of nearby and distant pyramidal cells.

The above discussion indicates that there is a solid theoretical basis for expecting a causal role of interneuron doublets in producing the 2-site synchrony of gamma oscillations. Now we shall present evidence that this theory is the case. In network simulations, using the chain model and without pyramidal $\rightarrow$ pyramidal connections (figure 9.8), tonic stimulating currents were delivered to interneurons with a 10% spread in amplitude and to pyramidal cells with a 13% spread in amplitude. Under control conditions, the phase lag between opposite ends of the chain was near zero. The simulation was then repeated with progressively smaller values of the pyramidal cell $\rightarrow$ interneuron AMPA conductance. (Under control conditions, this conductance was large enough for interneuron doublets to occur.)

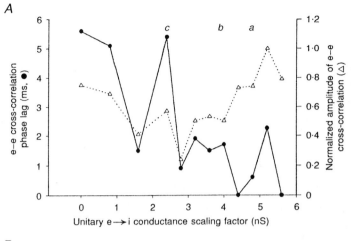

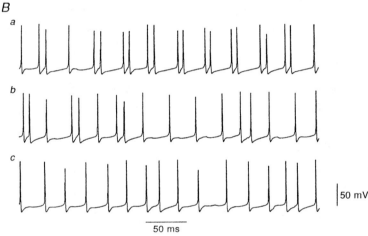

Figure 9.8
The model predicts that AMPA receptor-mediated pyramidal → interneuron synaptic connections, which induce the second spike of interneuron doublets, are necessary for synchronization to occur between the two sites. Simulations were done in the chain model with 5 cells groups, with tonic excitatory conductances to pyramidal cells and interneurons (not identical in each cell). The simulation was repeated with all parameters held constant, except for the unitary AMPA receptor-mediated conductance of pyramidal → interneuron ($e \to i$) connections. For each simulation, the cross-correlation between e-cell average signals (in Groups 1 and 5) was calculated, and we plot the mean phase lag (●) and amplitude (△). (A) As long as the $e \to i$ connection remains strong enough for interneuron doublets to occur (e.g., as in a and b, sample interneuron potentials plotted in B), the phase lag between sites remains less than 2.25 ms. Once doublets disappear (as in c), the phase lag between the two sites can fluctuate widely. (From Whittington, Stanford et al., 1997)

Two major effects were seen. First, as expected, the incidence of interneuron doublets decreased, and doublets finally disappeared. Second, the phase lag between oscillations at the ends of the chain fluctuated significantly once the interneuron AMPA conductance fell below a certain value (between points b and c in figure 9.8). Although not shown in this figure, individual cell groups in the chain could still oscillate with local synchrony.

Corresponding experiments were then performed, by evoking oscillations with 2-site stimuli (1.2 mm apart), while NBQX (20 μM) was washed into the bath (figure 9.9). This AMPA receptor-blocking drug should produce an action equivalent to the parameter change used in the simulations, but the action is not identical. NBQX eventually blocks the induced oscillations entirely; such block may result from blockade of kainate receptors, although this possibility has not been proven experimentally. It is necessary, therefore, to check that oscillations of reasonable amplitude are in fact occurring at points where data are collected. In addition, oscillations must not be evoked at intervals that are too short, so as to avoid the induction of epileptiform bursts or spreading depression. With these technical considerations in mind, it is clear that figure 9.9 shows a behavior in the slice similar to that in simulations: as AMPA receptors are progressively blocked, phase lags between the two sites become large (over 8 ms), but the increase in phase lag is not smooth.

What these data indicate is that interneuron network gamma, at least as long as interneuron axonal spreads are localized, is not able to synchronize tightly (~1 ms) on spatial scales longer than the interneuron axon spread. Long-range synchrony at gamma frequencies, at least that generated within a cortical structure, would appear to require firing of pyramidal cells in sufficient numbers and with sufficient synchrony to induce interneuron doublets.

Effects of Morphine on Gamma Oscillations in Vitro

Opiate drugs, including morphine, besides having addictive and analgesic properties, cloud the sensorium, impair performance in behavioral tasks, and cause amnesia (reviewed in Brust 1993). The cognitive effects of morphine, if not its other actions, might be explicable by an action on cortical structures. At the cellular level, morphine, by a presynaptic mechanism involving μ-receptors, diminishes the release of GABA at synapses on both principal neurons and interneurons in the hippocampus (Madison and Nicoll 1988; Capogna et al. 1993). In addition, enkephalin can hyperpolarize interneurons, apparently by an action on the neuronal membrane (Madison and Nicoll 1988; Masukawa and Prince 1982). It would be interesting to understand how these cellular mechanisms translate into population phenomena. We investigated the effects of morphine and some related compounds on tetanically induced gamma oscillations in the CA1 region in vitro (Whittington, Traub, et al. 1998).

Figure 9.10 illustrates the two major effects of morphine on in vitro gamma oscillations. First oscillation frequency may increase (e.g., with 100 μM morphine or 2 μM β-endorphin). In addition, sometimes small peaks appear in the autocorrelation of field potentials (e.g., with 100 μM morphine), suggesting that the local population is not entirely synchronized. Second, remarkably, the two sites do not synchronize in the presence of morphine or β-endorphin, even though the two sites do synchronize under control conditions. The 2-site desynchronizing effect of opiates is mediated by μ-receptors, as the effect is blocked by 10 μM cyprodime, a μ-receptor antagonist.

Why do these effects occur? As the tetanic stimulation induces such a strong depolarization (figure 9.5), one expects that the opiate-induced interneuron hyperpolarization would be, relatively speak-

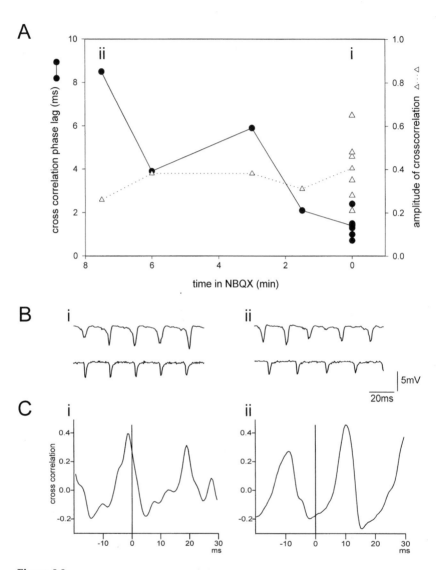

Figure 9.9
Experimental blockade of AMPA receptors prevents the two sites from oscillating synchronously, as predicted by the model. Population spikes can still occur at individual sites prior to abolition of the oscillation. Gamma oscillations were evoked by simultaneous 2-site tetanic stimulation (100 Hz, 200 ms) in CA1, with sites 1.2 mm apart. Extracellular field potentials were measured at each site, and cross-correlations calculated when the oscillation periods were nearly identical (to within

ing, insignificant. The opiate-induced reduction of IPSCs would be expected to increase oscillation frequency (see chapter 8, figure 9.5), so that this effect accords with intuition. What about the loss of 2-site synchrony? One would guess that reduction of IPSCs on pyramidal cells alone would make it more difficult for interneurons to entrain pyramidal cells, but of course, the local oscillation remains relatively synchronized. Simulations indicate that there is a narrow range of pyramidal cell IPSC size (when interneuron IPSCs remain normal), for which local oscillations are synchronized but for which 2-site synchrony is lost. Unfortunately, the corresponding experiment appears not to be technically feasible.

Finally, what might the effects be of reduced interneuron-interneuron IPSCs? Under control conditions, it will be recalled that interneurons fire as synchronized IPSPs relax under the influence of tonic depolarization (induced mainly by metabotropic receptors). Pyramidal cells fire at about the same time as the interneurons, and their synchronized output can induce a second interneuron spike to give the doublet. Because of conduction delays, the interneuron AMPA receptor-mediated EPSC is actually an envelope, spread out over some ms, of EPSCs originating in presynaptic neurons at different locations (an example of the simulated interneuronal g_{AMPA} is shown in control of figure 9.11c). Furthermore, for this EPSP to reach threshold, firing of pyramidal cells at the opposite site must occur, as 2-site stimulation can cause doublets, but 1-site stimulation does not. In morphine, however, with significantly reduced interneuronal

1 ms). Phase lags (●) and correlation amplitudes (△) are plotted as in Figure 9.8. NBQX (20 μM) was washed into the bath, and oscillations repeatedly evoked, under conditions expected to block progressively AMPA receptors. (A) Under control conditions, the phase lag is < 2.3 ms. As AMPA receptors are blocked, the phase lags fluctuate and are 8.5 ms just prior to loss of the oscillation. (B) Sample field potentials showing 2-site oscillations under control conditions (i) and just prior to loss of the oscillations (ii) (C) Sample cross-correlations for recordings i and ii. (From Whittington, Stanford et al., 1997)

a

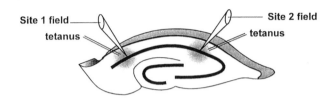

b

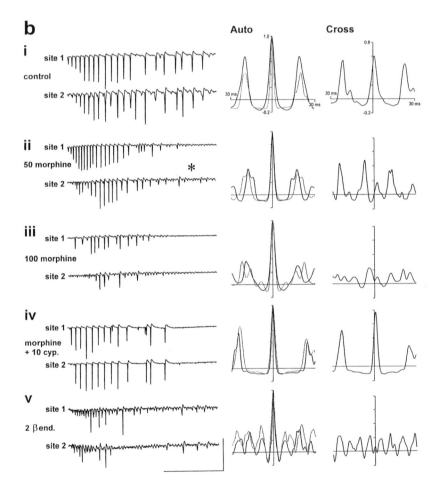

IPSCs, the pyramidal cell-induced EPSCs might induce not only doublets but also triplets. In disinhibited bursting interneurons, the timing of interneuron secondary spikes (those spikes after the first one) will not be an accurate indicator of the timing of presynaptic pyramidal cells; this firing of multiplets would contribute to loss of synchrony between the two sites. Interneuron bursting (but not single spikes) should be suppressed by blockade of AMPA receptors if this scheme is correct.

Figure 9.11 indicates that both simulations and experiments are consistent with this discussion, although the figure does not include a rigorous analysis of the sort used by Ermentrout and Kopell (1998) to analyze interneuron doublets. The traces in figure 9.11a, under control conditions, demonstrate again interneuron doublets after 2-site stimulation, while the morphine traces demonstrate the interneuron triplets that occur on some, but not all, waves. Figure 9.11b shows that, as predicted, the interneuron triplets are replaced by singlets in the presence of the AMPA receptor-blocker NBQX. These data, incidentally, provide further evidence that interneuron singlets are not phasically driven by the pyramidal cells. Finally, figure 9.11c shows in simulations that EPSCs in morphine are about the

Figure 9.10
Morphine, a drug that reduces GABA release, blocks 2-site synchronization, although individual sites can still oscillate with local synchrony. (a) Experimental arrangement for tetanically evoking oscillations at two separated sites in CA1 and recording of extracellular (field) potentials. In records below, we plot simultaneous field potentials at each site, autocorrelations at each site, and cross-correlations between the sites. (bi) Under control conditions, the frequency is 52 ± 2 Hz, and the phase lag is 1.0 ± 0.6 ms. (bii) 50 μM morphine in the bath leads to an increase in phase lag to 4.6 ± 0.7 ms. (biii) Further loss of 2-site synchrony with 100 μM morphine; each site continues to oscillate, although higher frequencies show up in the autocorrelation. (biv) Morphine (50 or 100 μM) added in the presence of 10 μM cyprodime (a selective μ-receptor antagonist) has no effect on the oscillations. (bv) The endogenous μ-receptor agonist β-endorphin (2 μM also disrupts 2-site synchrony, as well as speeding up the oscillations. (From Whittington, Traub et al., 1998 with permission of the National Academy of Sciences, U.S.A.)

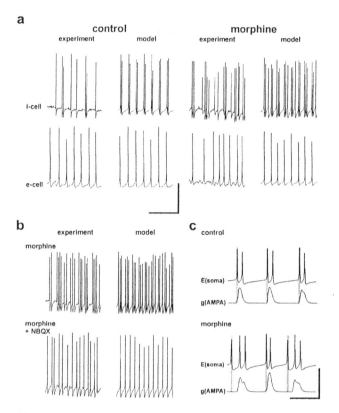

Figure 9.11
In the presence of morphine, tetanic stimulation leads to interneuron triplets, as well as singlets and doublets, which occur irregularly. Experiments were performed with tetanically evoked gamma oscillations, as in figure 9.10, under control conditions and with 50 μM morphine in the bath. Simulations were performed in a distributed-circuitry model with 120 pyramidal cells (e-cells) and 120 interneurons (i-cells), with tonic driving conductances to both cell types (not identical in each cell). The effects of morphine were simulated by reducing, relative to control conditions, unitary GABA$_A$ conductances by 75% onto pyramidal cells and by 86% onto interneurons (Madison and Nicoll, 1988). (a) Under control conditions, pyramidal cells fire rhythmic single action potentials, and interneurons often fire doublets. Experimental recordings are not simultaneous, but simulated recordings are. In the presence of morphine, pyramidal cells continue to fire singlets, but interneuron firing is irregular, with a mixture of triplets, doublets, and single spikes. (b) When the bath contains the AMPA receptor-blocker NBQX (20 μM), as well as morphine, interneuron firing is converted into a more regular pattern, with action potential

same amplitude as in control conditions, although more spread out in time, and of jittering onset relative to the first interneuron spike. However, in morphine, these EPSCs can lead to triplet firing because of reduced IPSPs in interneurons.

Thus, the morphine effects on in vitro gamma are explicable in a natural way by the known synaptic actions of morphine and the known physiology of the oscillations. It will be interesting to see if human studies lead to results that are consistent with opiate effects on long-range gamma synchrony.

Beta Activity enhanced in the Human EEG by Sedatives

Patients administered certain tranquilizing agents, including benzodiazepines (e.g., diazepam) and barbiturates, as well as abusing these agents often exhibit enhanced beta activity in their EEGs: the so-called beta buzz. An example is illustrated in figure 9.12. We have discussed in the previous chapter (see also Traub et al. 1996; Whittington, Jefferys, and Traub 1996) how these very compounds slow the frequency of gamma oscillations induced by metabotropic receptor activation of interneuron networks, with ionotropic glutamate receptors blocked. Suppose it were the case that these compounds slow gamma oscillations that are induced with normal glutamatergic transmission. It might follow that beta buzz results

singlets only. This pattern indicates that the later spike(s) in the interneuron doublets and triplets are AMPA receptor-driven but not the first spike. (c) Simulation of somatic potential (E) in an interneuron and the AMPA conductance, $g_{(AMPA)}$, to that interneuron, under control and morphine conditions. The amplitude of the AMPA conductance is about the same in the two conditions, although timing is irregular in morphine (as the two sites are not synchronized). Because IPSCs are smaller in interneurons in morphine and because EPSCs can be delayed, EPSCs are now able to evoke triplets where EPSCs in control conditions would evoke only doublets. In morphine, the combination of the irregular interneuronal firing pattern and the reduced ability of interneurons to entrain pyramidal cells, because pyramidal IPSCs are also reduced, contribute to the loss of 2-site synchrony. Calibrations: 50 mV, 100 ms (a and b); 80 mV/40 nS and 20 ms (c). (From Whittington, Traub et al., 1998, with permission of the National Academy of Sciences, U.S.A.)

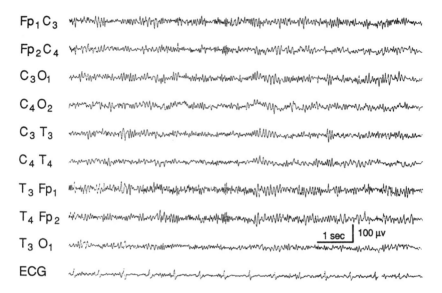

Figure 9.12
Diazepam leads to an increase in beta frequency activity in the human EEG. The EEG is from a 48-year-old man who was administered 10 mg of diazepam intravenously just prior to the recording. (From Glaze, 1990 with permission)

from slowing of normal background spontaneous oscillations in the cortex, which occur at frequencies usually filtered out in scalp EEG recordings. Alternatively, tranquilizing agents might increase the amplitude of either beta or gamma oscillations, which would have a direct effect on the EEG.

Figures 9.13 and 9.14 illustrate a) the experimental effect of diazepam (0.5 μM) on tetanically evoked gamma oscillations (see also Fox and Jefferys 1998; Faulkner et al., 1998), and b) the effect in a network simulation of doubling $g_{GABA(A)}$ of pyramidal cells and interneurons on gamma oscillations. In the experiment (figure 9.13), there is a striking prolongation of the oscillation (the reason for which is not clear), with minor effects on frequency and 2-site synchrony. In the simulation (figure 9.14), there are two effects to be noted: a small decrease in oscillation frequency and an increase in

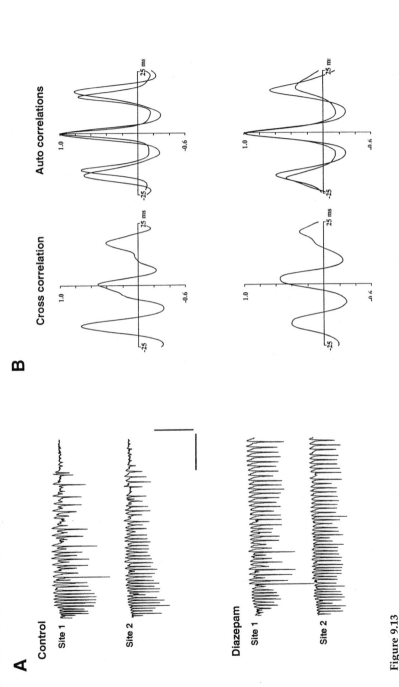

Figure 9.13

In the tetanically stimulated CA1 region in vitro, diazepam prolongs the gamma oscillation but has little effect on frequency. Two-site tetanically elicited oscillations were evoked under control conditions and in the presence of diazepam (0.5 μM). There is little effect of diazepam on frequency or 2-site phase lag, but there is a striking prolongation of the oscillation. Ionotropic glutamate receptors were not blocked in this experiment, in contrast to figure 8.5. (From Faulkner, Traub, and Whittington, 1998 with permission)

CONTROL $g_{GABA(A)}$ 32 Hz

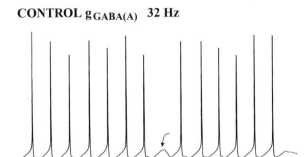

$g_{GABA(A)}$ x2   28 Hz

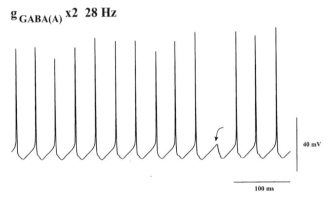

40 mV

100 ms

Figure 9.14
In network simulations, doubling of $g_{GABA(A)}$ on pyramidal cells and interneurons, such as would be induced by a suitable concentration of diazepam, leads to a minor slowing of oscillation frequency and to an increase in amplitude of synaptic potentials. Simulations were run in a network of 120 pyramidal cells and 120 interneurons, as with Figure 9.11. (Upper trace) Pyramidal cell from simulation under control conditions. Oscillation frequency is 32 Hz, and the phase lag between opposite ends of the array is near zero. (Lower trace) Pyramidal cell from a simulation in which unitary $GABA_A$ conductances were doubled, both on pyramidal cells and on interneurons. Oscillation frequency is now 28 Hz; the phase lag between opposite ends of the array remains near zero. Synaptic potential amplitude is increased relative to the control; this latter effect, most noticeable on waves without action potentials, would be expected to increase the amplitude of EEG waves if the effect were to occur in vivo. (R. D. Traub, unpublished data.)

oscillation amplitude (in the simulation, most evident in waves without action potentials). Two-site synchronization (not shown in the figure) was not altered by doubling $g_{GABA(A)}$. The increase in oscillation amplitude is a direct consequence of the larger $GABA_A$ conductances in a synchronized oscillatory system. We conclude, therefore, that gamma-prolonging effects, as well as (possibly) effects on frequency and on amplitude, could contribute to the beta buzz, assuming that the relevant site of action of tranquilizing drugs in producing the beta buzz is in the cortex, as seems most likely.

The Projection of Gamma Oscillations from One Brain Region to Another

We know that brief electrical stimulation of the CA1 region can cause, after a variable latent period, a train of gamma oscillations not time locked to the stimulus. This process, however, is not the only way that gamma oscillations can arise in the slice (and presumably also in vivo). Gamma oscillations can project in wave-by-wave fashion to the subiculum, a limbic structure that receives a monosynaptic input from CA1 pyramidal cells via axon collaterals running in the alveus (Tamamaki and Nojyo 1990). Furthermore, gamma oscillations in the CA1 region of the anesthetized guinea pig appear to be generated wave-by-wave in the entorhinal cortex (Charpak et al. 1995). This phenomenon is worth discussing in some detail, as it means that recording gamma oscillations at two sites A and B in vivo could have a number of interpretations: The oscillations are generated at A and project to B, or vice versa; the oscillations are generated in both A and B and are coupled; the oscillations are generated at C and project to both A and B; or A and B reside on a loop or cycle of oscillating structures; and so forth.

By way of background, the subiculum is a limbic structure that receives inputs from CA1, the entorhinal cortex, and multiple other temporal lobe structures (Van Hoesen et al. 1979), and that, in turn, projects to hypothalamus, septum, anterior thalamus, entorhinal cortex, cingulate and medial frontal cortices, amygdala, nucleus accumbens, and lateral dorsal thalamus (Rosene and Van Hoesen 1977), but without a recognized excitatory projection to CA1 pyramidal cells. The principal cells do not lie in a single layer as in hippocampus, nor are there the 6 layers of most other cortices. Rather, it is a transitional cortex (Lorente de Nó 1933). The physiological literature generally uses a simple classification into deep and superficial subicular principal cells. The principal cells fall into two functional (although not morphological) types: intrinsic bursting (IB) and regular spiking (RS) (Mattia et al. 1993; Stewart and Wong 1993; Taube 1993; Greene and Totterdell 1997), similar in pattern to many neocortical cells (Connors et al. 1982).

In terms of its functional properties, some neurons in the subicular complex, which includes the subiculum itself and adjacent regions, such as pre-and postsubiculum, are activated by head-direction, in contrast to the place-sensitive (but not direction-sensitive) properties of principal neurons in the hippocampus proper (Taube et al. 1990a,b; Goodridge and Taube 1997). Both sharp waves and theta rhythm appear in the subicular EEG in phase with similar events in the hippocampus (Chrobak and Buzsáki 1994; Buzsáki et al. 1986). Evidently, the subiculum is functionally, as well as anatomically, linked with the hippocampus. The simultaneous appearance of gamma rhythms in both structures may therefore have biological meaning.

A series of experiments has shown two interesting findings concerning the subiculum. First, the subiculum can express gamma oscillations in two distinct ways, either after local stimulation of the subiculum itself (endogenous oscillations) or projected from the CA1 region. Second, subicular gamma oscillations tend to be associated with population spike doublets, correlating with doublet firing of some of the principal neurons. In the following, we shall expand on these two findings.

Projection of Gamma Oscillations from CA1 to the Subiculum, but Not Vice Versa

Figure 9.15 (using data from Colling et al., 1998) illustrates a transverse dorsal hippocampal slice, containing a portion of subiculum (to the right of the distal end of CA1 s. pyramidale, indicated by the solid line). In the experiment, tetanic stimuli were delivered at the CA2 end of CA1 (★), while the response was monitored on successive trials at different locations along the CA1 pyramidal layer and into the subiculum. Gamma-frequency oscillations were evoked by the stimulus up to 400 μm away: this is the 1-site stimulation that we have been discussing. At larger distances from the stimulus—indeed, throughout the rest of CA1—no oscillations are evoked. Presumably, glutamate and other neuroactive substances released by the stimulus are confined to a definite locale, although we do not have direct experimental proof of this. Remarkably, however, the stimulus *does* lead to oscillations in the subiculum, 1.5 mm from the stimulus, and at the same frequency as oscillations near to the stimulus.

Pharmacological experiments were performed, applying blockers of $GABA_A$ receptors or of AMPA receptors either near to the CA1 stimulus or in the subiculum as it responded to CA1 stimulation. The results were as follows:

1. Blockade of $GABA_A$ receptors at the CA1 site prevents the occurrence of gamma oscillations at the CA1 site and, consequently at the subiculum site.

2. In contrast, blockade of $GABA_A$ receptors at the subiculum site has no effect on nearby oscillatory field potentials when CA1 is stimulated.

3. Blockade of AMPA and also kainate receptors at the CA1 site (as discussed above) also eventually blocks the oscillations at the CA1

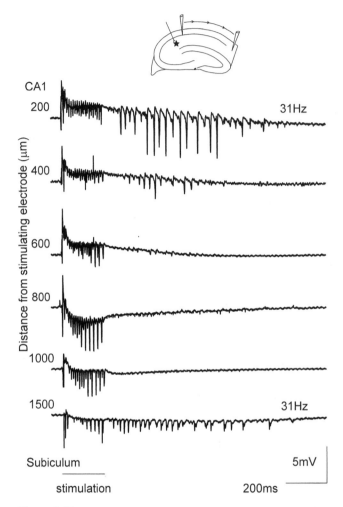

Figure 9.15
Localized tetanic stimulation of proximal CA1, near to CA2, induces gamma oscillations nearby, as well as in the subiculum, but not in intervening CA1. Schematic shows experimental arrangement: tetanic stimulation (100 Hz, 200 ms) was delivered in CA1 near the CA2 end (★), while the oscillatory response was measured in different trials with an extracellular recording electrode at various sites along s. pyramidale of CA1 and into the subiculum. Stimulation artifacts are shown in the recordings. Gamma oscillations appear 400 μM from the stimulation site, disappear, and again appear in the subiculum. These observations suggest that, in this protocol, subicular oscillations are driven by axonally conducted excitatory inputs, as a) intervening regions of CA1 are silent, after the stimulus artifact (sites 600, 800, and

site (for reasons not completely clear) and hence at the subiculum site.

4. Finally, blockade of AMPA receptors in the subiculum has no effect on the oscillations in CA1, but it does abolish the subicular oscillatory response.

These results can be economically interpreted: gamma oscillations evoked by a local stimulus require $GABA_A$ receptors to organize themselves, consistent with the critical role of interneurons. (The requirement for $GABA_A$ receptors also applies to oscillations evoked in the subiculum by nearby subicular stimulation.) Once a given region is oscillating, it can transmit or project a gamma frequency output over its axonal efferents to a synaptically connected region, utilizing AMPA receptors in the afferent synapses in the target region.

Consistent with this view, there is a phase lag from CA1 to subiculum when oscillations are evoked by CA1 stimulation (figure 9.16). The subiculum, as mentioned, can generate its own endogenous oscillations when locally stimulated, and the phase lag is reduced when both CA1 and subiculum are stimulated together. It is interesting that the 2.8 ms lag in the latter case is quite close to the axon conduction time from CA1 to subiculum (1.5 mm distance, ~0.5 mm/ms conduction velocity). The longer phase lag of 5.2 ms that occurs when only CA1 is stimulated may result from a combination of two processes: about 3 ms for axonal conduction and another 2.2 ms to force the postsynaptic cell to fire. When the subiculum is stimulated as well as CA1, the subicular cells should be strongly depolarized, and the synaptic recruitment time may then become negligible.

1000 μm) and as b) the spread of gamma activity to subiculum is prevented when AMPA receptors are blocked in the subiculum, while the spread is not prevented by blockade of $GABA_A$ receptors in the subiculum (see text). (From Colling et al., 1998 with permission of the American Physiological Society)

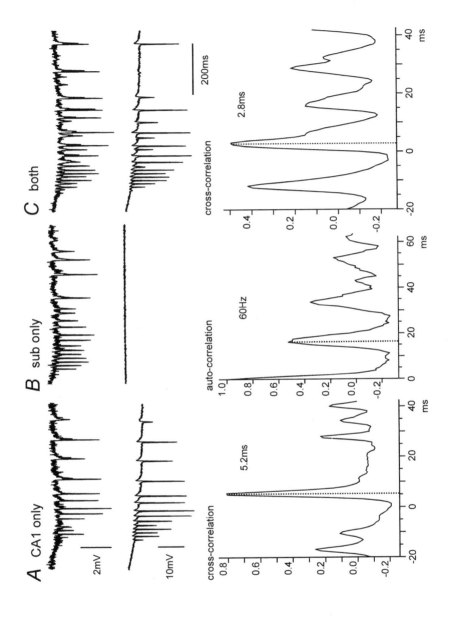

Fine Structure of Subicular Gamma Oscillations: Doublet Firing by Intrinsic Bursting Cells

As recorded in field potentials, gamma oscillations in subiculum, induced by CA1 oscillations, have a different fine structure than in CA1. In the subiculum, but not in CA1, gamma-frequency population spikes are often doublets (figure 9.17). At the cellular level, doublet population spikes can be seen to arise because IB cells—but not RS cells—fire in doublets during the oscillation (figure 9.18). This latter figure incidentally illustrates another finding: doublets in the subiculum are more common during a projected oscillation than during an endogenous oscillation.

Cellular Mechanisms of the Origin of Population Spike Doublets in the Subiculum

Where might IB doublets come from? There are at least three possibilities:

Figure 9.16
Phase differences between CA1 and subicular gamma oscillations. Oscillations were evoked by tetanic stimulation to CA1 alone, to the subiculum alone, or to both together. Extracellular potentials are shown for CA1 (above) and for the subiculum (below), without stimulation artifacts. (A) When gamma oscillations are projected from CA1 to subiculum, there is a phase lag of about 5 ms, explicable in part by axon conduction delays. (B) Stimulation of the subiculum alone can induce gamma oscillations. In contrast to projected gamma, locally induced gamma in the subiculum depends on $GABA_A$ receptors (see text). (C) Tetanic stimulation of CA1 and subiculum together leads to phase-locked oscillations in the two sites. The phase lag from CA1 to subiculum is less than when CA1 oscillates by itself: this is interpreted as implying that afferent EPSPs in subicular neurons, arriving from CA1, can trigger action potentials faster when the subicular neurons are depolarized (as they will be after subicular stimulation) than when the subicular neurons are at rest (as occurs when only CA1 is stimulated). (From Colling et al. 1998 with permission of the American Physiological Society)

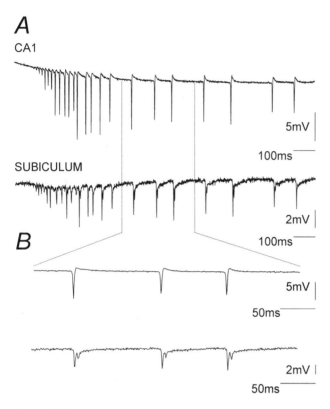

Figure 9.17
Tetanically induced oscillations in subiculum are often associated with double population spikes. (A) Simultaneous extracellular recordings from CA1 (s. pyramidale)
and subiculum. A 100 Hz, 200 ms tetanic stimulus was delivered to CA1, which
evokes a 62 Hz gamma oscillation nearby and a propagated oscillation in the subiculum (5 ms phase lag). Stimulus artifacts have been removed. (B) Expansion of
part of the record, showing the lag from CA1 to subiculum, as well as the double
population spikes in subiculum, but not in CA1. (Double population spikes can
occur in CA1 after particularly strong tetanic stimulation at beta frequency but not
at gamma frequency—see next chapter.) (From Stanford et al. 1998 with permission
of the American Physiological Society)

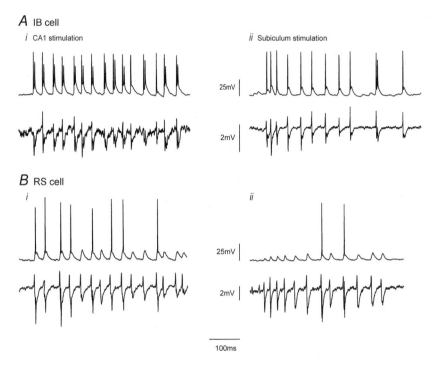

Figure 9.18
Subicular population spike doublets arise because of doublet-firing in intrinsic-bursting (IB) cells, rather than regular-spiking (RS) cells. Simultaneous intracellular (above) and extracellular recordings in the subiculum, (A) from an intrinsic-bursting cell and (B) from a regular-spiking cell. Oscillations were evoked by tetanic stimulation (100 Hz, 200 ms), either to CA1 (*i*, s. pyramidale), or to subiculum (*ii*). Doublets do occur in IB cells, more frequently after CA1 stimulation than after subicular stimulation. (From Stanford et al. 1998 with permission of the American Physiological Society)

1. a purely intrinsic mechanism might be operative, as can be seen with neocortical chattering cells (chapter 7, figures 7.7 and 7.8), which fire gamma-frequency bursts upon tonic depolarization.

2. IB cells might respond to gamma-frequency EPSPs (such as would impinge from oscillating CA1) with spike doublets.

3. IB spike doublets might appear as an emergent network property in gamma-oscillating subiculum due to recurrent excitation be-

tween the pyramidal cells: a synchronized pyramidal cell spike could evoke a second pyramidal cell spike, analogous to the way in which the second spike in an interneuron doublet is generated.

The data in figure 9.19A show that mechanism 1 is apparently wrong: injected steady depolarizing currents do not evoke spike doublets in intrinsic bursting subicular neurons, a result in accord with the findings of other investigators. On the other hand, injection of 40 Hz square-wave pulses (especially when the neuron is held hyperpolarized) can induce doublets (figure 9.19B). The results of figure 9.19A and B are replicated in a model bursting neuron as well. A

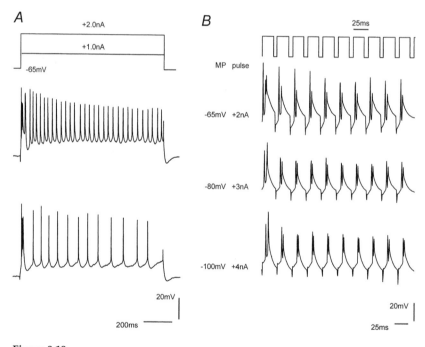

Figure 9.19
Phasic gamma-frequency inputs are required to induce gamma-frequency doublets in subicular intrinsically bursting neurons. (A) In subicular IB cells, somatic injection of tonic depolarizing currents leads to a brief burst, followed by a train of single spikes, but not to doublets. (B) Doublets can be induced, however, by a series of on/off current pulses. (From Stanford et al. 1998 with permission of the American Physiological Society)

likely mechanism is the recruitment during steady depolarization of K currents that tend to suppress doublet firing (which in the model requires participation of g_{Ca}). Periodic hyperpolarization can shut off a depolarization-activated K current and allow sufficient calcium current to be generated so as to induce the second spike in the doublet. In any case, the result of figure 9.19B indicates the plausibility of mechanism 2 above. Mechanism 3 is at least plausible as well, given that epileptogenesis can occur in the subiculum, implying the existence of recurrent synaptic excitation between the principal neurons.

Simulations of a subicular network of 120 intrinsically bursting principal cells and 120 interneurons (figure 9.20) are also consistent with both mechanisms 2 and 3. The protocol of stimulating the subiculum tetanically was modeled by tonically depolarizing both cell types, as in simulations of CA1 gamma oscillations. Provided that recurrent excitation is powerful enough, principal cell doublets can occur in these conditions (figure 9.20A). The protocol of stimulating CA1 was modeled by delivering 40 Hz EPSPs to the principal neurons, which also induced spike doublets, indeed more frequently than in the previous case (as in the experiments). As a check, we used both protocols simultaneously, and the network could gamma-oscillate under this condition as well.

What might be the significance of the doublets, or indeed of chattering, in the neocortex? This mode of cell firing presumably must be related to a synaptic action on target neurons. To investigate this possibility further, it will be necessary to identify the relevant targets, and examine postsynaptic actions when subicular cells (respectively cortical spiny cells) fire singlets at gamma-frequency verses firing doublets or bursts at gamma frequency.

Tetanically Induced Oscillations in Neocortical Slices

One question that runs through all of the data presented in this chapter is, do the results apply to the neocortex, for which there is

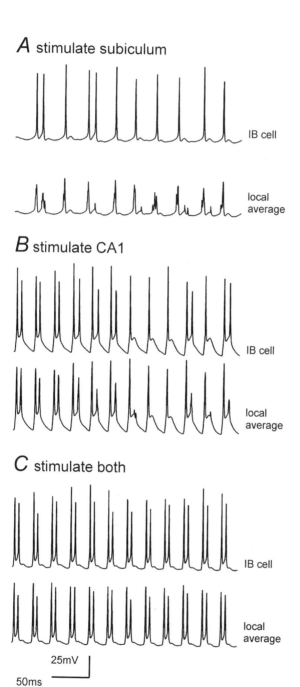

the most abundant experimental evidence suggesting a functional meaning for gamma oscillations? A first step in this direction is to demonstrate that tetanically evoked oscillations occur at all in neocortical slices and not just in hippocampal and subicular slices. Figure 9.21 shows, with intracellular and field potential recordings, that such oscillations (in this case 25 Hz) can be generated in a neocortical slice, consequent to a tetanic stimulus. The 25 Hz frequency is in the range observed in vivo in the sensorimotor cortex, although it is slower than what is usually found in visual cortex. Interestingly, the intracellular recording exhibits prominent EPSPs, presumably reflecting the dense recurrent excitatory connectivity of the cortex. It remains to be investigated what role the interneurons are playing in this oscillation, and the oscillation's long-range synchronization and other emergent properties.

In Conclusion

In this chapter, we have described a method for evoking gamma oscillations in the slice in such a way as to involve both principal cells and interneurons. We have shown, using closely coupled models and experiments, how first 2-site stimulation can, by a novel

Figure 9.20
Simulations illustrating how the same network (representing part of the subiculum) can generate gamma oscillations with principal cell doublets by two distinct mechanisms. (A) Tonic depolarization of both principal cells and interneurons induces gamma oscillations, as discussed previously; doublets are then generated by recurrent excitatory synaptic connections. This situation corresponds to oscillations induced in subiculum by subiculum stimulation. (B) When the cells are not tonically depolarized, but when principal cells are excited by gamma-frequency EPSPs, rhythmic doublets occur in the population, although as is true experimentally, a given neuron need not fire doublets on each wave. This corresponds to projected gamma from CA1. Note that, as in experiments, projected gamma leads to more doublets than does endogenous gamma. (C) The two mechanisms can work in harmony. (From Stanford et al. 1998 with permission of the American Physiological Society)

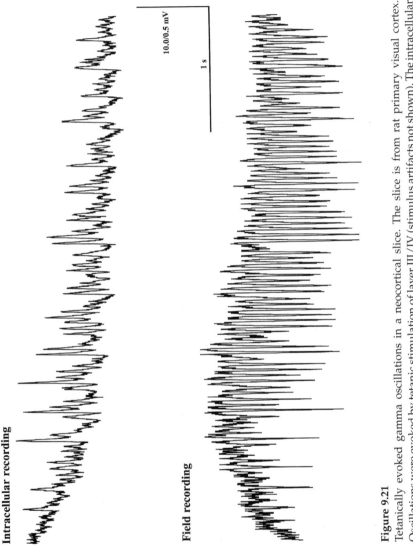

Figure 9.21
Tetanically evoked gamma oscillations in a neocortical slice. The slice is from rat primary visual cortex. Oscillations were evoked by tetanic stimulation of layer III/IV (stimulus artifacts not shown). The intracellular recording is from a principal neuron, hyperpolarized by passage of -0.3 nA current through the electrode. Oscillation frequency is about 25 Hz. (M. A. Whittington, unpublished data.)

mechanism, lead to tight synchronization when both stimuli are in CA1: interneuron spike doublets, the structure of which provides a feedback signal that tends to maintain synchrony. Second, we have seen that 2-site stimulation can lead to coupled oscillations with a phase lag when one stimulus is in CA1 and the other in subiculum or when CA1 alone is stimulated and oscillations are induced in subiculum. The structural difference between the two cases is that, in the first, axonal connections run in both directions, although not symmetrically, there being a larger pathway toward subiculum than toward CA2 (Tamamaki and Nojyo 1990). In the second, however, the axons run exclusively, or almost so, from CA1 to the target region. There is a remarkable agreement between model and experiment in terms of predicted phase relations of the cell types, of the firing patterns of interneurons, and of the inability of pure interneuron networks to synchronize on large spatial scales. Finally, the morphine data provide further (albeit indirect) evidence that long-range synchrony of gamma oscillations may really be of consequence to the brain for cognitive performance.

One physiological issue which remains unclear is what is the role in structuring a gamma oscillation of interneuron-interneuron synaptic interactions under conditions when many pyramidal cells are firing? In simulations, this role seems to be model-dependent and hence of uncertain biological significance. For example, in the Ermentrout/Kopell model (1998), interneuron-interneuron synaptic interactions are not necessary for 2-site synchrony to occur. In our networks that used distributed connectivity (for example, as used in the morphine simulations), the effects of interneuron-interneuron interactions can be minor, consisting of small (about 1 ms) phase differences. On the other hand, in the chain model (Traub et al. 1996), interneuron-interneuron connections are necessary in order to prevent loss of correlation between distant sites. This model-dependence of the role of interneuron-interneuron connections stands in distinct contrast to the role of interneuron doublets, which so far are required for long-range synchrony in all models in which gamma is generated autonomously. Of course, when pyramidal cells are silent, then interneuron-interneuron interactions are crucial for gamma to occur. In order to approach this type of question experimentally, it will be necessary to develop means for regulating $GABA_A$ conductances independently on pyramidal cells and on interneurons.

10

Gamma Oscillations in Networks of Interneurons and Pyramidal Cells in Vitro II: Synaptic Plasticity and the Switch to Beta Frequencies

The last two chapters have mostly concerned the mechanisms of synchronization—locally and over distance—of gamma frequency oscillations evoked by tetanic stimulation at one or two sites in the CA1 region in vitro. Although we have not emphasized this point, the intensity of tetanic stimulation used experimentally had been near to the threshold for eliciting oscillations at all. Remarkably, when more intense tetanic stimuli are employed, say at twice-threshold, a whole new range of oscillatory phenomena appear. There are both acute and chronic effects. Acutely, the intense stimulus is followed by a gamma oscillation having properties similar to gamma oscillations evoked by near-threshold stimuli, but the gamma oscillation, after some hundreds of ms, is succeeded by a slower oscillation at beta (10–25 Hz) frequency. Chronically, an intense tetanic stimulation, applied only one single time, affects properties of oscillations evoked by future near threshold stimuli. What exact effects are produced depends on whether the intense stimulus is applied to one site alone or to two sites simultaneously. The chronic effects last tens of minutes at least.

These results are of importance for two reasons. First, the synchronizing mechanisms for gamma and beta oscillations in this preparation are not identical. This lack of identity in turn implies that distinctive synaptic mechanisms are available to the brain to control separately the spatiotemporal patterns of one EEG frequency range vis-à-vis another frequency range. Second, if gamma oscillations truly are important for perception and cognition, as many have suggested (chapter 7), then beta oscillations and their associated synaptic plasticity are likely to be important for memory.

This chapter will be divided into two parts. First, we shall consider the phenomenology of the beta oscillation and its synaptic and cellular mechanisms. Then, we shall consider the synaptic plasticity that underlies the chronic effects of intense tetanic stimulation and how this plasticity can affect oscillatory synchrony in distinctive frequency regimes. The data in this chapter derive mainly from two papers: Whittington et al. (1997b) and Traub et al. (1999).

Phenomenology and Mechanisms of Beta Oscillations

Figure 10.1 illustrates the contrasting effects of threshold tetanic stimulation (A) and twice-threshold stimulation (B). (Single-site stimulation was used in A and two-site stimulation in B, but it is the intensity of stimulation, not the number of sites, that determines the temporal pattern of the immediately induced oscillation.) With threshold stimulation in this instance (A), the gamma oscillation slows progressively over about 1 second, breaking apart when the frequency reaches about 30 Hz. Doublets do not occur in the population spikes or in the intracellular (pyramidal cell) potentials. On the other hand, after twice-threshold stimulation (B), there is a period of gamma oscillation for about ½ second, followed by an abrupt switch to a beta oscillation, the latter continuing for about a second. During the beta phase, there are doublets in the population spikes and in pyramidal cell action potential trains. The intracellular recordings in both A and B illustrate the increase over time of pyramidal cell spike AHPs during the course of the gamma oscillation. Pyramidal cells remain depolarized during the beta phase.

Figure 10.2 illustrates some of the various combinations of a) number of sites stimulated (one or two) and b) stimulation intensity

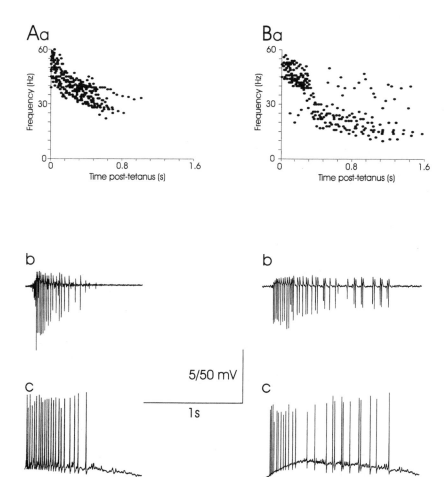

Figure 10.1

A gamma → beta frequency switch occurs with sufficiently strong tetanic stimulation. (A) Gamma oscillations were evoked 12 times at one site in the CA1 region (20 pulses of 50 μs duration, 100 Hz), with intensity near threshold for evoking an oscillation. a: instantaneous frequency plot for the 12 epochs. The frequency gradually declines to about 30 Hz, and the oscillation breaks up. b and c: example extracellular (b) and pyramidal-cell intracellular (c) recordings with stimulus artifact not shown. Spike doublets do not occur. (B) Oscillations were evoked 10 times at two sites in CA1 with intensity at twice threshold. (The gamma → beta frequency shift can also occur with 1-site twice-threshold stimulation, as shown in figure 10.2) a: instantaneous frequency plot for the 10 epochs shows a decline in gamma frequency to about 35 Hz and then an abrupt switch to beta frequency at about 10–25 Hz. b and c: example extracellular and intracellular (pyramidal cell) recordings, respectively, showing local synchrony of the beta oscillation (population spikes), along with occasional spike doublets in both extra-and intracellular recordings during the beta phase. (From Whittington, Traub, Faulkner et al. 1997 with permission of the National Academy of Sciences, U.S.A.)

The pattern of tetanus affects frequency and synchrony of oscillation

Beta frequencies are associated with EPSPs

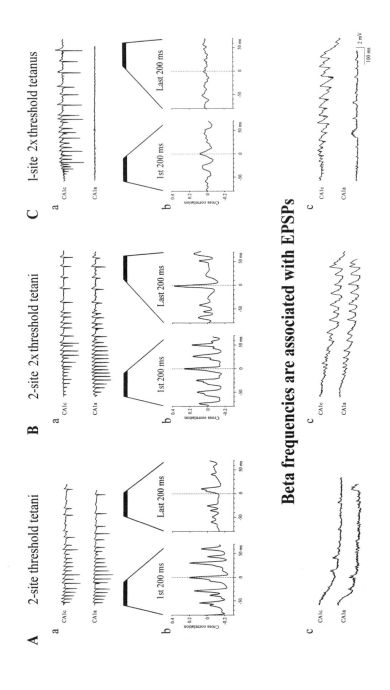

(threshold or twice-threshold). (Single-site threshold stimulation is illustrated in chapter 9, figure 9.2.) For three different stimulation protocols, the figure illustrates, first, field potentials at the two sites (CA3 and subicular ends of the CA1 region in vitro), second, cross-correlations of the field potentials for the first 200 ms and last 200 ms of the response, and third, intracellular potentials of two pyramidal cells, one at either site, which have been hyperpolarized by current injection so as to emphasize EPSPs and to diminish IPSPs.

A number of important points are shown in figure 10.2. First, gamma oscillations are evoked by either stimulus intensity and are synchronized between sites after either intensity when both sites are stimulated. Second, beta oscillations are evoked by twice-threshold stimuli at either one or two sites, and when both sites are stimulated, the beta oscillations synchronize between the sites. Finally, when twice-threshold stimulation is used, pyramidal cells in the site (or sites) receiving this intense stimulation develop EPSPs. The EPSPs take a few hundred ms to develop, occur at beta fre-

Figure 10.2
The gamma → beta frequency switch can occur after 1-site or 2-site stimulation. Beta oscillations are associated with EPSPs in pyramidal cells, and they are synchronized locally and also between the two sites after 2-site stimulation. Oscillations were evoked by tetanic stimulation at the CA3 end of CA1 (CA1c) or at both CA1c and the subicular end of CA1 (CA1a). Either threshold or twice-threshold stimuli were used. In each case, *a* shows field potentials at the two sites with stimulus artifact removed; *b* shows cross-correlations of the two field potentials, either for the first 200 ms of the response (left) or for the last 200 ms of the response (right); *c* shows intracellular recordings from two pyramidal cells, one at each site, hyperpolarized to about −80 mV by current injection. (A) 2-site threshold-intensity stimulation produces gamma activity that is synchronized between sites at first, but then synchrony is lost. There are few EPSPs in the pyramidal cells, and these EPSPs are not rhythmic. (B) 2-site twice-threshold stimulation induces synchronized gamma and also beta oscillation. Large, rhythmical EPSPs occur at both sites, at beta frequency, and in synchrony. (C) 1-site twice-threshold tetanus induces gamma → beta activity, along with large rhythmical EPSPs, at that site only. The small EPSPs at the other site indicate the presence of excitatory synaptic connections from the CA3 end of CA1 to the subicular end. (From Whittington et al., 1997b with permission of the National Academy of Sciences, U.S.A.)

quency, are synchronized between sites when 2-site stimuli are used, and can reach 5 mV in amplitude. These EPSPs can not be an epiphenomenon of increased synchrony during the beta phase: population spikes during the beta phase are actually smaller than during the gamma phase. When threshold stimulation is used to evoke a gamma oscillation, some EPSPs do occur, but they are rarer than in the beta oscillation, smaller, and are not rhythmic.

Figure 10.3 provides quantitative support for comments made above on spike AHPs and EPSPs. Starting after about 5 or 8 periods (roughly 150 ms for a gamma oscillation with period about 25 ms), spike AHPs begin to increase. The increase continues over about 8 periods and then levels off. Spike AHPs increase with comparable time course whether or not beta oscillations occur, that is, with threshold or twice-threshold stimuli. Note, however, that initial spike AHPs are smaller after twice-threshold stimuli, perhaps reflecting a greater activation of metabotropic glutamate receptors. In contrast to the AHP recovery, recurring EPSPs are observed only when there is a shift to beta frequency. The time courses for the increases of AHPs and of EPSPs are comparable. These data suggest that the generation of the EPSPs and the occurrence of the beta oscillation are somehow causally related. We shall argue below that this causal relationship is indeed the case. But first let us show some of the properties of the EPSPs.

Figure 10.4 illustrates some of the factors responsible for the EPSPs and some of their consequences. First (A), when EPSPs are present, pyramidal cells can fire in doublets, although doublets need not occur often or regularly in any particular pyramidal cell. Simulations indicate that the second action potential in a pyramidal cell doublet is synaptically elicited via AMPA receptors by the synchronous firing (population spike) of the general pyramidal cell ensemble. In a sense, this process is analogous to the generation of interneuron spike doublets after 2-site tetanic stimulation, but there are differences in detail. The pyramidal cell → pyramidal cell con-

AHP recovery during oscillation

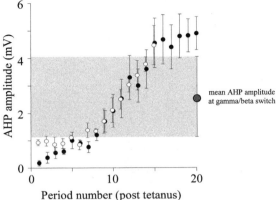

mean AHP amplitude
at gamma/beta switch

EPSP potentiation during oscillation

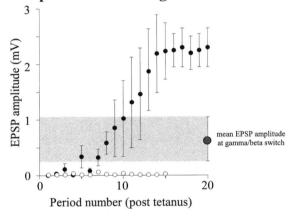

mean EPSP amplitude
at gamma/beta switch

○ Oscillation with no frequency shift (n = 6)
● Oscillation with gamma/beta frequency shift (n = 6)

Figure 10.3
During the gamma → beta transition, pyramidal-cell spike AHPs recover, in addition to the appearance of EPSPs. Oscillations were evoked by 2-site stimulation in CA1, with intensity that evoked a gamma → beta transition (●, n = 6) or gamma oscillation alone (○, n = 6), while recording from a pyramidal cell. The spike AHP increased whether or not the transition took place (above), but EPSPs increased only when there was a transition. It is unlikely that the beta oscillation itself caused the EPSPs as population spikes during beta tend to be smaller than during gamma; rather, it is the EPSPs that cause beta, as shown below. Error bars show standard error of the mean. Shaded areas show the range of AHP and EPSP sizes just prior to the gamma → beta transition when such transition occurred. (From Whittington, Traub, Faulkner et al 1997 with permission of the National Academy of Sciences, U.S.A.)

EPSPs contribute to beta frequency oscillations

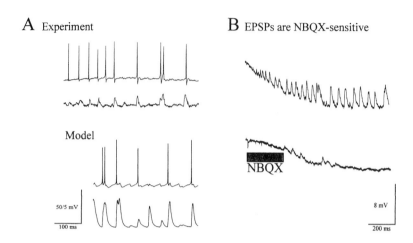

A Experiment

Model

50/5 mV

100 ms

B EPSPs are NBQX-sensitive

NBQX

8 mV

200 ms

Action potentials are required to generate EPSPs

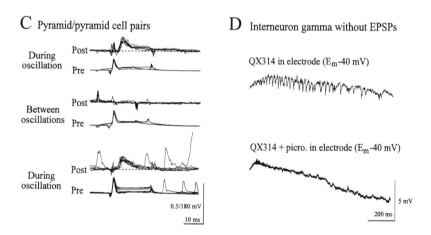

C Pyramid/pyramid cell pairs

During oscillation   Post

Pre

Between oscillations   Post

Pre

During oscillation   Post

Pre

0.5/180 mV

10 ms

D Interneuron gamma without EPSPs

QX314 in electrode (E_m -40 mV)

QX314 + picro. in electrode (E_m -40 mV)

5 mV

200 ms

Figure 10.4
AMPA receptor-mediated EPSPs are associated with pyramidal cell spike doublets during beta; functional synaptic coupling between pyramidal cells increases during the oscillation; postsynaptic cell firing is required for EPSP generation; IPSP-

nection, even in its potentiated state, appears to be weaker than the pyramidal cell → basket cell connection; additionally, pyramidal cells appear to have synaptic inputs from fewer other pyramidal cells than do basket cells. For these reasons, doublet firing in pyramidal cells during beta is intermittent. In simulations, when recurrent pyramidal cell → pyramidal cell connections become powerful enough to elicit doublets regularly, then bursts begin to occur as well, even though the recurrent connections are in the basal dendrites and not in apical dendrites, which are known to be susceptible to bursting.

Second (figure 10.4B), the EPSPs are largely, if not exclusively, mediated by AMPA receptors. The upper trace shows EPSPs in a pyramidal cell, hyperpolarized by current injection after a tetanic stimulation intense enough to elicite beta oscillations. The lower

mediated gamma continues throughout the gamma and beta oscillations. Oscillations were evoked (unless stated otherwise) with 2-site, twice-threshold stimulation. (A) Experiment shows two nearby pyramidal cells, upper one with membrane potential −70 mV, the lower one being hyperpolarized by current injection to −79 mV. This shows synchrony between EPSPs in one cell and spikes (or spike doublets) in a nearby cell. The simulation shows similar result, using the chain model of 40 pyramidal cells and 40 interneurons, including $e \rightarrow e$ synaptic connections. (B) A pyramidal cell was hyperpolarized to about −85 mV during a gamma → beta transition (above), showing the EPSPs. Lower trace shows the same cell and stimulation conditions, but the AMPA receptor-blocker NBQX was pressure-ejected (bar), abolishing the EPSPs. (C) Simultaneous recordings of two pyramidal cells. The presynaptic cell (lower traces, a cell in CA1c) was forced to fire by current injection, while the postsynaptic response was observed in another pyramidal cell (upper traces, cell in CA1a). Membrane potential was −65 to −70 mV. During the oscillation, but not between oscillations, action potentials in one cell evoked EPSPs in the other cell. (D) Pyramidal cell recorded with the Na$^+$ channel blocker QX314 in the electrode, with depolarizing current passed to keep the membrane potential at about −55 mV, enhancing IPSP amplitude. Oscillations were evoked by twice-threshold intensity stimuli. With QX314 in the electrode, the cell does not fire. In these cases, EPSPs do not develop in the recorded cell. A gamma-frequency oscillation still occurs; that the potential waves are IPSPs is shown by the recording in the lower trace, in which the electrode also contained picrotoxin (200 μM and in which oscillations are abolished. These data indicate that an underlying inhibitory gamma oscillation persists during the beta oscillation. (From Whittington, Traub, Faulkner et al. 1997 with permission of the National Academy of Sciences, U.S.A.)

trace shows the same cell during an oscillation evoked by the same stimulus, but this time (bar) the AMPA receptor-blocker, NBQX, was pressure-ejected onto stratum oriens, leading to almost complete suppression of the EPSPs.

Third (figure 10.4C), the EPSPs reflect a change in functional connectivity between CA1 pyramidal cells during the oscillation. This change was shown by impaling two pyramidal cells (*Pre*, or presynaptic, and *Post*, or postsynaptic) and evoking a series of oscillations. The Pre cell was induced to fire with a current pulse delivered every 200 ms. The cells were unlikely to be monosynaptically connected, as—during control conditions and between oscillations—firing in the Pre cell did not elicit an EPSP in the Post cell. Nevertheless, during the oscillation, in 2 out of 15 pairs, firing of the Pre cell would induce EPSPs in the Post cell. This observation implies that the Pre cell must induce firing in an intercalated pyramidal cell during the oscillation, the intercalated cell(s) in turn connecting to the Post cell. This firing, however, is not present in the time between oscillations when (we presume) the EPSPs are not sufficiently large.

The functional pyramidal/pyramidal connectivity so expressed during beta oscillations may be a result of enhanced glutamate release, owing to metabotropic glutamate receptor activation. This phenomenon at any rate has been shown to occur at excitatory synapses on CA1 stratum oriens/alveus interneurons (McBain, DiChiara, and Kauer 1994). (It should be noted, however, that presynaptic metabotropic glutamate receptor activation, perhaps of subtypes mGluR2 or mGluR3, has been shown to decrease GABA release onto CA3 pyramidal cells [Poncer, Shinozaki, and Miles 1995].)

Finally (figure 10.4D), EPSPs will not develop in a particular neuron if that neuron is prevented from firing during the oscillation, either by hyperpolarization (not shown) or by impaling it with an electrode containing the Na^+ channel blocker, QX314. Interestingly (and, we believe, crucially to the mechanism responsible for beta oscillations), gamma frequency IPSPs continue in neurons that do not exhibit EPSPs. This fact suggests that the interneuron network continues to produce synchronized IPSPs at gamma frequency while the pyramidal cells are exhibiting beta.

In simulations, increases in $g_{K(AHP)}$ and in recurrent pyramidal/ pyramidal EPSPs are sufficient to induce a switch from gamma to beta frequency. Here, we are assuming that the slow Ca^{2+}-mediated AHP is suppressed by metabotropic glutamate receptors during the gamma oscillation, along with faster spike AHPs, and that this Ca^{2+}-mediated AHP recovers with a similar time course to the faster spike AHPs. An increase in membrane leak conductance, toward the end of the gamma oscillation, would be expected to exert a similar effect. Thus, in a distributed network model (as in chapter 9, figure 9.3), we can choose parameters (GABA$_A$ conductances, pyramidal cell → interneuron and pyramidal cell → pyramidal cell AMPA conductances, together with tonic driving conductances) that lead to a synchronized gamma oscillation. Then, simply by increasing $g_{K(AHP)}$ and the AMPA conductance of unitary pyramidal/ pyramidal EPSCs in tandem, while changing no other parameters, the system is induced to switch to a synchronized beta oscillation (figure 10.5). Several details are worthy of note in this simulation, which agree with experiment. First, gamma oscillations—evident as synaptic potentials—persist during the beta phase (compare figure 10.4D); second, the pyramidal cell sometimes fires in doublets (compare also figure 10.1); and third, interneurons sometimes fire in bursts, attributable to doublet-firing by the pyramidal cells. Similar interneuron bursting during beta has been recorded experimentally (figure 10.6).

We have seen (figure 10.4) that pressure ejection of NBQX, following a tetanic stimulus that normally would induce gamma followed by beta, abolishes the usual development of beta-associated EPSPs within individual pyramidal cells. Figure 10.7 shows that pressure

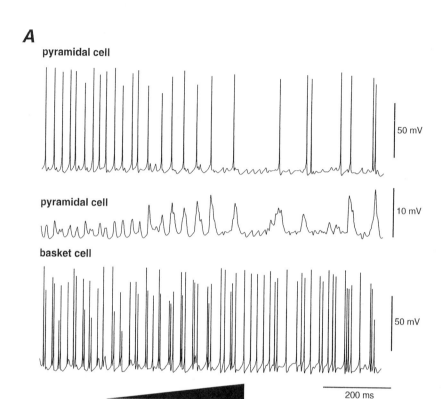

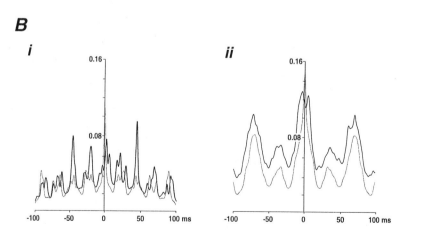

ejection of NBQX also prevents the occurrence of the beta oscillation itself, as measured with extracellular recordings. While pressure-ejected NBQX would also block AMPA receptors on nearby inter-neurons, it is difficult to see how this ejection would suppress pyramidal cell firing or destroy local synchrony; indeed, we have seen that pyramidal cells can become phase locked by interneuron network gamma oscillations when both AMPA and NMDA recep-tors are blocked (chapter 8, figure 8.10). Furthermore, beta oscilla-tions (that are synchronized locally, at any rate) can occur in the presence of joro toxin, which blocks certain AMPA receptors on in-terneurons (Traub, Whittington et al., 1999). For these reasons, we believe that it is the block of pyramidal/pyramidal EPSPs that pro-duces the loss of synchronized beta oscillations, so providing evi-dence that EPSP induction helps to cause synchrony of the beta oscillation.

Figure 10.5
Increases in $g_{K(AHP)}$, along with the recurrent EPSPs, suffice to account for the gamma → beta transition (simulation). Simulation in distributed network of 3,072 pyramidal cells and 384 interneurons (as for figure 8.13). To generate network oscillations, tonic excitatory conductances were delivered to pyramidal cells and interneurons. Max-imal $g_{K(AHP)}$ conductance began at 0.25 × its standard value, but over the time in-terval shown by the ramp, increased to its standard value. Recurrent pyramidal cell/pyramidal cell EPSCs began with a peak value for the unitary conductance of 0.55 nS, but increased 4.6-fold over the time shown by the ramp. (A) Pyramidal cell from the left part of the array, a hyperpolarized pyramidal cell from the right part (to show the growth of population EPSPs), and a basket cell. A transition from gamma to beta oscillations occurs. The EPSPs show that the beta oscillations are synchronized (as do average pyramidal cell voltages, not shown). The basket cell fires singlets and doublets during gamma, but it fires in a complex, more irregular pattern during beta, sometimes in triplets and quadruplets. Pyramidal cells fire occasional doublets, as shown, although some pyramidal cells do not fire doublets. (B) For average pyramidal cell voltages, we plot autocorrelations (hatched) and 2-site cross-correlations (solid) for gamma (i) and for beta (ii). The gamma oscillation is at 52 Hz, with 1.7 ms lag between sites; the beta oscillation is at a mean of about 14 Hz and is also synchronized between sites. Note also the gamma peak during the beta oscillation. (From Traub, Whittington et al., 1999 with permission)

intracellular

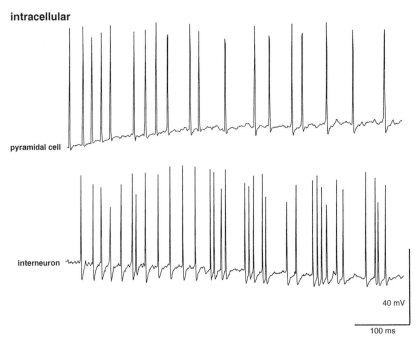

Figure 10.6
Firing patterns during gamma and beta oscillations (experiment). Two-site twice-threshold tetanic stimulation was used to evoke gamma followed by beta oscillations. The stimulus artifacts are not shown. The pyramidal cell fires regular single spikes during gamma. Firing during beta is more irregular, and there are subthreshold membrane fluctuations between spikes. The interneuron (not recorded simultaneously) fires single spikes and a doublet during gamma. During the beta phase, the firing pattern is more complex and includes a triplet and a quadruplet, similar to the simulated interneuron (figure 10.5). (From Traub, Whittington et al., 1999 with permission)

If it is true that simultaneous increases in $g_{K(AHP)}$ and EPSPs together account for the gamma→beta transition, along with a persistent tonic excitatory conductance to both pyramidal cells and interneurons, what is expected to happen when a single one of these parameters is increased, while the other is held constant, or increases insufficiently? Figure 10.8 illustrates a simulation performed similarly to the one in figure 10.5, with maximum $g_{K(AHP)}$ conduc-

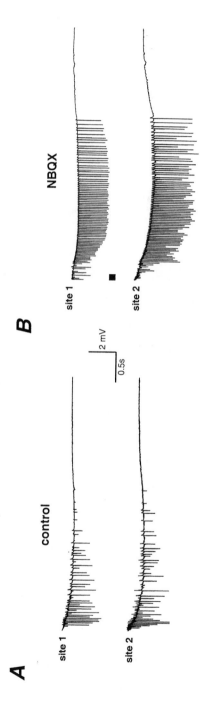

Figure 10.7

Blockade of AMPA receptors prevents the gamma → beta transition. Two-site twice-threshold tetanic stimuli were delivered to the same slice (recordings between sites are concurrent in each case, and stimulation artifacts are not shown). Under control conditions (A), a gamma → beta oscillation was evoked. Cross-correlation of the signals showed that the gamma oscillation was tightly synchronized, with phase lag near 0 (not shown). When the stimulus was repeated (B), but with the AMPA receptor-blocker NBQX (20 μM) having been puffed on (■), only gamma is evoked. The reason for the prolongation of the gamma is not known. Cross-correlation of the initial gamma signals showed a 5.6 ms phase lag, consistent with expectation (see Chapter 9). (From Traub, Whittington et al., 1999 with permission)

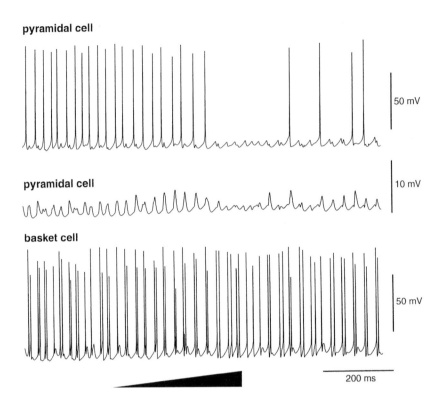

pyramidal cell

pyramidal cell   10 mV

basket cell

50 mV

50 mV

200 ms

Figure 10.8
Increase of $g_{K(AHP)}$ alone, without sufficient recurrent EPSPs, is predicted to lead to nonsynchronized beta activity (simulation). The simulation is identical to that of figure 10.5, except that over the period of the ramp, unitary EPSCs are increased only 2-fold, rather than 4.6-fold, while $g_{K(AHP)}$ increases as before. Individual pyramidal cells slow their firing rate to the beta range, but the firing is not synchronized. Note that in the hyperpolarized pyramidal cell (middle trace), the EPSPs are about the same size during beta as during gamma, even though unitary EPSCs have doubled—pyramidal cell firing has separated into different clusters. Note also the lack of triplets and quadruplets in the interneuron during the beta phase. (From Traub, Whittington et al., 1999 with permission)

tance increasing 4-fold over a 400 ms time interval. In figure 10.8, however, unitary pyramidal/pyramidal EPSCs increase only 2-fold, rather than 4.6-fold as in figure 10.5. In figure 10.8, individual pyramidal cell firing slows to beta frequency, but pyramidal cell firing is less synchronized than in the gamma phase. Note that the EPSPs in the hyperpolarized cell are about the same size during the beta phase as they are during the gamma phase, even though unitary EPSCs are twice as large. This, and other similar, simulations suggest that there is a critical EPSC amplitude required for the beta switch to occur, other things (such as K^+ conductances) being equal. Note also in figure 10.8 that pyramidal cell doublets do not occur when EPSCs are too small and that interneurons do not fire in bursts without the pyramidal cell doublets.

It is possible that figure 10.8 captures the situation that occurs when gamma oscillations are evoked by near-threshold intensity tetanic stimuli: K^+ conductances increase, without EPSPs reaching a critical size; pyramidal cell firing slows while synchrony is lost; and at the level of field potentials, the evoked response fades away. This sequence of events can occur, we suspect, even if metabotropic receptor-induced depolarizations are maintained.

Figure 10.9 illustrates a situation converse to that of figure 10.8. In figure 10.9, conditions of driving conductances, etc. are set to produce a gamma oscillation as in figure 10.5. Then, over a 400 ms interval, unitary pyramidal/pyramidal EPSCs are increased 4.2–fold, while K^+ conductances are held constant. In this case, a series of bursts occurs that resembles an epileptic afterdischarge. Similar periodic bursting can arise experimentally, as the figure demonstrates. In the experimental case, however, it is difficult to be certain if it is excessive increases in EPSCs or insufficient increases in K^+ conductance(s), alone or in combination, that are responsible for the afterdischarge. Conceivably, other parameters, not yet identified, change as well.

As an aside, we should note that there are two types of synchronized oscillations in the in vitro CA3 region that have some

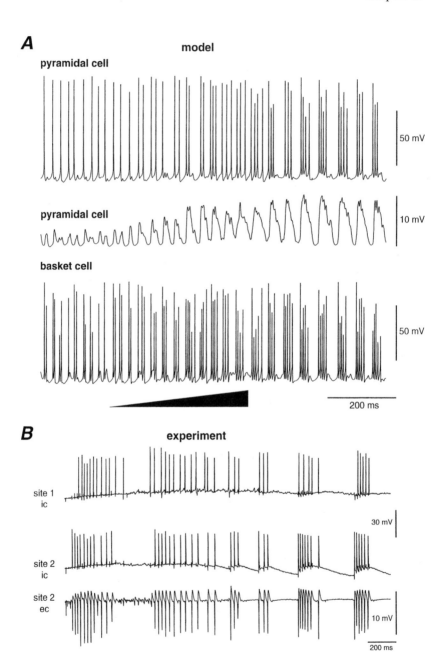

phenomenological resemblance to the beta oscillation in CA1 (figure 5.12). First, there is the 7–27 Hz oscillation induced by activation of metabotropic glutamate receptors with ACPD (60–100 μM) (Taylor, Merlin, and Wong 1995), and second, these are the oscillations evoked by carbachol (about 50 μM) (MacVicar and Tse 1989; Williams and Kauer 1997). In both of these latter cases, AMPA receptors are required for synchronization, and the intracellular potential waves resemble EPSPs capped by one or two action potentials or by brief bursts. NMDA receptors are not required, and strikingly, and unlike gamma oscillations, neither are GABA$_A$ receptors. These phenomena have been discussed in chapter 5. We note once more that recurrent excitatory synaptic connections between CA3 pyramidal cells are powerful and numerically relatively frequent, even in the absence of potentiation, unlike CA1.

Chronic Effects Induced in the Hippocampal Slice by Strong Tetanic Stimulation: Synaptic Plasticity and Altered Synchronization Properties of Oscillations Induced by Normal Stimuli

We have discussed how a twice-threshold tetanic stimulus—either at one site or two—evokes a gamma → beta oscillation, along with pyramidal cell EPSPs, and have argued that the EPSPs are causally related to the gamma → beta switch, while K$^+$ conductance(s) must

Figure 10.9
Increase in recurrent EPSPs without sufficient increase in $g_{K(AHP)}$ is predicted to lead to synchronized epileptiform afterdischarges. (A) The simulation of figure 10.5 was again repeated, but this time $g_{K(AHP)}$ did not change during the time shown by the ramp, while unitary pyramidal cell/pyramidal cell EPSCs increased 4.2-fold. Instead of developing a beta phase with pyramidal cell singlets and doublets, a series of epileptiform bursts is generated at about 20 Hz. (B) similar firing patterns are sometimes seen experimentally, although the underlying mechanisms are not known. The epileptiform bursts in this example are also slower (about 4 Hz) than in the simulation. Symbol ic, intracellular; ec, extracellular. (From Traub, Whittington et al., 1999 with permission)

also increase prior to beta in order to prevent an epileptic afterdis-charge. Interestingly, a single application of a twice-threshold teta-nus to CA1 induces lasting effects as well; these effects can be observed in the oscillatory response to threshold-intensity stimu-lation. The nature of the effects depends on whether one site or two sites receive the twice-threshold stimulus. The latter effect is con-ceptually the simpler, and we shall discuss it first.

A single episode of 2-site twice-threshold stimulation has a long-lasting enhancing effect on the occurrence and synchroniza-tion of beta oscillations. This basic observation is illustrated in figure 10.10, with the long-lasting nature of the effect being shown in more detail in figure 10.11A. The protocol used to examine this phenomenon (figure 10.11A) was to examine the form and ampli-tude of the cross-correlation function, calculated from the last 200 ms of field potentials at sites 1 and 2. The field potentials were re-sponses to simultaneous 2-site threshold stimuli, what might be considered test stimuli used to probe the properties of the net-work. The last 200 ms of the signals are epochs during which beta oscillations might occur. Beta oscillations never occur immediately after the tetanic stimulus; if they are to occur at all in our experi-mental protocols, it will be following a period of gamma oscilla-tion. After control oscillations were elicited by 2-site threshold (i.e., test) stimuli, a single conditioning stimulus was given at the time marked by the arrow (↑).

Of course, the control stimuli, having only threshold intensity, failed to evoke beta so that the cross-correlation amplitude (last 200 ms of the signals) is small. When the conditioning stimulus is twice-threshold, but at a single site, later test stimuli do not evoke syn-chronized beta (open circles: small cross-correlation amplitude). On the other hand, if the single conditioning stimulus is twice-threshold, but at two sites, then later test stimuli now evoke syn-chronized beta oscillations (field potentials ②, cross-correlation of last 200 ms below). We emphasize that these same test stimuli do not normally evoke synchronized beta oscillations. The effect of this conditioning stimulus on evoked beta oscillations lasts at least 90 minutes.

How is one to understand the lasting effects of a 2-site twice-threshold stimulus on later evoked oscillations? It was shown in Whittington et al. (1997b) that such a stimulus has lasting effects on EPSPs, in that later test stimuli (2-site, threshold intensity) remain associated with enhanced functional synaptic connectivity between CA1 pyramidal cells. The most straightforward interpretation of these data is then that some hundreds of ms after a tetanic stimulus that evokes an oscillation, K^+ conductances will increase and terminate the oscillation unless EPSPs are large enough. EPSPs will be large enough if the immediately preceding tetanus was itself large enough or possibly even if a 2-site tetanus in the last 90 minutes was large enough, owing to plastic changes in recurrent pyramidal/pyramidal connections. With large enough EPSPs, a 2-site synchronized beta oscillation will occur.

A single episode of 1-site twice-threshold stimulation has a long-lasting suppressing effect on the 2-site synchronization of gamma oscillations. To show this effect, the same protocol as described immediately above was used, but now with examination of the first 200 ms of the evoked oscillation during the gamma phase (figure 10.11B). When the conditioning stimulus is 2-site twice-threshold, synchronized gamma oscillations are evoked (large cross-correlation amplitude), as shown previously (figure 10.2). When the conditioning stimulus is 1-site twice-threshold, then, of course, 2-site synchrony does not exist—the other site not oscillating at all (field potentials ②). What is remarkable, however, is that following this 1-site twice-threshold conditioning stimulus, later test stimuli (2-site threshold) now fail to evoke 2-site synchrony of gamma, test stimuli that normally would evoke synchrony of gamma between the two sites. This suppression of gamma synchrony lasts at least 45 minutes.

A   2-site threshold stimulus

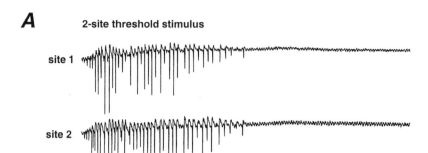

B   2-site 2 x threshold stimulus

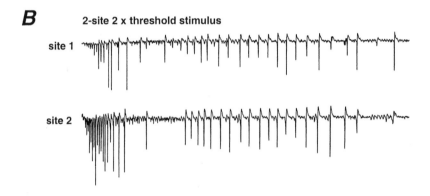

C   2-site threshold stimulus

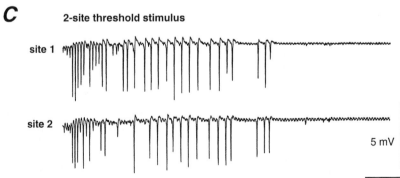

How should one interpret such a suppression of 2-site gamma synchrony? As discussed in the previous chapter, interneuron doublets are necessary in our experimental preparation for long-range synchrony of gamma oscillations. Could the conditioning stimulus (1 site, twice-threshold) somehow produce a long-lasting state, in which interneuron doublets are suppressed? Such a state could arise, in principle, if excitation of interneurons at site 1 by pyramidal cells at site 2 were to be suppressed and, likewise, if excitation of interneurons at site 2 by pyramidal cells at site 1 were to be depressed. In such a case, 2-site stimulation of the slice would be equivalent, from the point of view of the interneurons, to 1-site stimulation, and after 1-site stimulation, interneurons are not excited sufficiently to generate doublets (chapter 9; figures 10.2 and 10.3). There are precedents for the regulation of interneuron EPSPs onto CA1 hippocampal interneurons in s. radiatum and lacunosum/moleculare (McMahon and Kauer 1997; Desai et al. 1994). One could even imagine an anti-Hebbian long-term depression (LTD)-like mechanism: after a strong stimulation, say, of site 1, pyramidal cells at site 1 should fire rapidly, but their postsynaptic targets in site 2 might not be firing rapidly. Similarly, interneurons in site 1 should be firing rapidly, but their excitatory afferents from site 2 should be silent. In either case, one could imagine that synaptic depression would occur.

Figure 10.10
A single instance of 2-site twice-threshold stimulation allows later 2-site *threshold* stimuli to induce oscillations with gamma and beta phases. Simultaneous field potential recordings with stimulus artifacts not shown. (A) A 2-site threshold tetanic stimulation evokes gamma oscillation at the two sites. (B) A 2-site twice-threshold tetanic stimulation evokes gamma followed by beta. (C) after the single administration of the twice-threshold stimulus (B), a 2-site threshold stimulus evokes gamma followed by beta. (A series of 2-site threshold tetani, applied every 4 minutes as in these experiments, does not lead to gamma followed by beta.) (From Traub, Whittington et al., 1999 with permission)

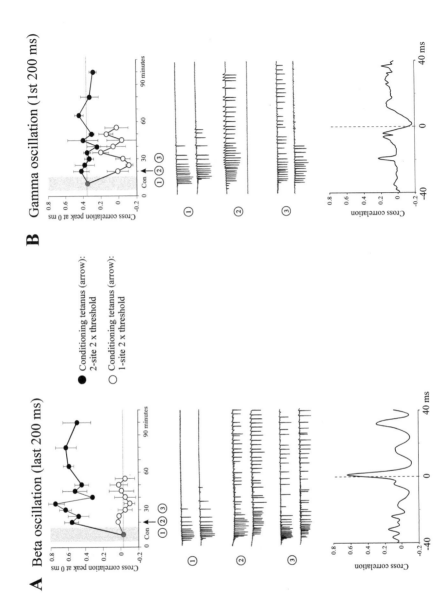

This notion was first tested in simulations (figure 10.12). The parameters of the simulation in figure 10.5 were used (i.e., parameters in which 2-site-synchronized gamma would occur), except that the conductance of unitary pyramidal cell→interneuron excitatory synapses was reduced 10-fold for connections that crossed the midline of the array. In effect, we reduced the interaction between parts of the array that is mediated by long-range pyramidal cell → interneuron connections. What this parameter change accomplishes, as expected, is to eliminate interneuron doublets and to abolish the tight synchrony between the two halves of the array.

Next, we tested the hypothesis experimentally by evoking oscillations while recording from a s. pyramidale interneuron (figure 10.13). Under test conditions, 2-site threshold tetani evoked gamma

Figure 10.11
A strong 2-site tetanus allows later weak 2-site tetani to induce synchronized beta oscillations (as in figure 10.10); while a strong 1-site tetanus *prevents* later weak 2-site tetani from inducing synchronized gamma oscillations. Field potentials were measured at the 2 sites in CA1 during tetanically evoked oscillations, and cross-correlations calculated, either for the beta phase (last 200 ms of the response, A) or for the gamma phase (first 200 ms of the response, B). The amplitude of these cross-correlations at 0 ms is plotted in the graphs above. Field potentials at the two sites are shown for times ① (control = Con), ② (conditioning stimulus, ↑, • points for A and ○ points for B), and ③ (later test stimuli, • points for A and ○ points for B). The cross-correlation at time 3 is plotted below. Control (Con) runs were for oscillations evoked by 2-site threshold stimulation, which evoked negligible beta synchrony (A) and strong gamma synchrony (B). (A) For the • points at ↑, a 2-site twice-threshold stimulus was given, evoking a synchronized beta oscillation (cross-correlation amplitude about 0.6). Later test stimuli were 2-site threshold intensity, with the beta synchrony continuing to be observed for > 90 minutes. For the ○ points, the stimulus at ↑ was 1-site twice-threshold, which failed to evoke synchronized beta oscillations. In this case, the same test stimuli (2-site threshold) never evoked synchronized beta. (B) For the • points, the stimulus at ↑ was 2-site twice-threshold, evoking synchronized gamma oscillations, just as do later test stimuli of 2-site threshold intensity. For the ○ points, however, the stimulus at ↑ was 1-site twice-threshold. Later test stimuli (2-site threshold) evoke gamma oscillations in which the cross-correlation amplitude (at 0 ms) is much reduced and may even be negative (as in the example from ③, plotted lower right). (From Whittington, Traub, Faulkner et al., 1997 with permission of the National Academy of Sciences, U.S.A.)

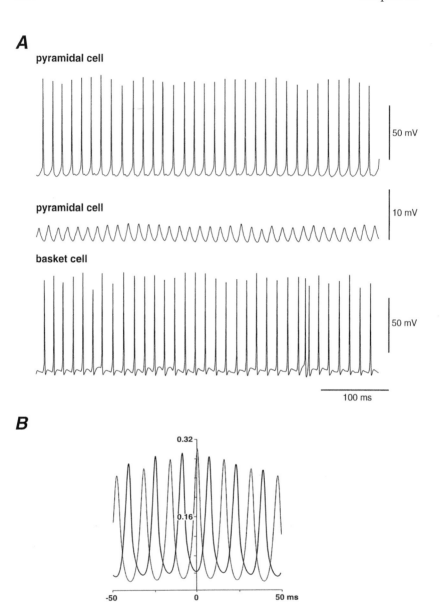

Figure 10.12

Depression of long-range pyramidal cell → interneuron synaptic connections is predicted to disrupt long-range synchrony of gamma oscillations. The stimulation is the same as for the gamma portion of the simulation in figure 10.5 but for one difference: synaptic conductances are reduced 90% for a left-half pyramidal cell

oscillations that were synchronized between the two sites; doublets in the interneuron occurred. After a series of 1-site twice-threshold stimuli at the site opposite to that of the interneuron, oscillation-associated EPSPs in the interneuron were progressively suppressed, and doublets in the interneuron no longer occurred after 2-site threshold tetani. While the mean phase lag between sites in this example remained small (2 ms), the cross-corrrelation is disorganized, owing to the variable phase relations between interneuron spikes at one site and population spikes at the opposite site.

In conclusion, we suggest that the most economical hypothesis to explain the long-term effects of a 1-site twice threshold stimulus is that such a stimulus desynchronizes gamma oscillations in response to later test stimuli because long-range synaptic excitation of interneurons is suppressed, and interneurons can no longer fire doublets.

To summarize some of the results presented in this chapter, the mechanisms of gamma oscillations and beta oscillations are not identical. EPSPs between pyramidal cells appear to be critical for beta, but not for gamma after tetanic stimulation, at least in the CA1 region in slices. Interneuron network gamma activity may, however, be a substrate on top of which beta oscillations are superimposed. One effect of the EPSPs between pyramidal cells is pyramidal cell spike doublets that occur in some of the neurons. Intense stimuli evoke pyramidal-cell EPSPs acutely (within a few hundred ms of

connecting to a right-half interneuron or for a right-half pyramidal cell connecting to a left-half interneuron. (A) Firing patterns for a pyramidal cell in the left half (top), a hyperpolarized pyramidal cell in the right half (middle), and a basket cell in the left half (lower). There is a regular firing pattern, but the interneuron fires almost no doublets because its AMPA receptor mediated synaptic input is almost the same as if the left half were oscillating alone (compare with figure 9.3). (B) Analysis of average pyramidal cell voltages, autocorrelation (hatched) for signal from the left half of the array and cross-correlation (solid) of signals from the two halves. As expected for a gamma oscillation without interneuron doublets, there is a phase lag between the two halves, 5.6 ms in this case. (From Traub, Whittington et al., 1999 with permission)

A Control: 2-site threshold stimulation

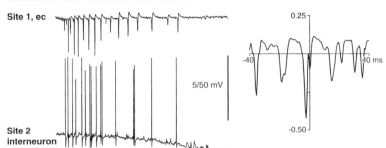

B Conditioning: 1-site 2 x threshold stimulation

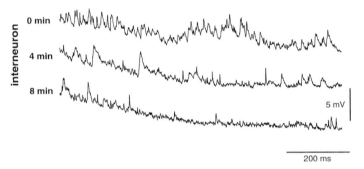

C Test: 2-site threshold stimulation

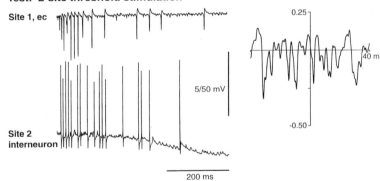

the stimulus), hence an acute beta oscillation, but they also produce lasting changes in pyramidal cell/pyramidal cell connections, so that later normal stimuli can also now evoke EPSPs amd beta oscillations. Localized intense stimuli lead to a lasting desynchronization of gamma oscillations between two sites when one of the sites has been intensely stimulated and the other has not. The mechanism appears to involve a diminution of synaptic excitation of interneurons.

It is difficult to avoid the idea that gamma/beta oscillations (perhaps related to perception) are intimately related to synaptic plasticity when these oscillations are evoked by strong stimuli and hence that gamma/beta oscillations are related to memory. That the memory manifests itself by changes in the long-term synchrony of the oscillations themselves is fascinating.

Figure 10.13
Intense tetanic stimulation of a single site leads to reduction of EPSPs in an interneuron and to loss of interneuron doublets. Recordings are all from the same slice, with an extracellular (*ec*) recording electrode at site 1 and an intracellular recording of an interneuron at site 2 (same cell throughout the figure). Stimulus artifacts not shown. (A) Gamma oscillation induced by 2-site threshold stimulation. Interneuron doublets occur. Cross-correlation of the two signals (right) produces a negative-going peak at -2 ms because one signal is upgoing and the other downgoing. (B) The interneuron at site 2 was hyperpolarized to -75 mV, near GABA$_A$ reversal potential, by passage of -0.3 nA current. Successive oscillations induced by twice-threshold stimulation of the opposite site lead to EPSPs in the interneuron that are progressively reduced in amplitude and in frequency. (C) A subsequent 2-site threshold tetanus-evoked oscillation is no longer associated with interneuron doublets. The variable phase relations of population spikes and action potentials lead to a disorganized appearance of the cross-correlation (right). (From Traub, Whittington et al., 1999 with permission)

11   Conclusions: Are Gamma Oscillations Significant for Brain Function?

In this monograph, we have reviewed topics relevant to gamma and beta oscillations in vitro and to their basic underpinning mechanisms. Underpinning mechanisms include the electrophysiological properties of single neurons, synaptic connectivity between neurons and details on unitary synaptic actions, and certain collective neuronal phenomena that are easier to analyze than gamma oscillations themselves, including synchronized epileptiform bursts.

As for the gamma oscillations, we discussed oscillations generated by pharmacologically isolated networks of interneurons, how pyramidal cells can participate as well as interneurons and how tight synchrony can emerge over distances of several mm. Tight synchrony occurs when pyramidal cells can synaptically evoke interneuron doublets, that is, a second spike shortly after the first interneuron spike arising from tonic depolarization at the end of a gamma cycle. We further covered the synaptic transfer of gamma activity from one region to another; the induction of synaptic plasticity in recurrent excitatory collaterals between pyramidal cells, and also to interneurons when oscillations are induced by strong stimuli and how this plasticity can in turn influence synchronization. In addition, we looked at how the synchronizing mechanisms of beta oscillations are somewhat different than for gamma oscillations. We have tried to place the in vitro work in the context of some fundamental observations on gamma oscillations in vivo. This

entire field is moving rapidly, and however this monograph is concluded, justice can not be done to important work ongoing in a
number of laboratories.

A cardinal question to be addressed experimentally is whether in
vivo gamma mechanisms correspond to any of the in vitro oscillation paradigms so far investigated. It is useful to list some of the
reasons why this matter will not be easy to determine:

1. In any in vivo structure (say the neocortex or hippocampus),
there are far more neurons than in the corresponding slice, and
many more structures are connected together in vivo than can be
obtained in vitro.

2. As a consequence of 1, there are huge numbers of neurons in
vivo whose activities are not accessible to the experimenter. This
means that the oscillating neurons will be subjected to barrages of
inputs of unknown time course and synaptic actions; even if these
parameters were known, interpreting the data would be immensely
complicated, for conceptual reasons.

3. Numerous neuromodulatory systems are active in vivo that are
lost in slices.

4. It is technically difficult in vivo to perform multiple intracellular
recordings and to apply drugs that modify membrane properties or
alter synaptic actions. Is this cause for despair? Hardly. One need
only accept that the bridge from slice to whole animal is rarely
crossed in a single step. Having accepted this limitation, one notices
that there are many lifetimes' worth of interesting problems to address. Patience is required.

Possible Functions of Gamma Oscillations

In trying to make sense of the cellular physiology of gamma oscillations, it is useful to have two things. First, one must have
faith that the oscillations will some day be shown to be crucial for

brain function, despite their sometime evanescence and their occurrence in certain brain regions and not others. And second, one needs a set of hypotheses on what the purpose of gamma oscillations might be.

With respect to this latter question, three hypotheses that have been considered are as follows. The first is coincidence detection (Abeles 1982; König et al. 1996). Most unitary EPSPs are of insufficient amplitude to discharge a neuron, especially a pyramidal cell. Hence, if a pyramidal cell is to fire at all, one imagines that a number of EPSPs must occur that are temporally coincident to within some time resolution determined by the cell's membrane properties, as well as by IPSPs. (This need not be the case, however, if the cell is tonically depolarized, as it can then fire without phasic EPSPs.) During a gamma oscillation, the temporal pattern of population IPSPs and EPSPs would favor the discharge of postsynaptic neurons. What happens in in vitro systems, however, is probably better called gamma oscillation transfer, or projection, a term describing the population phenomenon, rather than coincidence detection, a term that misleadingly focuses attention on a single neuron. When gamma oscillations are induced in one region, they can induce gamma oscillations in a connected region. This process has been observed for CA1 to subiculum in vitro (Colling et al., 1998; Stanford et al., 1998); for CA3 to CA1 in vitro (Fisahn et al. 1998), and also for projections from entorhinal cortex to CA1 in vivo (Charpak et al. 1995).

The second hypothesis is synaptic plasticity. The phenomenology and mechanisms of synaptic plasticity induced by gamma oscillations—themselves induced by intense stimulation—have been reviewed in the previous chapter. Oscillation-induced synaptic plasticity is intriguing because it could tie together, in principle, a phenomenon linked to perception (the gamma oscillation itself) to a phenomenon linked to memory (changes in synaptic conductances). This form of plasticity suggests a readout mechanism as well: whether or not two sites synchronize, at either gamma or beta frequency. Nevertheless, it remains to be shown that oscillation-induced synaptic plasticity occurs in vivo.

A third hypothesis is phase encoding. Information can be encoded, and computation performed, in the brain by selecting *which* neurons are to participate in an operation and by determining *how much* they are to participate. The how-much signal can, in turn, be represented in a number of ways, including the mean firing rate of the neuron or the phase of firing relative to an ongoing clock signal produced by a neuronal population oscillation (Hopfield 1995; O'Keefe and Recce 1993).

One can picture regulation of phase in at least two ways. First, the mean driving currents to a population of principal neurons might be distributed over some range. One expects that the firing phases of the principal neurons, relative to the gamma oscillation (which depends in large part on the interneurons), will be distributed in a manner corresponding to the driving currents, the most driven cells being phase-advanced. And, indeed, in a variety of network models, this expectation is what happens, provided that recurrent excitation between pyramidal cells is not too strong (Traub, Jefferys, and Whittington 1997; chapter 8, figure 8.11).

Second, one can suppose that the driving currents to the population of pyramidal cells are uniform, but one particular principal cell is biased, either positively or negatively, with corresponding phase advance or delay, respectively. This mechanism also works in simulations without recurrent pyramidal cell/pyramidal cell excitation, but interestingly, experiments show that phase delay, while possible without recurrent excitation, is prevented when recurrent excitation is present (chapter 8, figure 8.12; Burchell et al. 1998).

How is one to interpret the manner in which recurrent excitation interferes with phase encoding? Significant recurrent excitation only develops when a certain fraction of the population is firing approximately synchronously. Let us suppose that k pyramidal cells must fire before recurrent EPSPs become large enough to influence firing in other pyramidal cells. Then it should be possible to phase advance (approximately) the first k-1 cells. If one tries to phase advance more cells than this, the recurrent EPSPs will force the remaining cells to fire, interfering with a smooth distribution of phases. On the other hand, phase delay of a single pyramidal cell—call it P—should be difficult when recurrent excitation is present and most of the cells are firing because the synchronous firing of the population will tend to force P to fire, independent (within reason) of its bias current.

Clinical Significance of Synchronized Gamma Oscillations

In the preface, we mentioned an hypothesis that helps to motivate our interest in oscillations: while local synchronization of thalamocortical oscillations can occur in slow-wave sleep (Steriade, Contreras, et al. 1996), the synchronization of gamma oscillations over distance is necessary (if not sufficient) for the normal function of the waking brain. If this hypothesis turns out to be correct, two areas in which gamma oscillations will be clinically relevant are a) dementing illnesses (Ribary et al. 1991; Sheer 1989) and b) anesthesia (Whittington et al. 1996; Faulkner et al., 1998).

With respect to dementia, loss of cholinergic input to the neocortex and limbic system has been postulated to contribute to the pathophysiology of Alzheimer's disease (Appel 1981). It seems likely that a cholinergic input to the hippocampus, acting via muscarinic receptors, contributes to the generation of gamma rhythms (Fisahn et al. 1998). With respect to anesthesia, we have discussed in previous chapters how benzodiazepines, barbiturates, and opiates influence gamma oscillations in in vitro preparations (see also Whittington, Jefferys, and Traub 1996; Whittington, Traub, Faulkner et al. 1998; Faulkner et al. 1998). These agents, alone and in combination, also produce a variety of clinical effects, including sedation, anesthesia, and amnesia. We would like to think that this connection is not a coincidence.

Final Thoughts

How can we be sure that gamma oscillations are necessary for brain function at all? One can imagine at least two possibilities. First, there may perhaps be human "experiments of nature," walking about and functioning normally, in whom 40 Hz brain oscillations are simply absent, either because of a mutation or because of some nonlethal neuropathological insult. A chance magnetoencephalographic recording in such an individual might suffice, then, in principle, to demonstrate that gamma oscillations are not necessary for cognition. Something of this sort happened in the case of REM sleep. It was hypothesized (Crick and Mitchison 1983) that REM sleep was required for memory consolidation. Yet, rare individuals have been found who, because of neuropathology, have normal cognition but in whom REM sleep is virtually absent (Osorio and Daroff 1980; Daroff and Osorio 1984), casting grave doubts on the original hypothesis.

Second, it may be possible to develop transgenic mice or other species in which gamma oscillations are either absent or severely disrupted. Behavioral studies of such genetically altered individuals could provide important clues concerning the function of the oscillations. In order to know which genes to target so as to produce the requisite mice—and have the animals survive—one probably needs to understand a great deal about the cellular mechanisms of the oscillations. This understanding is an important motivation for the type of research discussed in our monograph.

References

Abdul-Ghani M A, Valiante T A, Carlen P L, Pennefather P S (1996) Metabotropic glutamate receptors coupled to IP3 production mediate inhibition of I_{AHP} in rat dentate granule cells.*J. Neurophysiol.* 76: 2691–2700.

Abeles M (1982) Role of the cortical neuron. Integrator or coincidence detector. *Israel J. Med. Sci.* 18: 83–92.

Adrian E D (1942) Olfactory reactions in the brain of the hedgehog.*J. Physiol.* 100: 459–473.

Adrian E D (1950) The electrical activity of the mammalian olfactory bulb. *Electroenceph. Clin. Neurophysiol.* 2: 377–388.

Agmon A, Connors B W (1989) Repetitive burst-firing neurons in the deep layers of mouse somatosensory cortex. *Neurosci. Lett.* 99: 137–141.

Alaluf S, Mulvihil E R, McIlhinney R A (1995) Rapid agonist mediated phosphorylation of the metabotropic glutamate 1α by protein kinase C in permanently transfected BHK cells. *FEBS Lett.* 367: 301–305.

Alford S, Frenguelli B G, Schofield J G, Collingridge G L (1993) Characterization of Ca^{2+} signals induced in hippocampal CA1 neurones by the synaptic activation of NMDA receptors. *J. Physiol.* 469: 693–716.

Ali A B, Deuchars J, Pawelzik H, Thomson A M (1998) CA1 pyramidal to basket and bistratified cell EPSPs: dual intracellular recordings in rat hippocampal slices. *J. Physiol.* 507: 201–218.

Ali A B, Thomson A M (1998) Facilitating pyramid to horizontal oriens-alveus interneurone inputs: dual intracellular recordings in slices of rat hippocampus. *J. Physiol.*: 185–200.

Alonso A, Llinás R R (1989) Subthreshold Na^{+}-dependent theta-like rhythmicity in stellate cells of entorhinal cortex layer II. *Nature* 342: 175–177.

Alvarez P, Zola-Morgan S, Squire L R (1995) Damage limited to the hippocampal region produces long-lasting memory impairment in monkeys. *J. Neurosci.* 15: 3796–3807.

Amit D J (1989) *Modeling Brain Function. The World of Attractor Neural Networks.* Cambridge University Press, Cambridge, U.K.

Amitai Y, Friedman A, Connors B W, Gutnick M J (1993) Regenerative activity in apical dendrites of pyramidal cells in neocortex. *Cereb. Cortex* 3: 26–38.

Amzica F, Steriade M (1995) Short-and long-range neuronal synchronization of the slow (< 1 Hz) cortical oscillation. *J. Neurophysiol.* 73: 20–38.

Andersen P, Silfvenius H, Sundberg S, Sveen O, Wigström H (1978) Functional characteristics of unmyelinated fibres in the hippocampal cortex. *Brain Res.* 144: 11–18.

Anderson C M, Jefferys J G R (1997) Disinhibition in CA3 triggers epileptic activity more easily in the ventral hippocampus. *Soc. Neurosci. Abstr.* 23: 2154.

Anderson W W, Swartzwelder H S, Wilson W A (1987) The NMDA receptor antagonist 2–amino-5–phosphonovalerate blocks stimulus train-induced epileptogenesis but not epileptiform bursting in the rat hippocampal slice. *J. Neurophysiol.* 57, 1–21.

Andreasen M, Lambert J D C (1995) Regenerative properties of pyramidal cell dendrites in area CA1 of the rat hippocampus. *J. Physiol.* 483: 421–441.

Appel S H (1981) A unifying hypothesis for the cause of amyotrophic lateral sclerosis, parkinsonism and Alzheimer's disease. *Ann. Neurol.* 10:499–505.

Aram J A, Michelson H B, Wong R K S (1991) Synchronized GABAergic IPSPs recorded in the neocortex after blockade of synaptic transmission mediated by excitatory amino acids. *J. Neurophysiol.* 65: 1034–1041.

Arancio O, Korn H, Gulyas A, Freund T, Miles R (1994) Excitatory synaptic connections onto rat hippocampal inhibitory cells may involve a single transmitter release site. *J. Physiol.* 481: 395–405.

Ascher P, Bregestovski P, Nowak L (1988) N-methyl-D-aspartate-activated channels of mouse central neurones in magnesium-free solutions. *J. Physiol.* 399: 207–226.

Avoli M (1990) Epileptiform discharges and a synchronous GABAergic potential induced by 4–aminopyridine in the rat immature hippocampus. *Neurosci. Lett.* 117: 93–98.

Avoli M (1996) GABA-mediated synchronous potentials and seizure generation. *Epilepsia* 37: 1035–1042.

Avoli M, Drapeau C, Louvel J, Pumain R, Olivier A, Villemure J-G (1991) Epileptiform activity induced by low extracellular magnesium in the human cortex maintained in vitro. *Ann. Neurol.* 30: 589–596.

Avoli M, Louvel J, Kurcewicz I, Pumain R, Barbarosie M (1996) Extracellular free potassium and calcium during synchronous activity induced by 4–aminopyridine in the juvenile rat hippocampus. *J. Physiol.* 493: 707–717.

Avoli M, Psarropoulou C, Tancredi V, Fueta Y (1993) On the synchronous activity induced by 4–aminopyridine in the CA3 subfield of juvenile rat hippocampus. *J. Neurophysiol.* 70: 1018–1029.

Azouz R, Gray C M, Nowak L G, McCormick D A (1997) Physiological properties of inhibitory interneurons in cat striate cortex. *Cerebral Cortex* 7: 534–545.

Azouz R, Jensen M S, Yaari Y (1994) Muscarinic modulation of intrinsic burst firing in rat hippocampal neurons. *Eur. J. Neurosci.* 6: 961–966.

Azouz R, Jensen M S, Yaari Y (1996) Ionic basis of spike after-depolarization and burst generation in adult rat hippocampal CA1 pyramidal cells. *J. Physiol.* 492: 211–223.

Bal T, McCormick D A (1993) Mechanisms of oscillatory activity in guinea-pig nucleus reticularis thalami *in vitro:* a mammalian pacemaker. *J. Physiol.* 468: 669–691.

Bal T, von Krosigk M, McCormick D A (1995a) Synaptic and membrane mechanisms underlying synchronized oscillations in the ferret lateral geniculate nucleus *in vitro.* *J. Physiol.* 483: 641–663.

Bal T, von Krosigk M, McCormick D A (1995b) Role of the ferret perigeniculate nucleus in the generation of synchronized oscillations *in vitro. J. Physiol.* 483: 665–685.

Barrie J M, Freeman W J, Lenhart M D (1996) Spatiotemporal analysis of prepyriform, visual, auditory, and somesthetic surface EEGs in trained rabbits. *J. Neurophysiol.* 76: 520–539.

Barth D S, MacDonald K D (1996) Thalamic modulation of high-frequency oscillating potentials in auditory cortex. *Nature* 383: 78–81.

Basar-Eroglu C, Strüber D, Schürmann M, Stadler M, Basar E (1996) Gamma-band responses in the brain: a short review of psychophysiological correlates and functional significance. *Int. J. Psychophysiol.* 24: 101–112.

Bashir Z I, Bortolotto Z A, Davies C H, Berretta N, Irving A J, Seal A J, Henley J M, Jane D E, Watkins J C, Collingridge G L (1993) Induction of LTP in the hippocampus needs synaptic activation of glutamate metabotropic receptors. *Nature* 363: 347–350.

Baskys A, Malenka R C (1991) Agonists at metabotropic glutamate receptors presynaptically inhibit EPSCs in neonatal rat hippocampus. *J. Physiol.* 444: 687–701.

Baude A, Nusser Z, Roberts J D B, Mulvihill E, McIlhinney R A J, Somogyi P (1993) The metabotropic glutamate receptor (mGluR1α) is concentrated at perisynaptic membrane of neuronal subpopulations as detected by immunogold reaction. *Neuron* 11: 771–787.

Baude A, Nusser Z, Molnár E, McIlhinney R A J, Somogyi P (1995) High-resolution immunogold localization of AMPA type glutamate receptor subunits at synaptic and non-synaptic sites in rat hippocampus. *Neuroscience* 69: 1031–1055.

Behrends J C, ten Bruggencate G (1993) Cholinergic modulation of synaptic inhibition in the guinea pig hippocampus in vitro: excitation of GABAergic interneurons and inhibition of GABA-release. *J. Neurophysiol.* 69: 626–629.

Bekenstein J W, Lothman E W (1993) Dormancy of inhibitory interneurons in a model of temporal lobe epilepsy. *Science* 259: 97–100.

Benardo L S, Masukawa L M, Prince D A (1982) Electrophysiology of isolated hippocampal pyramidal dendrites. *J. Neurosci.* 2: 1614–1622.

Ben-Ari Y, Cherubini E, Corradetti R, Gaiarsa J-L (1989) Giant synaptic potentials in immature rat CA3 hippocampal neurones. *J. Physiol.* 416: 303–325.

Benson D M, Blitzer R D, Landau E M (1988) An analysis of the depolarization produced in guinea-pig hippocampus by cholinergic receptor stimulation. *J. Physiol.* 404: 479–496.

Bernard C, Wheal H V (1994) Model of local connectivity patterns in CA3 and CA1 areas of the hippocampus. *Hippocampus* 4: 497–529.

Bernardo K L, Woolsey T A (1987) Axonal trajectories between mouse somatosensory thalamus and cortex. *J. Comp. Neurol.* 258 542–564.

Bianchi R, Wong R K S (1994) Carbachol-induced synchronized rhythmic bursts in CA3 neurons of guinea pig hippocampus in vitro. *J. Neurophysiol.* 72: 131–138.

Bianchi R, Wong R K S (1995) Excitatory synaptic potentials dependent on metabotropic glutamate receptor activation in guinea-pig hippocampal pyramidal cells. *J. Physiol.* 487: 663–676.

Bochet P, Audinat E, Lambolez B, Crépel F, Rossier J, Iino M, Tsuzuki K, Ozawa S (1994) Subunit composition at the single-cell level explains functional properties of a glutamate-gated channel. *Neuron* 12: 383–388.

Boddeke H W, Best R, Boeijinga P H (1997) Synchronous 20 Hz rhythmic activity in hippocampal networks induced by activation of metabotropic glutamate receptors in vitro. *Neuroscience* 76: 653–658.

Bortolotto Z A, Collingridge G L (1993) Characterisation of LTP induced by the activation of glutamate metabotropic receptors in area CA1 of the hippocampus. *Neuropharmacology* 32: 1–9.

Bortolotto Z A, Collingridge G L (1995) On the mechanism of long-term potentiation induced by (1S,3R)-1–aminocyclopentane-1,3–dicarboxylic acid (ACPD) in rat hippocampal slices. *Neuropharmacology* 34: 1003–1014.

Bouyer J J, Montaron M F, Rougeul A (1981) Fast fronto-parietal rhythms during combined focused attentive behaviour and immobility in cat: cortical and thalamic localizations. *Electroenceph. Clin. Neurophysiol.* 51: 244–252.

Bouyer J J, Montaron M F, Vahnée J M, Albert M P, Rougeul A (1987) Anatomical localization of cortical beta rhythms in cat. *Neuroscience* 22: 863–869.

Bragin A, Csicsvári J, Penttonen M, Buzsáki G (1997) Epileptic afterdischarge in the hippocampal-entorhinal system: current source density and unit studies. *Neuroscience* 76: 1187–1203.

Bragin A, Jandó G, Nádasdy Z, Hetke J, Wise K, Buzsáki G (1995) Gamma (40–100 Hz) oscillation in the hippocampus of the behaving rat. *J. Neurosci.* 15: 47–60.

Bressler S L, Freeman W J (1980) Frequency analysis of olfactory system EEG in cat, rabbit, and rat. *Electroenceph. Clin. Neurophysiol.* 50: 19–24.

Brett B, Barth D S (1997) Subcortical modulation of high-frequency (gamma band) oscillating potentials in auditory cortex. *J. Neurophysiol.* 78: 573–581.

Bringuier V, Frégnac Y, Baranyi A, Debanne D, Shulz D E (1997) Synaptic origin and stimulus dependency of neuronal oscillatory activity in the primary visual cortex of the cat. *J. Physiol.* 500: 751–774.

Brodal A (1981) *Neurological Anatomy in Relation to Clinical Medicine.* Oxford University Press.

Brosch M, Bauer R, Eckhorn R (1995) Synchronous high-frequency oscillations in cat area 18. *Eur. J. Neurosci.* 7: 86–95.

Brown R E, Reymann K G (1995) Metabotropic glutamate receptor agonists reduce paired-pulse depression in the dentate gyrus of the rat in vitro. *Neurosci. Lett.* 196: 17–20.

Brust J C M (1993) *Neurological Aspects of Substance Abuse.* Butterworth-Heinemann, Boston.

Buckle P J, Haas H L (1982) Enhancement of synaptic transmission by 4–aminopyridine in hippocampal slices of the rat. *J. Physiol.* 326: 109–122.

Buhl E H, Cobb S R, Halasy K, Somogyi P (1995) Properties of unitary IPSPs evoked by anatomically identified basket cells in the rat hippocampus. *Eur. J. Neurosci.* 7: 1989–2004.

Buhl E H, Halasy K, Somogyi P (1994) Diverse sources of hippocampal unitary inhibitory postsynaptic potentials and the number of synaptic release sites. *Nature* 368: 823–828.

Buhl E H, Han Z-S, Lörinczi Z, Stezhka V V, Karnup S V, Somogyi P (1994) Physiological properties of anatomically identified axo-axonic cells in the rat hippocampus. *J. Neurophysiol.* 71: 1289–1307.

Buhl E H, Szilágyi T, Halasy K, Somogyi P (1996) Physiological properties of anatomically identified basket and bistratified cells in the CA1 area of the rat hippocampus in vitro. *Hippocampus* 6: 294–305.

Burchell T R, Faulkner H J, Whittington M A (1998) Gamma frequency oscillations gate temporally coded afferent inputs in the rat hippocampal slice. *Neurosci. Lett.*, 255: 1–4.

Burke J P, Hablitz J J (1994) Metabotropic glutamate receptor activation decreases epileptiform activity in rat neocortex. *Neurosci. Lett.* 174: 29–33.

Burnashev N, Monyer H, Seeburg P H, Sakmann B (1992) Divalent ion permeability of AMPA receptor channels is dominated by the edited form of a single subunit. *Neuron* 8: 189–198.

Bush P C, Sejnowski T J (1996) Inhibition synchronizes sparsely connected cortical neurons within and between columns in realistic network models. *J. Comput. Neurosci.* 3: 91–110.

Buzsáki G (1986) Hippocampal sharp waves: their origin and significance. *Brain Res.* 398, 242–252.

Buzsáki G (1989) Two-stage model of memory trace formation: a role for "noisy" brain states. *Neuroscience* 31: 551–570.

Buzsáki G, Czopf J, Kondákor I, Kellényi L (1986) Laminar distribution of hippocampal rhythmic slow activity (RSA) in the behaving rat current-source density analysis. Effects of urethane and atropine. *Brain Res.* 365: 125–137.

Buzsáki G, Eidelberg E (1982) Direct afferent excitation and long-term potentiation of hippocampal interneurons. *J. Neurophysiol.* 48: 597–607.

Buzsáki G, Gage F H, Czopf J, Björklund A (1987) Restoration of rhythmic slow activity (θ) in the subcortically denervated hippocampus by fetal CNS transplants. *Brain Res.* 400: 334–347.

Buzsáki G, Leung L-W S and Vanderwolf C H (1983) Cellular bases of hippocampal EEG in the behaving rat. *Brain Res.* 287: 139–171.

Buzsáki G, Penttonen M, Nádasdy Z, Bragin A (1996) Pattern and inhibition-dependent invasion of pyramidal cell dendrites by fast spikes in the hippocampus *in vivo. Proc. Natl. Acad. Sc. USA* 93: 9921–9925.

Caeser M, Brown D A, Gähwiler B H, Knöpfel T (1993) Characterization of a calcium-dependent current generating a slow afterdepolarization of CA3 pyramidal cells in rat hippocampal slice cultures. *Eur. J. Neurosci.* 5: 560–569.

Cahusac P M B (1994) Cortical layer-specific effects of the metabotropic glutamate receptor agonist 1S,3R-ACPD in rat primary somatosensory cortex *in vivo. Eur. J. Neurosci.* 6: 1505–1511.

Callaway J C, Ross W N (1995) Frequency-dependent propagation of sodium action potentials in dendrites of hippocampal CA1 pyramidal neurons. *J. Neurophysiol.* 74: 1395–1403.

Capogna M, Gähwiler B H, Thompson S M (1993) Mechanism of μ-opioid receptor-mediated presynaptic inhibition in the rat hippocampus *in vitro. J. Physiol.* 470: 539–558.

Carslaw H S, Jaeger J C (1959) *Conduction of Heat in Solids,* 2nd edition. Oxford University Press.

Castillo P E, Malenka R C, Nicoll R A (1997) Kainate receptors mediate a slow post-synaptic current in hippocampal CA3 neurons. *Nature* 388: 182–186.

Chamberlin N L, Traub R D, Dingledine R (1990) Spontaneous EPSPs initiate burst-firing in rat hippocampal neurons bathed in high potassium. *J. Neurophysiol.* 64: 1000–1008.

Charpak S, Gähwiler B (1991) Glutamate mediates a slow synaptic response in hippocampal slice cultures. *Proc. R. Soc. Lond. B* 243: 221–226.

Charpak S, Gähwiler B, Do KQ, Knöpfel T (1990) Potassium conductances in hippocampal neurons blocked by excitatory amino-acid transmitters. *Nature* 347: 765–767.

Charpark, S. Paré D, Llinás R (1995) The entorhinal cortex entrains fast CA1 hippocampal oscillations in the anaesthetized guinea-pig: role of the monosynaptic component of the perforant path. *Eur. J. Neurosci.* 7: 1548–1557.

Chavis P, Shinozaki H, Bockaert J, Fagni L (1994) The metabotropic glutamate receptor types 2/3 inhibit L-type calcium channels via a pertussis toxin-sensitive G protein in cultured cerebellar granule cells. *J. Neurosci.* 14: 7067–7076.

Chen Q X, Kay A R, Stelzer A, Kay A R, Wong R K S (1990) CABA$_A$-receptor function is regulated by phosphorylation in acutely dissociated guinea-pig hippocampal neurones. *J. Physiol.* 420: 207–221.

Chen Q X, Wong R K S (1991) Intracellular Ca^{2+} suppressed a transient potassium current in hippocampal neurons. *J. Neurosci.* 11: 337–343.

Chen Q X, Wong R K S (1995) Suppression of GABA$_A$ receptor responses by NMDA application in hippocampal neurones acutely isolated from the adult guinea-pig. *J. Physiol.* 482: 353–362.

Chen W R, Midtgaard J, Shepherd G M (1997) Forward and backward propagation of dendritic impulses and their synaptic control in mitral cells. *Science* 278: 463–467.

Cherubini E, Gaiarsa J L, Ben-Ari Y (1991) GABA: an excitatory transmitter in early postnatal life. *Trends Neurosci.* 14: 515–519.

Choi S, Lovinger D M (1996) Metabotropic glutamate receptor modulation of voltage-gated calcium channels involves multiple receptor subtypes in cortical neurons. *J. Neurosci.* 16: 36–45.

Christian E P, Dudek F E (1988) Electrophysiological evidence from glutamate microapplications for local excitatory circuits in the CA1 area of rat hippocampal slices. *J. Neurophysiol.* 59: 110–123.

Christie B R, Eliot L S, Ito K-I, Miyakawa H, Johnston D (1995) Different Ca^{2+} channels in soma and dendrites of hippocampal pyramidal neurons mediate spike-induced Ca^{2+} influx. *J. Neurophysiol.* 73: 2553–2557.

Chrobak J J, Buzsáki G (1994) Selective activation of deep layer (V–VI) retrohippocampal cortical neurons during hippocampal sharp waves in the behaving rat. *J. Neurosci.* 14: 6160–6170.

Chrobak J J, Buzsáki G (1998) Gamma oscilllations in the entorhinal cortex of the freely behaving rat. *J. Neurosci.* 18: 388–398.

Cobb S R, Buhl E H, Halasy K, Paulsen O, Somogyi P (1995) Synchronization of neuronal activity in hippocampus by individual GABAergic interneurons. *Nature* 378: 75–78.

Cobb S R, Halasy K, Vida I, Nyiri G, Tamás G, Buhl E H, Somogyi P (1997) Synaptic effects of identified interneurones innervating both interneurones and pyramidal cells in the rat hippocampus. *Neuroscience* 79: 629–648.

Cohen G A, Doze V A, Madison D V (1992) Opioid inhibition of GABA release from presynaptic terminals of rat hippocampal interneurons. *Neuron* 9: 325–335.

Colbert C M, Johnston D (1996) Axonal action-potential initiation and Na^+ channel densities in the soma and axon initial segment of subicular pyramidal neurons. *J. Neurosci.* 16: 6676–6686.

Cole A E, Nicoll R A (1984) Characterization of a slow cholinergic post-synaptic potential recorded *in vitro* from rat hippocampal pyramidal cells. *J. Physiol.* 352: 173–188.

Colling S B, Stanford I M, Traub R D, Jefferys J G R (1998) Limbic gamma rhythms. I. Phase-locked oscillations in hippocampal CA1 and subiculum. *J. Neurophysiol* 80: 155–161.

Colquhoun D, Jonas P, Sakmann B (1992) Action of brief pulses of glutamate on AMPA/kainate receptors in patches from different neurones of rat hippocampal slices. *J. Physiol.* 458: 261–287.

Colwell S A (1975) Thalamocortical-corticothalamic reciprocity: a combined anterograde-retrograde trace technique. *Brain Res.* 92: 443–449.

Connors B W, Gutnick M J and Prince D A (1982) Electrophysiological properties of neocortical neurons in vitro. *J. Neurophysiol.* 48: 1302–1320.

Constanti A, Bagetta G (1991) Muscarinic receptor activation induces a prolonged post-stimulus afterdepolarization with a conductance decrease in guinea-pig olfactory cortex neurones in vitro. *Neurosci. Lett.* 131: 27–32.

Contreras D, Curró Dossi R, Steriade M (1992) Bursting and tonic discharges in two classes of reticular thalamic neurons. *J. Neurophysiol.* 68: 973–977.

Contreras D, Steriade M (1996) Spindle oscillation in cats: the role of corticothalamic feedback in a thalamically generated rhythm. *J. Physiol.* 490: 159–179.

Contreras D, Timofeev I, Steriade M (1996) Mechanisms of long-lasting hyperpolarizations underlying slow sleep oscillations in cat corticothalamic networks. *J. Physiol.* 491: 251–264.

Craig A D Jr, Wiegand S J, Price J L (1982) The thalamo-cortical projection of the nucleus submedius in the cat. *J. Compar. Neurol.* 206: 28–48.

Crépel V, Aniksztejn L, Ben-Ari Y, Hammond C (1994) Glutamate metabotropic receptors increase a Ca^{2+}-activated nonspecific cationic current in CA1 hippocampal neurons. *J. Neurophysiol.* 72: 1561–1569.

Crépel V, Khazipov R, Ben-Ari Y (1997) Blocking $GABA_A$ inhibition reveals AMPA- and NMDA-receptor-mediated polysynaptic responses in the CA1 region of the rat hippocampus. *J. Neurophysiol.* 77: 2071–2082.

Crick F, Mitchison G (1983) The function of dream sleep. *Nature* 304: 111–114.

Daroff R B, Osorio I (1984) The function of dreaming. *Neurology* 34: 1271.

Davies C H, Davies S N, Collingridge G L (1990) Paired-pulse depression of monosynaptic GABA-mediated inhibitory postsynaptic responses in rat hippocampus. *J. Physiol.* 424: 513–531.

Debanne D, Guérineau N C, Gähwiler B H, Thompson S M (1997) Action potential propagation gated by an axonal I_A-like K^+ conductance in hippocampus. *Nature* 389: 286–289.

Desai M A, McBain C J, Kauer J A, Conn P J (1994) Metabotropic glutamate receptor-induced disinhibition is mediated by reduced transmission at excitatory synapses onto interneurons and inhibitory synapses onto pyramidal cells. *Neurosci. Lett.* 181: 78–82.

Deschênes M (1981) Dendritic spikes induced in fast pyramidal tract neurons by thalamic stimulation. *Exper. Brain Res.* 43: 304–308.

Desmedt J E, Tomberg C (1994) Transient phase-locking of 40 Hz electrical oscillations in prefrontal and parietal human cortex reflects the process of conscious somatic perception. *Neuroscience Lett.* 168: 126–129.

Destexhe A, Babloyantz A (1992) Cortical coherent activity induced by thalamic oscillations. In: Taylor J G, Caianello E R, Cotterill R M J, Clark J W (eds.), *Neural Network Dynamics*, Springer Verlag, Berlin, pp. 234–249.

Destexhe A, Contreras D, Sejnowski T J, Steriade M (1994) A model of spindle rhythmicity in the isolated thalamic reticular nucleus. *J. Neurophysiol.* 72: 803–818.

Deuchars J, Thomson A M (1996) CA1 pyramid-pyramid connections in rat hippocampus *in vitro*: dual intracellular recordings with biocytin filling. *Neuroscience* 74: 1009–1018.

Dichter M, Spencer W A (1969) Penicillin-induced interictal discharges from the cat hippocampus. I. Characteristics and topographical features. *J. Neurophysiol.* 32: 649–662.

Dickinson P S, Marder E (1989) Peptidergic modulation of a multioscillator system in the lobster. I. Activation of the cardiac sac motor pattern by the neuropeptides proctolin and red pigment-concentrating hormone. *J. Neurophysiol.* 61: 833–844.

Dingledine R, Hynes M A, King G L (1986) Involvement of N-methyl-D-aspartate receptors in epileptiform bursting in the rat hippocampal slice. *J. Physiol.* 380: 175–189.

Dodge F A Jr, Cooley J W (1973) Action potential of the motoneuron. *IBM J. Res. Dev.* 17: 219–229.

Domann R, Uhlig S, Dorn T, Witte O W (1991) Participation of interneurons in penicillin-induced epileptic discharges. *Exp. Brain Res.* 83: 683–686.

Donoghue J P, Sanes J N, Hatsopoulos N G, Gaál G (1998) Neural discharge and local field potential oscillations in primate motor cortex during voluntary movements. *J. Neurophysiol* 79: 159–173.

Draguhn A, Traub R D, Schmitz D, Jefferys J G R (1998) Electrical coupling underlies high-frequency oscillations in the hippocampus *in vitro*. *Nature* 394: 189–192.

Dutar P, Nicoll R A (1988a) A physiological role for GABA$_B$ receptors in the central nervous system. *Nature* 332: 156–158.

Dutar P, Nicoll R A (1988b) Classification of muscarinic responses in hippocampus in terms of receptor subtypes and second-messenger systems: electrophysiological studies in vitro. *J. Neurosci.* 8: 4214–4224.

Eccles J C, Libet B, Young R R (1958) The behaviour of chromatolysed motoneurones studied by intracellular recording. *J. Physiol.* 143: 11–40.

Eckhorn R, Bauer R, Jordan W, Brosch M, Kruse W, Munk M, Reitboeck H J (1988) Coherent oscillations: a mechanism of feature linking in the visual cortex? *Biol. Cybern.* 60: 121–130.

Eckhorn R, Frien A, Bauer R, Woelbern T, Kehr H (1993) High frequency (60–90 Hz) oscillations in primary visual cortex of awake monkey. *NeuroReport* 4: 243–246.

Eckhorn R, Obermüeller A (1993) Single neurons are differently involved in stimulus-specific oscillations in cat visual cortex. *Exp. Brain Res.* 95: 177–182.

Elliott E M, Malouf A T, Catterall W A (1995) Role of calcium channel subtypes in calcium transients in hippocampal CA3 neurons. *J. Neurosci.* 15: 6433–6444.

Engel A K, König P, Kreiter A K, Singer W (1991) Interhemispheric synchronization of oscillatory neuronal responses in cat visual cortex. *Science* 252: 1177–1179.

Engel A K, Kreiter A K, König P, Singer W (1991) Synchronization of oscillatory neuronal responses between striate and extrastriate visual cortical areas of the cat. *Proc. Natl. Acad. Sci. USA* 88: 6048–6052.

Ermentrout G B, Kopell N (1998) Fine structure of neural spiking and synchronization in the presence of conduction delays. *Proc. Natl. Acad. Sci. USA* 95: 1259–1264.

Faulkner H J, Traub R D, Whittington M A (1998) Disruption of synchronous gamma oscillations in the rat hippocampal slice: a common mechanism of anaesthetic drug action. *Br. J. Pharmacol.* 125: 483–492.

Federico P, MacVicar B A (1996) Imaging the induction and spread of seizure activity in the isolated brain of the guinea pig: the roles of GABA and glutamate receptors. *J. Neurophysiol.* 76: 3471–3492.

Fisahn A, Pike F G, Buhl E H, Paulsen O (1998) Cholinergic induction of network oscillations in the hippocampus *in vitro*. *Nature* 394: 186–189.

Fisher M E (1961) Critical probabilities for cluster size and percolation problems. *J. Math. Phys.* 2: 620–627.

Fisher R, Johnston D (1990) Differential modulation of single voltage-gated calcium channels by cholinergic and adrenergic agonists in adult hippocampal neurons. *J. Neurophysiol.* 64: 1291–1302.

Fleidervish I, Astman N, Gutnick M J (1997) PKC activation increases persistent Na$^+$ current at subthreshold potentials in neocortical neurons. *Abstr. Soc. Neurosci.* 23: 1472.

Fleidervish I, Friedman A, Gutnick M J (1996) Slow inactivation of Na$^+$ current and slow cumulative spike adaptation in mouse and guinea-pig neocortical neurones in slices. *J. Physiol.* 493: 83–97.

Forsythe I D, Westbrook G L (1988) Slow excitatory postsynaptic currents mediated by N-methyl-D aspartate receptors on cultured mouse central neurones. *J. Physiol.* 396: 515–533.

Forsythe I D, Westbrook G L, Mayer M L (1988) Modulation of excitatory synaptic transmission by glycine and zinc in cultures of mouse hippocampal neurons. *J. Neurosci.* 8: 3733–3741.

Forti M, Michelson H B (1998) Synaptic connectivity of distinct hilar interneuron subpopulations. *J. Neurophysiol.* 79: 3229–3237.

Fox J E, Jefferys J G R (1998) The effect of diazepam and propofol on gamma activity recorded from the CA1 region of the rat hippocampal slice. *Eur. J. Neurosci.* 10 Suppl 10: 39.

Fox S E, Ranck J B Jr (1975) Localization and anatomical identification of theta and complex spike cells in the dorsal hippocampal formation of rats. *Exper. Neurol.* 49: 299–313.

Fraser D D, MacVicar B A (1996) Cholinergic-dependent plateau potential in hippocampal CA1 pyramidal neurons. *J. Neurosci.* 16: 4113–4128.

Freeman W J (1974) Average transmission distance from mitral-tufted to granule cells in olfactory bulb. *Electroenceph. clin. Neurophysiol.* 36: 609–618.

Freeman W J (1978) Spatial properties of an EEG event in the olfactory bulb and cortex. *Electroenceph. Clin. Neurophysiol.* 44: 586–605.

Freeman W J, Schneider W (1982) Changes in spatial patterns of rabbit olfactory EEG with conditioning to odors. *Psychophysiol.* 19: 44–56.

Freund T F, Antal M (1988) GABA-containing neurons in the septum control inhibitory interneurons in the hippocampus. *Nature* 336: 170–173.

Freund T F, Buzsáki G (1996) Interneurons of the hippocampus. *Hippocampus* 6: 347–470.

Freund T F, Meskenaite V (1992) γ-Aminobutyric acid-containing basal forebrain neurons innervate inhibitory interneurons in the neocortex. *Proc. Natl. Acad. Sci. USA* 89: 738–742.

Frien A, Eckhorn R, Bauer R, Woelbern T, Kehr H (1994) Stimulus-specific fast oscillations at zero phase between visual areas V1 and V2 of awake monkey. *NeuroReport* 5: 2273–2277.

Fukuda T, Aika Y, Heizmann C W, Kosaka T (1996) Dense GABAergic input on somata of parvalbumin-immunoreactive GABAergic neurons in the hippocampus of the mouse. *Neurosci. Res.* 26: 181–194.

Fumitaka K, Baughman R W (1997) Distinct muscarinic receptor subtypes suppress excitatory and inhibitory synaptic responses in cortical neurons. *J. Neurophysiol.* 77: 709–716.

Gähwiler B H (1980) Excitatory action of opioid peptides and opiates on cultured hippocampal pyramidal cells. *Brain Res.* 194: 193–203.

Galambos R (1992) A comparison of certain gamma band (40-Hz) brain rhythms in cat and man. In: Baçar E and Bullock T H (eds), *Induced Rhythms in the Brain*. Birkhäuser, Boston, pp. 201–216.

Galambos R, Makeig S, Talmachoff P (1981) A 40 Hz auditory potential recorded from the human scalp. *Proc. Natl. Acad. Sci. USA* 78: 2643–2647.

Galey D, Simon H, Le Moal M (1977) Behavioral effects of lesions in the A10 dopaminergic area of the rat. *Brain Res.* 124: 83–97.

Galvan M, Grafe P, ten Bruggencate G (1982) Convulsive actions of 4–aminopyridine on the guinea-pig olfactory cortex slice. *Brain Res.* 241: 75–86.

Garaschuk O, Hanse E, Konnerth A (1998) Developmental profile and synaptic origin of early network oscillations in the CA1 region of rat neonatal hippocampus. *J. Physiol.* 507: 219–236.

Geiger J R P, Melcher T, Koh D-S, Sakmann B, Seeburg P H, Jonas P, Monyer H (1995) Relative abundance of subunit mRNAs determines gating and Ca^{2+} permeability of AMPA receptors in principal neurons and interneurons in rat CNS. *Neuron* 15: 193–204.

Gereau R W IV, Conn P J (1995a) Roles of specific metabotropic glutamate receptor subtypes in regulation of hippocampal CA1 pyramidal cell excitability. *J. Neurophysiol.* 74: 122–129.

Gereau R W IV, Conn P J (1995b) Multiple presynaptic metabotropic glutamate receptors modulate excitatory and inhibitory synaptic transmission in hippocampal area CA1. *J. Neurosci.* 15: 6879–6889.

Ghose G M, Freeman R D (1992) Oscillatory discharge in the visual system: does it have a functional role? *J. Neurophysiol.* 68: 1558–1574.

Gilbert C D, Wiesel T N (1983) Clustered intrinsic connections in cat visual cortex. *J. Neurosci.* 3: 1116–1133.

Gilbert C D, Wiesel T N (1989) Columnar specificity of intrinsic horizontal and corticocortical connections in cat visual cortex. *J. Neurosci.* 9: 2432–2442.

Glaze D G (1990) Drug effects. In: Daly D D, Pedley T A (eds.), *Current Practice of Clinical Electroencephalography*, 2nd edition. Raven Press, New York, pp. 489–512.

Golomb D, Rinzel J (1993) Dynamics of globally coupled inhibitory neurons with heterogeneity. *Phys. Rev. E* 48: 4810–4814.

Goodridge J P, Taube J S (1997) Interaction between the postsubiculum and anterior thalamus in the generation of head direction cell activity. *J. Neurosci.* 17: 9315–9330.

Gray C M (1994) Synchronous oscillations in neuronal systems: mechanisms and functions. *J. Comput. Neurosci.* 1: 11–38.

Gray C M, Engel A K, König P, Singer W (1990) Stimulus-dependent neuronal oscillations in cat visual cortex: receptive field properties and feature dependence. *Eur. J. Neurosci.* 2: 607–619.

Gray C M, Engel A K, König P, Singer W (1992) Synchronization of oscillatory neuronal responses in cat striate cortex: temporal properties. *Visual Neurosci.* 8: 337–347.

Gray C M, König P, Engel A K, Singer W (1989) Oscillatory responses in cat visual cortex exhibit inter-columnar synchronization which reflects global stimulus properties. *Nature* 338: 334–337.

Gray C M, McCormick D A (1996) Chattering cells: superficial pyramidal neurons contributing to the generation of synchronous oscillations in the visual cortex. *Science* 274: 109–113.

Gray C M, Singer W (1989) Stimulus-specific neuronal oscillations in orientation columns of cat visual cortex. *Proc. Natl. Acad. Sci.* 86: 1698–1702.

Gray C M, Skinner J E (1988) Centrifugal regulation of neuronal activity in the olfactory bulb of the waking rabbit as revealed by reversible cryogenic blockade. *Exp. Brain Res.* 69: 378–386.

Gray C M, Viana Di Prisco G (1997) Stimulus-dependent neuronal oscillations and local synchronization in striate cortex of the alert cat. *J. Neurosci.* 17: 3239–3253.

Greene J R T, Totterdell S (1997) Morphology and distribution of electrophysiologically defined classes of pyramidal and nonpyramidal neurons in rat ventral subiculum in vitro. *J. Comp. Neurol.* 380: 395–408.

Griniasty M, Tsodyks M V, Amit D J (1993) Conversion of temporal correlations between stimuli to spatial correlations between attractors. *Neural Comput.* 5, 1–17.

Gu J G, Albuquerque C, Lee C J, MacDermott A B (1996) Synaptic strengthening through activation of Ca^{2+}-permeable AMPA receptors. *Nature* 381: 793–796.

Guérineau N C, Bossu J-L, Gähwiler B H, Gerber U (1995) Activation of a nonselective cationic conductance by metabotropic glutamatergic and muscarinic agonists in CA3 pyramidal neurons of the rat hippocampus. *J. Neurosci.* 15: 4395–4407.

Guérineau N C, Bossu J-L, Gähwiler B H, Gerber U (1997) G-protein-mediated desensitization of metabotropic glutamatergic and muscarinic responses in CA3 cells in rat hippocampus. *J. Physiol.* 500: 487–496.

Guérineau N C, Gähwiler B H, Gerber U (1994) Reduction of resting K^+. current by metabotropic glutamate and muscarinic receptors in rat CA3 cells: mediation by G-proteins. *J. Physiol.* 474: 27–33.

Gulyás A I, Miles R, Hájos N, Freund T F (1993) Precision and variability in postsynaptic target selection of inhibitory cells in the hippocampal CA3 region. *Eur. J. Neurosci.* 5: 1729–1751.

Gulyás A I, Miles R, Sik A, Tóth K, Tamamaki N, Freund T F (1993) Hippocampal pyramidal cells excite inhibitory neurons through a single release site. *Nature* 366: 683–687.

Gutfreund Y, Yarom Y, Segev I (1995) Subthreshold oscillations and resonant frequency in guinea-pig cortical neurons: physiology and modelling. *J. Physiol.* 483: 621–640.

Gutnick M J, Prince D A (1972) Thalamocortical relay neurons: antidromic invasion of spikes from a cortical epileptogenic focus. *Science* 176: 424–426.

Hablitz J J (1984) Picrotoxin-induced epileptiform activity in the hippocampus: role of endogenous versus synaptic factors. *J. Neurophysiol.* 51: 1011–1027.

Halasy K, Buhl E H, Lőrinczi Z, Tamás G, Somogyi P (1996) Synaptic target selectivity and input of GABAergic basket and bistratified interneurons in the CA1 area of the rat hippocampus. *Hippocampus* 6: 306–329.

Hallanger A E, Wainer B H (1988) Ultrastructure of ChAT-immunoreactive synaptic terminals in the thalamic reticular nucleus of the rat. *J. Comp. Neurol.* 278:486–497.

Hanse E, Durand G M, Garaschuk O, Konnerth A (1997) Activity-dependent wiring of the developing hippocampal neuronal circuit. *Sem. Cell Develop. Biol.* 8: 35–42.

Hansel D, Mato G, Meunier C (1995) Synchrony in excitatory neural networks. *Neural Comput.* 7: 307–337.

Harris-Warrick R M, Marder E, Selverston A I, Moulins M (1992) *Dynamic Biological Networks. The Stomatogastric Nervous System.* MIT Press, Cambridge, MA.

Haverkampf K, Lübke J, Jonas P (1997) Single-channel properties of native AMPA receptors depend on the putative subunit composition. *Soc. Neurosci. Abstr.* 23: 1204.

Hersch S M, White E L (1981) Thalamocortical synapses with corticothalamic projection neurons in mouse SmI cortex: electron microscopic demonstration of a monosynaptic feedback loop. *Neurosci. Lett.* 24: 207–210.

Hestrin S. Nicoll R A. Perkel D J. Sah P (1990) Analysis of excitatory synaptic action in pyramidal cells using whole-cell recording from rat hippocampal slices. *J. Physiol.* 422: 203–225.

Hestrin S (1993) Different glutamate receptor channels mediate fast excitatory synaptic currents in inhibitory and excitatory cortical neurons. *Neuron* 11: 1083–1091.

Heyer C B, Llinás R (1977) The control of rhythmic firing in normal and axotomized cat spinal motoneurones. *J. Neurophysiol.* 40: 480–488.

Hirsch M W, Smale S (1974) *Differential Equations, Dynamical Systems and Linear Algebra.* Academic Press, New York.

Hodgkin A L, Huxley A F (1952) A quantitative description of membrane current and its application to conduction and excitation in nerve. *J. Physiol.* 117: 500–544.

Hoffman D A, Magee J C, Colbert C M, Johnston D (1997) K^+ channel regulation of signal propagation in dendrites of hippocampal pyramidal neurons. *Nature* 387: 869–875.

Hoffman W H, Haberly L B (1989) Bursting induces persistent all-or-none EPSPs by an NMDA-dependent process in piriform cortex. *J. Neurosci.* 9: 206–215.

Hollrigel G S, Soltesz I (1997) Slow kinetics of miniature inhibitory postsynaptic currents during early postnatal development in granule cells of the dentate gyrus. *J. Neurosci.* 17: 5119–5128.

Hopfield J J (1995) Pattern recognition computation using action potential timing for stimulus representation. *Nature* 376: 33–36.

Horikawa J, Tanahashi A, Suga N (1994) After-discharges in the auditory cortex of the mustached bat: no oscillatory discharges for binding auditory information. *Hearing Res.* 76: 45–52.

Houser C R, Vaughn J E, Barber R P, Roberts E (1980) GABA neurons are the major cell type of the nucleus reticularis thalami. *Brain Res.* 200: 341–354.

Huang Q, Zhou D, Chase K, Gusella J F, Aronin N, DiFiglia M (1992) Immunohistochemical localization of the D1 dopamine receptor in rat brain reveals its axonal transport, pre-and postsynaptic localization, and prevalence in the basal ganglia, limbic system, and thalamic reticular nucleus. *Proc. Natl. Acad. Sci. USA* 89: 11988–11992.

Huguenard J R, Hamill O P, Prince D A (1988) Developmental changes in Na^+ conductances in rat neocortical neurons: appearance of a slowly inactivating component. *J. Neurophysiol.* 59: 778–795.

Huguenard J R, Hamill O P, Prince D A (1989) Sodium channels in dendrites of rat cortical pyramidal neurons. *Proc. Natl. Acad. Sci. USA* 86: 2473–2477.

Huguenard J R, McCormick D A (1992) Simulation of the currents involved in rhythmic oscillations in thalamic relay neurons. *J. Neurophysiol.* 68: 1373–1383.

Huguenard J R, Prince D A (1991) Slow inactivation of a TEA-sensitive K current in acutely isolated rat thalamic relay neurons. *J. Neurophysiol.* 66: 1316–1328.

Iino M, Koike M, Isa T, Ozawa S (1996) Voltage-dependent blockage of Ca^{2+}-permeable AMPA receptors by joro spider toxin in cultured rat hippocampal neurones. *J. Physiol.* 496: 431–437.

Iino M, Ozawa S, Tsuzuki K (1990) Permeation of calcium through excitatory amino acid receptor channels in cultured rat hippocampal neurones. *J. Physiol.* 424: 151–165.

Innocenti G M (1980) The primary visual pathway through the corpus callosum: morphological and functional aspects in the cat. *Arch. Ital. Biol.* 118: 124–188.

Ishizuka N, Weber J, Amaral D G (1990) Organization of intrahippocampal projections originating from CA3 pyramidal cells in the rat. *J. Compar. Neurol.* 295: 580–623.

Ives A E, Jefferys J G R (1990) Synchronization of epileptiform bursts induced by 4-aminopyridine in the in-vitro hippocampal slice preparation. *Neurosci. Lett.* 112: 239–245.

Jacobson S, Trojanowski J Q (1975) Corticothalamic neurons and thalamocortical terminal fields: an investigation in rat using horseradish peroxidase and autoradiography. *Brain Res.* 85: 385–401.

Jaffe D B, Johnston D, Lasser-Ross N, Lisman J E, Miyakawa H, Ross W N (1992) The spread of Na^+ spikes determines the pattern of dendritic Ca^{2+} entry into hippocampal neurons. *Nature* 357: 244–246.

Jaffe D B, Ross W N, Lisman J E, Lasser-Ross N, Miyakawa H, Johnston D (1994) A model for dendritic Ca^{2+} accumulation in hippocampal pyramidal neurons based on fluorescence imaging measurements. *J. Neurophysiol.* 71: 1065–1077.

Jagadeesh B, Gray C M, Ferster D (1992) Visually evoked oscillations of membrane potential in cells of cat visual cortex. *Science* 257: 552–554.

Jahnsen H, Llinás R (1984) Ionic basis for the electro-responsiveness and oscillatory properties of guinea-pig thalamic neurones *in vitro*. *J. Physiol.* 349: 227–247.

Jahr C E, Stevens C F (1990) Voltage dependence of NMDA-activated macroscopic conductances predicted by single-channel kinetics. *J. Neurosci.* 10: 3178–3182.

Jefferys J G R (1979) Initiation and spread of action potentials in granule cells maintained *in vitro* in slices of guinea-pig hippocampus. *J. Physiol.* 289: 375–388.

Jefferys J G R (1989) Chronic epileptic foci in vitro in hippocampal slices from rats with the tetanus toxin epileptic syndrome. *J. Neurophysiol.* 62: 458–468.

Jefferys J G R, Empson R M, Prusiner S B, Whittington M A (1994) Scrapie infection of transgenic mice leads to network dysfunction of neurons in cortical and hippocampal slices. *Neurobiol. Dis.* 1: 25–30.

Jefferys J G R, Haas H L (1982) Synchronized bursting of CA1 hippocampal pyramidal cells in the absence of synaptic transmission. *Nature* 300: 448–450.

Jefferys J G R, Traub R D, Whittington M A (1996) Neuronal networks for induced "40 Hz" rhythms. *Trends Neurosci.* 19: 202–208.

Jensen M S, Azouz R, Yaari Y (1993) Variant firing patterns in rat hippocampal pyramidal cells modulated by extracellular potassium. *J. Neurophysiol.* 71: 831–839.

Jensen M S, Azouz R, Yaari Y (1996) Spike after-depolarization and burst generation in adult rat hippocampal CA1 pyramidal cells. *J. Physiol.* 492: 199–210.

Jensen M S, Yaari Y (1997) Role of intrinsic burst firing, potassium accumulation, and electrical coupling in the elevated potassium model of hippocampal epilepsy. *J. Neurophysiol.* 77: 1224–1233.

Johnston D, Brown T H (1981) Giant synaptic potential hypothesis for epileptiform activity. *Science* 211: 294–297.

Johnston D, Magee J C, Colbert C M, Christie B R (1996) Active properties of neuronal dendrites. *Ann. Rev. Neurosci.* 19: 165–186.

Joliot M, Ribary U, Llinás R (1994) Human oscillatory brain activity near 40 Hz coexists with cognitive temporal binding. *Proc. Natl. Acad. Sci. USA* 91: 11748–11751.

Jonas P, Monyer H (in press) *Ionotropic Glutamate Receptors in the CNS. Handbook of Experimental Pharmacology*, Springer-Verlag, Berlin.

Jonas P, Racca C, Sakmann B, Seeburg P H, Monyer H (1994) Differences in Ca^{2+} permeability of AMPA-type glutamate receptor channels in neocortical neurons caused by differential GluR-B subunit expression. *Neuron* 12: 1281–1289.

Jones M S, Barth D S (1997) Sensory-evoked high-frequency (gamma-band) oscillating potentials in somatosensory cortex of the unanesthetized rat. *Brain Res.* 768: 167–176.

Jouvenceau A, Dutar P, Billard J M (1995) Presynaptic depression of inhibitory postsynaptic potentials by metabotropic glutamate receptors in rat hippocampal CA1 pyramidal cells. *Eur. J. Pharmacol.* 281: 131–139.

Jung H-Y, Mickus T, Spruston N (1997) Prolonged sodium channel inactivation contributes to dendritic action potential attenuation in hippocampal pyramidal neurons. *J. Neurosci.* 17: 6639–6646.

Kamiya H, Shinozaki H, Yamamoto C (1996) Activation of metabotropic glutamate receptor type 2/3 suppresses transmission at rat hippocampal mossy fibre synapses. *J. Physiol.* 493: 447–455.

Kamondi A, Acsády L, Wang X-J, Buzsáki G (1998) Theta oscillations in somata and dendrites of hippocampal pyramidal cells in vivo: activity-dependent phase-precession of action potentials. *Hippocampus* 8: 244–261.

Kandel E R, Spencer W A (1961) Electrophysiology of hippocampal neurons. II. Afterpotentials and repetitive firing. *J. Neurophysiol.* 24: 243–259.

Kapoor R, Smith K J, Felts P A, Davies M (1993) Internodal potassium currents can generate ectopic impulses in mammalian myelinated axons. *Brain Res.* 611: 165–169.

Karst H, Joëls, Wadman W J (1993) Low-threshold calcium current in dendrites of the adult rat hippocampus. *Neurosci. Lett.* 164: 154–158.

Kato F, Morin-Surun M-P, Denavit-Saubié M (1996) Coherent inspiratory oscillation of cranial nerve discharges in perfused neonatal cat brainstem *in vitro*. *J. Physiol.* 497: 539–549.

Katsumaru H, Kosaka T, Heizmann C W, Hama K (1988) Gap junctions on GABAergic neurons containing the calcium-binding protein parvalbumin in the rat hippocampus (CA1 region). *Exp. Brain Res.* 72: 363–370.

Kawaguchi Y (1997) Selective cholinergic modulation of cortical GABAergic cell subtypes. *J. Neurophysiol.* 78: 1743–1747.

Kawaguchi Y, Hama K (1987) Two subtypes of non-pyramidal cells in rat hippocampal formation identified by intracellular recording and HRP injection. *Brain Res.* 411: 190–195.

Kawasaki H, Avoli M (1996) Excitatory effects induced by carbachol on bursting neurons of the rat subiculum. *Neurosci. Lett.* 219: 1–4.

Kay A R (1991) Inactivation kinetics of calcium current of acutely dissociated CA1 pyramidal cells of the mature guinea pig hippocampus. *J. Physiol.* 437: 27–48.

Kay A R, Wong R K S (1986) Isolation of neurons suitable for patch-clamping from adult mammalian central nervous systems. *J. Neurosci. Meth.* 16: 227–238.

Kay A R, Wong R K S (1987) Calcium current activation kinetics in pyramidal neurones of the CA1 region of the mature guinea pig hippocampus. *J. Physiol.* 392: 603–616.

Keller A, White E L (1989) Triads: a synaptic network component in the cerebral cortex. *Brain Res.* 496: 105–112.

Ketchum K L, Haberly L B (1993) Synaptic events that generate fast oscillations in piriform cortex. *J. Neurosci.* 13: 3980–3985.

Khazipov R, Leinekugel X, Khalilov I, Gaiarsa J L, Ben-Ari Y (1997) Synchronization of GABAergic interneuronal network in CA3 subfield of neonatal rat hippocampal slices. *J. Physiol.* 498: 763–772.

Khazipov R, Ragozzino D, Bregestovski P (1995) Kinetics and Mg^{2+} block of N-methyl-D-aspartate receptor channels during postnatal development of hippocampal CA3 pyramidal neurons. *Neuroscience* 69: 1057–1065.

Kisvárday Z F, Beaulieu C, Eysel U T (1993) Network of GABAergic large basket cells in cat visual cortex (area 18): implication for lateral disinhibition. *J. Compar. Neurol.* 327: 398–415.

Kisvárday Z F, Eysel U T (1993) Functional and structural topography of horizontal inhibitory connections in cat visual cortex. *Eur. J. Neurosci.* 5: 1558–1572.

Kisvárday Z F, Martin K A C, Friedlander M J, Somogyi P (1987) Evidence for interlaminar inhibitory circuits in the striate cortex of the cat. *J. Comp. Neurol.* 260: 1–19 1987.

Klink R, Alonso A (1993) Ionic mechanisms for the subthreshold oscillations and differential electroresponsiveness of medial entorhinal cortex layer II neurons. *J. Neurophysiol.* 70: 144–157.

Klink R, Alonso A (1997a) Muscarinic modulation of the oscillatory and repetitive firing properties of entorhinal cortex layer II neurons. *J. Neurophysiol.* 77: 1813–1828.

Klink R, Alonso A (1997b) Ionic mechanisms of muscarinic depolarization in entorhinal cortex layer II neurons. *J. Neurophysiol.* 77: 1829–1843.

Klishin A, Tsintsadze T, Lozovaya N, Krishtal O (1995) Latent N-methyl-D-aspartate receptors in the recurrent excitatory pathway between hippocampal CA1 pyramidal neurons: Ca^{2+}-dependent activation by blocking A_1 adenosine receptors. *Proc. Natl. Acad. Sci. USA* 92: 12431–12435.

Kneisler T B, Dingledine R (1995) Synaptic input from CA3 pyramidal cells to dentate basket cells in rat hippocampus. *J. Physiol.* 487: 125–146.

Knöpfel T, Gähwiler B H (1992) Activity-induced elevations of intracellular calcium concentration in pyramidal and nonpyramidal cells of the CA3 region of rat hippocampal slice cultures. *J. Neurophysiol.* 68: 961–963.

Knöpfel T, Vranesic I, Gähwiler B, Brown D A (1990) Muscarinic and β-adrenergic depression of the slow Ca^{2+}-activated potassium conductance in hippocampal CA3 pyramidal cells is not mediated by a reduction of depolarization-induced cytosolic Ca^{2+} transients. *Proc. Natl. Acad. Sci. USA* 87: 4083–4087.

Knowles W D, Schwartzkroin P A (1981) Local circuit synaptic interactions in hippocampal brain slices. *J. Neurosci.* 1: 318–322.

Knowles W D, Traub R D, Strowbridge BW (1987) The initiation and spread of epileptiform bursts in the *in vitro* hippocampal slice. *Neuroscience* 21: 441–455.

Koch C, Segev I, eds. (1998) *Methods in Neuronal Modeling. From Ions to Networks*, 2nd edition. MIT Press, Cambridge, MA.

König P, Engel A K, Roelfsema P R, Singer W (1995) How precise is neuronal synchronization? *Neural Comput.* 7: 469–485.

König P, Engel A K, Singer W (1995) Relation between oscillatory activity and long-range synchronization in cat visual cortex. *Proc. Natl. Acad. Sci. USA* 92: 290–294.

König P, Engel A K, Singer W (1996) Integrator or coincidence detector? The role of the cortical neuron revisited. *Trends Neurosci.* 19: 130–137.

König P, Schillen T B (1991) Stimulus-dependent assembly formation of oscillatory responses: I. Synchronization. *Neural Comput.* 3: 155–166.

Kopell N (1988) Toward a theory of modelling central pattern generators. In: Cohen A (ed.) *Neural Control of Rhythmic Movements in Vertebrates*. Wiley, New York, pp. 369–413.

Korn S J, Giacchino J L, Chamberlin N L, Dingledine R (1987) Epileptiform burst activity induced by potassium in the hippocampus and its regulation by GABA-mediated inhibition. *J. Neurophysiol.* 57: 325–340.

Kosaka T (1983a) Gap junctions between non-pyramidal cell dendrites in the rat hippocampus (CA1 and CA3 regions). *Brain Res.* 271: 157–161.

Kosaka T (1983b) Neuronal gap junctions in the polymorph layer of the rat dentate gyrus. *Brain Res.* 277: 347–351.

Kultas Ilinsky K, Ribak C E, Peterson G M, Oertel W H (1985) A description of the GABAergic neurons and axon terminals in the motor nuclei of the cat thalamus. *J. Neurosci.* 5: 1346–1369.

Kuno M, Llinás R (1970a) Enhancement of synaptic transmission by dendritic potentials in chromatolysed motoneurones of the cat. *J. Physiol.* 210: 807–821.

Kuno M, Llinás R (1970b) Alterations of synaptic action in chromatolysed motoneurones of the cat. *J. Physiol.* 210: 823–838.

Lacaille J-C, Mueller A L, Kunkel D D, Schwartzkroin P A (1987) Local circuit interactions between oriens/alveus interneurons and CA1 pyramidal cells in hippocampal slices: electrophysiology and morphology. *J. Neurosci.* 7: 1979–1993.

Lacaille J-C, Schwartzkroin P A (1988a) Stratum lacunosum-moleculare interneurons of hippocampal CA1 region. I. Intracellular response characteristics, synaptic responses, and morphology. *J. Neurosci.* 8: 1400–1410.

Lacaille J-C, Schwartzkroin P A (1988b) Stratum lacunosum-moleculare interneurons of hippocampal CA1 region. II. Intrasomatic and intradendritic recordings of local circuit synaptic interactions. *J. Neurosci.* 8: 1411–1424.

Lacaille J-C, Williams S (1990) Membrane properties of interneurons in stratum oriens-alveus of the CA1 region of rat hippocampus *in vitro*. *Neuroscience* 36: 349–359.

Lambert N A, Borroni A M, Grover L M, Teyler T J (1991) Hyperpolarizing and depolarizing $GABA_A$ receptor-mediated dendritic inhibition in area CA1 of the rat hippocampus. *J. Neurophysiol.* 66: 1538–1548.

Lambert N A, Harrison N L, Teyler T J (1991) Evidence for μ opiate receptors on inhibitory terminals in area CA1 of rat hippocampus. *Neurosci. Lett.* 124: 101–104.

Lamsa K, Kaila K (1997) Ionic mechanisms of spontaneous GABAergic events in rat hippocampal slices exposed to 4-aminopyridine. *J. Neurophysiol.* 78: 2582–2591.

Land P W, Buffer S A Jr, Yaskosky J D (1995) Barreloids in adult rat thalamus: three-dimensional architecture and relationship to somatosensory cortical barrels. *J. Comp. Neurol.* 355: 573–588.

Laurent G, Davidowitz H (1994) Encoding of olfactory information with oscillating neural assemblies. *Science* 265: 1872–1875.

Laurent G, Wehr M, Davidowitz H (1996) Temporal representations of odors in an olfactory network. *J. Neurosci.* 16: 3837–3847.

Lebeda F J, Hablitz J J, Johnston D (1982) Antagonism of GABA-mediated responses by d-tubocurarine in hippocampal neurons. *J. Neurophysiol.* 48: 622–632.

Lee W-L, Hablitz J J (1989) Involvement of non-NMDA receptors in picrotoxin-induced epileptiform activity in the hippocampus. *Neurosci. Lett.* 107: 129–134.

Lee W-L, Hablitz J J (1990) Effect of APV and ketamine on epileptiform activity in the CA1 and CA3 regions of the hippocampus. *Epilepsy Res.* 6: 87–94.

Lee K H, McCormick D A (1995) Acetylcholine excites GABAergic neurons of the ferret perigeniculate nucleus through nicotinic receptors. *J. Neurophysiol.* 73: 2123–2128.

Leinekugel X, Medina I, Khalilov I, Ben-Ari Y, Khazipov R (1997) Ca^{2+} oscillations mediated by the synergistic excitatory actions of $GABA_A$ and NMDA receptors in the neonatal hippocampus. *Neuron* 18: 243–255.

Leinekugel X, Tseeb V, Ben-Ari Y, Bregestovski P (1995) Synaptic $GABA_A$ activation induces Ca^{2+} rise in pyramidal cells and interneurons from rat neonatal hippocampal slices. *J. Physiol.* 487: 319–329.

Leitch B, Laurent G (1996) GABAergic synapses in the antennal lobe and mushroom body of the locust olfactory system. *J. Compar. Neurol.* 372: 487–514.

Lester R, Jahr C (1990) Quisqualate receptor-mediated depression of calcium currents in hippocampal neurons. *Neuron* 4: 741–749.

Leung L S (1987) Hippocampal electrical activity following local tetanization. I. Afterdischarges. *Brain Res.* 419: 173–187.

Leung L S, Yim C Y (1991) Intrinsic membrane potential oscillations in hippocampal neurons in vitro. *Brain Res.* 553: 261–274.

Li X-G, Somogyi P, Tepper J M, Buzsáki G (1992) Axonal and dendritic arborization of an intracellularly labeled chandelier cell in the CA1 region of rat hippocampus. *Exp. Brain Res.* 90: 519–525.

Li X-G, Somogyi P, Ylinen A, Buzsáki G (1993) The hippocampal CA3 network: an in vivo intracellular labeling study. *J. Compar. Neurol.* 338: 1–29.

Liao D, Hessler N A, Malinow R (1995) Activation of postsynaptically silent synapses during pairing-induced LTP in CA1 region of hippocampal slice. *Nature* 375: 400–404.

Lindström S, Wróbel A (1990) Frequency dependent corticofugal excitation of principal cells in the cat's dorsal lateral geniculate nucleus. *Exp. Brain Res.* 79: 313–318.

Liu Y B, Disterhoft J F, Slater N T (1993) Activation of metabotropic glutamate receptors induces long-term depression of GABAergic inhibition in hippocampus. *J. Neurophysiol.* 69: 1000–1004.

Livingstone M S (1996) Oscillatory firing and interneuronal correlations in squirrel monkey striate cortex. *J. Neurophysiol.* 75: 2467–2485.

Livingstone M S, Hubel D H (1982) Thalamic inputs to cytochrome oxidase-rich regions in monkey visual cortex. *Proc. Natl. Acad. Sci. USA* 79: 6098–6101.

Llinás R R, Grace A A, Yarom Y (1991) *In vitro* neurons in mammalian cortical layer 4 exhibit intrinsic oscillatory activity in the 10-to 50-Hz range. *Proc. Natl. Acad. Sci. USA* 88: 897–901. (Published erratum in *Proc. Natl. Acad. Sci. USA* (1991) 88: 3510.)

Llinás R, Nicholson C (1971) Electrophysiological properties of dendrites and somata in alligator Purkinje cells. *J. Neurophysiol.* 34: 532–551.

Llinás R R, Paré D (1991) Of dreaming and wakefulness. *Neuroscience* 44: 521–535.

Llinás R, Ribary U (1993) Coherent 40-Hz oscillation characterizes dream state in humans. *Proc. Natl. Acad. Sci. USA* 90: 2078–2081.

Llinás R, Sugimori M (1980a) Electrophysiological properties of *in vitro* Purkinje cell somata in mammalian cerebellar slices. *J. Physiol.* 305: 171–195.

Llinás R, Sugimori M (1980b) Electrophysiological properties of *in vitro* Purkinje cell dendrites in mammalian cerebellar slices. *J. Physiol.* 305: 197–213.

Lopez L, Sannita W G (1997) Magnetically recorded oscillatory responses to luminance stimulation in man. *Electroenceph. Clin. Neurophysiol.* 104: 91–95.

Lorente de Nó R (1933) Studies on the structure of the cerebral cortex I. The area entorhinalis. *J. Psychol. Neurol.* 45: 381–438.

Lorente de Nó R (1934) Studies on the structure of the cerebral cortex II. Continuation of the study of the Ammonic system. *J. Psychol. Neurol.* 46: 113–177.

Lujan R, Nusser Z, Roberts J D, Shigemoto R, Somogyi P (1996) Perisynaptic location of metabotropic glutamate receptors mGluR1 and mGluR5 on dendrites and dendritic spines in the rat hippocampus. *Eur. J. Neurosci.* 8: 1488–1500.

Lujan R, Roberts J D, Shigemoto R, Ohishi H, Somogyi P (1997) Differential plasma membrane distribution of metabotropic glutamate receptors mGluR1 α, mGluR2 and mGluR5, relative to neurotransmitter release sites. *J. Chem. Neuroanat.* 13: 219–241.

Lüthi A, Gähwiler B H, Gerber U (1997) 1S,3R-ACPD induces a region of negative slope conductance in the steady-state current-voltage relationship of hippocampal pyramidal cells. *J. Neurophysiol.* 77: 221–228.

Lytton W W, Sejnowski T J (1991) Simulations of cortical pyramidal neurons synchronized by inhibitory interneurons. *J. Neurophysiol.* 66: 1059–1079.

Maccaferri G, Mangoni M, Lazzari A, DiFrancesco D (1993) Properties of the hyperpolarization-activated current in rat hippocampal CA1 pyramidal cells. *J. Neurophysiol.* 69: 2129–2136.

Maccaferri G, McBain C J (1996) The hyperpolarization-activated current I_h and its contribution to pacemaker activity in rat CA1 hippocampal stratum oriens-alveus interneurones. *J. Physiol.* 497: 119–130.

Macchi G, Bentivoglio M, Minciacchi D, Molinari M (1986) The organization of thalamic connections. *Rev. Neurol. Paris* 142: 267–282.

MacDonald K D, Brett B, Barth D S (1996) Inter-and intra-hemispheric spatiotemporal organization of spontaneous electrocortical oscillations. *J. Neurophysiol.* 76: 423–437.

MacDonald K D, Fifkova E, Jones M S, Barth D S (1998) Focal stimulation of the thalamic reticular nucleus induces focal gamma waves in cortex. *J. Neurophysiol.* 79: 474–477.

MacDonald R L, Olsen R W (1994) $GABA_A$ receptor channels. *Annu. Rev. Neurosci.* 17: 569–602.

MacLeod K, Laurent G (1996) Distinct mechanisms for synchronization and temporal patterning of odor-encoding neural assemblies. *Science* 274: 976–980.

MacVicar B A, Tse F W Y (1989) Local neuronal circuitry underlying cholinergic rhythmical slow activity in CA3 area of rat hippocampal slices. *J. Physiol.* 417: 197–212.

Madison D V, Nicoll R A (1984) Control of the repetitive discharge of rat CA1 pyramidal neurones *in vitro*. *J. Physiol.* 354: 319–331.

Madison D V, Nicoll R A (1988) Enkephalin hyperpolarizes interneurones in the rat hippocampus. *J. Physiol.* 398: 123–130.

Magee J C, Christofi G, Miyakawa H, Christie B, Lasser-Ross N, Johnston D (1995) Subthreshold synaptic activation of voltage-gated Ca^{2+} channels mediates a localized Ca^{2+} influx into the dendrites of hippocampal pyramidal neurons. *J. Neurophysiol.* 74: 1335–1342.

Magee J C., Johnston D (1995) Characterization of single voltage-gated Na^+ and Ca^{2+} channels in apical dendrites of rat CA1 pyramidal neurons. *J. Physiol.* 487: 67–90.

Mainen Z F, Carnevale N T, Zador A M, Claiborne B J, Brown T H (1996) Electrotonic architecture of hippocampal CA1 pyramidal neurons based on three-dimensional reconstructions. *J. Neurophysiol.* 76: 1904–1923.

Mainen Z F, Joerges J, Huguenard J R, Sejnowski T J (1995) A model of spike initiation in neocortical pyramidal neurons. *Neuron* 15: 1427–1439.

Major G, Larkman A U, Jonas P J, Sakmann B, Jack J J B (1994) Detailed passive cable models of whole-cell recorded CA3 pyramidal neurons in rat hippocampal slices. *J. Neurosci.* 14: 4613–4638.

Malenka R C, Nicoll R A (1993) NMDA-receptor-dependent synaptic plasticity: multiple forms and mechanisms. *Trends Neurosci.* 16: 521–527.

Manzoni O, Bockaert J (1995) Metabotropic glutamate receptors inhibiting excitatory synapses in the CA1 area of rat hippocampus. *Eur. J. Neurosci.* 7: 2518–2523.

Manzoni T, Caminiti R, Spidalieri G, Morelli E (1979) Anatomical and functional aspects of the associative projections from somatic area SI to SII. *Exper. Brain Res.* 34: 453–470.

Marder E, Calabrese R L (1996) Principles of rhythmic motor pattern generation. *Physiol. Rev.* 76: 687–717.

Markram H, Helm P J, Sakmann B (1995) Dendritic calcium transients evoked by single back-propagating action potentials in rat neocortical pyramidal neurons. *J. Physiol.* 485: 1–20.

Markram H, Lübke J, Frotscher M, Sakmann B (1997) Regulation of synaptic efficacy by coincidence of postsynaptic APs and EPSPs. *Science* 275: 213–215.

Martin L J, Blackstone C D, Huganir R L, Price D L (1992) Cellular localization of a metabotropic glutamate receptor in rat brain. *Neuron* 9: 259–270.

Martina M, Jonas P (1997) Functional differences in Na^+ channel gating between fast-spiking interneurones and principal neurones of rat hippocampus. *J. Physiol.* 505: 593–603.

Mason A (1993) Electrophysiology and burst-firing of rat subicular pyramidal neurons in vitro: a comparison with area CA1. *Brain Res.* 600: 174–178.

Mason A, Nicoll A, Stratford K (1991) Synaptic transmission between individual pyramidal neurons of the rat visual cortex *in vitro*. *J. Neurosci.* 11: 72–84.

Masukawa L M, Prince D A (1982) Enkephalin inhibition of inhibitory input to CA1 and CA3 pyramidal neurons in the hippocampus. *Brain Res.* 249: 271–280.

Masukawa L M, Prince D A (1984) Synaptic control of excitability in isolated dendrites of hippocampal neurons. *J. Neurosci.* 4: 217–227.

Mattia D, Hwa GGC, Avoli M (1993) Membrane properties of rat subicular neurons in vitro. *J. Neurophysiol.* 70: 1244–1248.

Mayer M L, Westbrook G L, Guthrie P B (1984). Voltage-dependent block by Mg^{2+} of NMDA responses in spinal cord neurones. *Nature* 309: 261–263.

McBain C J, DiChiara T J, Kauer J A (1994) Activation of metabotropic glutamate receptors differentially affects two classes of hippocampal interneurons and potentiates excitatory synaptic transmission. *J. Neurosci.* 14: 4433–4445.

McBain C, Dingledine R (1992) Dual-component miniature excitatory synaptic currents in rat hippocampal CA3 pyramidal neurons. *J. Neurophysiol.* 68: 16–27.

McBain C, Dingledine R (1993) Heterogeneity of synaptic glutamate receptors on CA3 stratum radiatum interneurones of rat hippocampus. *J. Physiol.* 462: 373–392.

McCormick DA (1993) Actions of acetylcholine in the cerebral cortex and thalamus and implications for function. *Prog. Brain Res.* 98: 303–308.

McCormick D A, Connors B W, Lighthall J W and Prince D A (1985) Comparative electrophysiology of pyramidal and sparsely spiny stellate neurons of the neocortex. *J. Neurophysiol.* 54: 782–806.

McCormick D A, Nowak L G (1996) Possible cellular mechanisms for arousal-induced higher frequency oscillations: acetylcholine and ACPD induce repetitive burst firing in visual cortical neurons. *Abstr. Soc. Neurosci.* 22: 644.

McCormick D A, Prince D A (1986) Mechanisms of action of acetylcholine in the guinea-pig cerebral cortex *in vitro. J. Physiol.* 375: 169–194.

McCormick D A, Prince DA (1987) Actions of acetylcholine in the guinea-pig and cat medial and lateral geniculate nuclei, *in vitro. J. Physiol.* 392: 147–165.

McCormick D A, von Krosigk M (1992) Corticothalamic activation modulates thalamic firing through glutamate "metabotropic" receptors. *Proc. Natl. Acad. Sci.* 89: 2774–2778.

McCormick D A, Wang Z, Huguenard J (1993) Neurotransmitter control of neocortical neuronal activity and excitability. *Cerebral Cortex* 3: 387–398.

McGuinness N, Anwyl R, Rowan M (1991) The effects of trans-ACPD on long-term potentiation in the rat hippocampal slice. *NeuroReport* 2: 688–690.

McLean H A, Rovira C, Ben-Ari Y, Gaiarsa J-L (1995) NMDA-dependent GABA$_A$-mediated polysynaptic potentials in the neonatal rat hippocampal CA3 region. *Eur. J. Neurosci.* 7: 1442–1448.

McMahon L L, Kauer J A (1997) Hippocampal interneurons express a novel form of synaptic plasticity. *Neuron* 295–305.

Meier C L, Dudek F E (1996) Spontaneous and stimulation-induced synchronized burst afterdischarges in the isolated CA1 of kainate-treated rats. *J. Neurophysiol.* 76: 2231–2239.

Menon V, Freeman W J, Cutillo B A, Desmond J E, Ward M F, Bressler S L, Laxer K D, Barbaro N, Gevins A S (1996) Spatio-temporal correlations in human gamma band electrocorticograms. *Electroenceph. Clin. Neurophysiol.* 98: 89–102.

Menschik D E, Finkel L H (1998) Neuromodulatory control of hippocampal function: Towards a model of Alzheimer's disease. *Artif. Intell. Med.* 13: 99–121.

Merlin L R, Taylor G W, Wong R K S (1995) Role of metabotropic glutamate receptor subtypes in the patterning of epileptiform activities in vitro. *J. Neurophysiol.* 74: 896–900.

Merlin L R, Wong R K S (1997) Role of group I metabotropic glutamate receptors in the patterning of epileptiform activities in vitro. *J. Neurophysiol.* 78: 539–544.

Mesher R A, Schwartzkroin P A (1980) Can CA3 epileptiform burst discharge induce bursting in normal CA1 hippocampal neurons? *Brain Res.* 183: 472–476.

Metherate R, Cox C L, Ashe J H (1992) Cellular bases of neocortical activation: modulation of neural oscillations by the nucleus basalis and endogenous acetylcholine. *J. Neurosci.* 12: 4701–4711.

Michelson H B, Wong RKS (1991) Excitatory synaptic responses mediated by GABA$_A$ receptors in the hippocampus. *Science* 253: 1420–1423.

Michelson H B, Wong R K S (1994) Synchronization of inhibitory neurones in the guinea pig hippocampus *in vitro. J. Physiol.* 477: 35–45.

Migliore M, Cook E P, Jaffe D B, Turner D A, Johnston D (1995) Computer simulations of morphologically reconstructed CA3 hippocampal neurons.*J. Neurophysiol.* 73: 1157–1168.

Miles R (1990a) Synaptic excitation of inhibitory cells by single CA3 hippocampal pyramidal cells of the guinea-pig *in vitro. J. Physiol.* 428: 61–77.

Miles R (1990b) Variation in strength of inhibitory synapses in the CA3 region of guinea-pig hippocampus *in vitro. J. Physiol.* 431: 659–676.

Miles R, Poncer J-C (1993) Metabotropic glutamate receptors mediate a post-tetanic excitation of guinea-pig hippocampal inhibitory neurones. *J. Physiol.* 463: 461–473.

Miles R, Tóth K, Gulyás A I, Hajos N, Freund T F (1996) Differences between somatic and dendritic inhibition in the hippocampus. *Neuron* 16: 815–823.

Miles R, Traub R D, Wong R K S (1988) Spread of synchronous firing in longitudinal slices from the CA3 region of the hippocampus. *J. Neurophysiol.* 60: 1481–1496.

Miles R, Wong R K S (1983) Single neurones can initiate synchronized population discharge in the hippocampus. *Nature* 306: 371–373.

Miles R, Wong RKS (1984) Unitary inhibitory synaptic potentials in the guinea-pig hippocampus *in vitro. J. Physiol.* 356: 97–113.

Miles R, Wong R K S (1986) Excitatory synaptic interactions between CA3 neurones in the guinea-pig hippocampus. *J. Physiol.* 373: 397–418.

Miles R, Wong R K S (1987a) Inhibitory control of local excitatory circuits in the guinea-pig hippocampus. *J. Physiol.* 388: 611–629.

Miles R, Wong R K S (1987b) Latent synaptic pathways revealed after tetanic stimulation in the hippocampus. *Nature* 329: 724–726.

Miles R., Wong R K S, Traub R D (1984) Synchronized afterdischarges in the hippocampus: contribution of local synaptic interaction. *Neuroscience* 12: 1179–1189.

Misgeld D, Bijak M, Brunner H, Dembowsky K (1992) K-dependent inhibition in the dentate-CA3 network of guinea pig hippocampal slices. *J. Neurophysiol.* 68: 1548–1557.

Misgeld U, Frotscher M (1986) Postsynaptic-GABAergic inhibition of non-pyramidal neurons in the guinea-pig hippocampus. *Neuroscience* 19: 193–206.

Mitani A, Shimokouchi M, Itoh K, Nomura S, Kudo M, Mizuno N (1985) Morphology and laminar organization of electrophysiologically identified neurons in the primary auditory cortex in the cat. *J. Comp. Neurol.* 235: 430–447.

Mittman T, Linton S M, Schwindt P, Crill W (1997) Evidence for persistent Na^+ current in apical dendrites of rat neocortical neurons from imaging of Na^+-sensitive dye. *J. Neurophysiol.* 78: 1188–1192.

Miyakawa H, Ross W N, Jaffe D, Callaway J C, Lasser-Ross N, Lisman J E, Johnston D (1992) Synaptically activated increases in Ca^{2+} concentration in hippocampal CA1 pyramidal cells are primarily due to voltage-gated Ca^{2+} channels. *Neuron* 9: 1163–1173.

Miyashita Y (1988) Neuronal correlate of visual associative long-term memory in the primate temporal cortex. *Nature* 335: 817–820.

Miyashita Y, Chang H S (1988) Neuronal correlate of pictorial short-term memory in the primate temporal cortex. *Nature* 331: 68–70.

Mody I, Lambert J D, Heinemann U (1987) Low extracellular magnesium induces epileptiform activity and spreading depression in rat hippocampal slices. *J. Neurophysiol.* 57: 869–888.

Mogul D J, Fox A P (1991) Evidence for multiple types of Ca^{2+} channels in acutely isolated hippocampal CA3 neurones of the guinea-pig. *J. Physiol.* 433: 259–281.

Monn J A, Valli M J, Johnson B G, Salhoff C R, Wright R A, Howe T, Bond A, Lodge D, Spangle L A, Paschal J W, Campbell J B, Griffey K, Tizzano J P, Schoepp D D (1996) Synthesis of the four isomers of 4–aminopyrrolidine-2,4–dicarboxylate: identification of a potent, highly selective, and systemically-active agonist for metabotropic glutamate receptors negatively coupled to adenylate cyclase. *J. Med. Chem.* 39: 2990–3000.

Montaron M F, Bouyer J J, Rougeul A, Buser P (1984) Unit activity in the ventral tegmental area and the state of focused attention in the normal awake cat. *C.R. Acad. Sci. III* 298: 229–236.

Monyer H, Jonas P (1995) Polymerase chain reaction analysis of ion channel expression in single neurons of brain slices. In: Sakmann B, Neher E (eds.), *Single-Channel Recording*, 2nd edition. Plenum, New York, pp. 357–373.

Moore S D, Madamba S G, Schweitzer P, Siggins G R (1994) Voltage-dependent effects of opioid peptides on hippocampal CA3 pyramidal neurons *in vitro*. *J. Neurosci.* 14: 809–820.

Morin F, Beaulieu C, Lacaille J-C (1996) Membrane properties and synaptic currents evoked in CA1 interneuron subtypes in rat hippocampal slices. *J. Neurophysiol.* 76: 1–16.

Moss S J, Gorrie G H, Amato A, Smart T G (1995) Modulation of $GABA_A$ receptors by tyrosine phosphorylation. *Nature* 377: 344–348.

Moss S J, Smart T G, Blackstone C D, Huganir R L (1992) Functional modulation of GABA$_A$ receptors by cAMP-dependent protein phosphorylation. *Science* 257: 661–665.

Mulle C, Marariaga A, Deschênes M (1986) Morphology and electrophysiological properties of reticularis thalami neurons in cat: in vivo study of a thalamic pacemaker. *J. Neurosci.* 6: 2134–2145.

Muller R U, Stead M, Pach J (1996) The hippocampus as a cognitive graph. *J. Gen. Physiol.* 107: 663–694.

Müller W, Misgeld U (1986) Slow cholinergic excitation of guinea pig hippocampal neurons is mediated by two muscarinic receptor subtypes. *Neurosci. Lett.* 67: 107–112.

Müller W, Misgeld U (1990) Inhibitory role of dentate hilus neurons in guinea pig hippocampal slice. *J. Neurophysiol.* 64: 141–147.

Müller W, Misgeld U (1991) Picrotoxin-and 4–aminopyridine-induced activity in hilar neurons in the guinea pig hippocampal slice. *J. Neurophysiol.* 65: 141–147.

Munk M H J, Nowak L G, Nelson J I, Bullier J (1995) Structural basis of cortical synchronization II. Effects of cortical lesions. *J. Neurophysiol.* 74: 2401–2414.

Munk M H J, Roelfsema P R, König P, Engel A K, Singer W (1996) Role of reticular activation in the modulation of intracortical synchronization. *Science* 272: 271–274.

Murakoshi T, Guo J-Z, Ichinose T (1993) Electrophysiological identification of horizontal synaptic connections in rat visual cortex in vitro. *Neurosci. Lett.* 163: 211–214.

Murthy V N, Fetz E E (1992) Coherent 25– to 35–Hz oscillations in the sensorimotor cortex of awake behaving monkeys. *Proc. Natl. Acad. Sci. USA* 89: 5670–5674.

Murthy V N, Fetz E E (1996a) Oscillatory activity in sensorimotor cortex of awake monkeys: synchronization of local field potentials and relation to behavior. *J. Neurophysiol.* 76: 3949–3967.

Murthy V N, Fetz E E (1996b) Synchronization of neurons during local field potential oscillations in sensorimotor cortex of awake monkeys. *J. Neurophysiol.* 76: 3968–3982.

Naber P A, Witter M P (1998) Subicular efferents are mostly organized as parallel projections; a double labelling retrograde tracing study in the rat. *J. Comp. Neurol.* 393: 284–297.

Nelson S, Toth L, Sheth B, Sur M (1994) Orientation selectivity of cortical neurons during intracellular blockade of inhibition. *Science* 265: 774–777.

Neuenschwander S, Singer W (1996) Long-range synchronization of oscillatory light responses in the cat retina and lateral geniculate nucleus. *Nature* 379: 728–733.

Noebels J L, Prince D A (1978) Development of focal seizures in cerebral cortex: role of axon terminal bursting. *J. Neurophysiol.* 41: 1267–1281.

Numann R, Wong R K S (1984) Voltage-clamp study on GABA response desensitization in single pyramidal cells dissociated from the hippocampus of adult guinea pigs. *Neurosci. Lett.* 47: 289–294.

Nuñez A, Amzica F, Steriade M (1992a) Voltage-dependent fast (20–40 Hz) oscillations in long-axoned neocortical neurons. *Neuroscience* 51: 7–10.

Nuñez A, Amzica F, Steriade M (1992b) Intrinsic and synaptically generated delta (1–4 Hz) rhythms in dorsal lateral geniculate neurons and their modulation by light-induced fast (30–70 Hz) events. *Neuroscience* 51: 269–284.

O'Dell T J, Alger B E (1991) Single calcium channels in rat and guinea-pig hippocampal neurons. *J. Physiol.* 436: 739–767.

Ohara P T, Sefton A J, Lieberman A R (1980) Mode of termination of afferents from the thalamic reticular nucleus in the dorsal lateral geniculate nucleus of the rat. *Brain Res.* 197: 503–506.

Ohishi, H, Nomura S, Ding Y Q, Shigemoto R, Wada E, Kinoshita A, Li J L, Neki A, Nakanishi S, Mizuno N (1995) Presynaptic localization of a metabotropic glutamate receptor, mGluR7, in the primary afferent neurons: an immunohistochemical study in the rat. *Neurosci. Lett.* 202: 85–88.

Ohishi H, Ogawa-Meguro R, Shigemoto R, Kaneko T, Nakanishi S, Mizuno N (1994) Immunohistochemical localization of metabotropic glutamate receptors, mGluR2 and mGluR3, in rat cerebellar cortex. *Neuron* 13: 55–66.

O'Keefe J (1993) Hippocampus, theta, and spatial memory. *Curr. Opin. Neurobiol.* 3: 917–924.

O'Keefe J, Recce M L (1993) Phase relationship between hippocampal place units and the EEG theta rhythm. *Hippocampus* 3: 317–330.

O'Mara S M, Rowan M, Anwyl R (1995) Metabotropic glutamate receptors can mediate long-term depression of synaptic transmission in the dentate gyrus of rat hippocampal slices independently of NMDA receptor activation. *J. Physiol.* 483: 71P–72P.

Osorio I, Daroff R B (1980) Absence of REM and altered NREM sleep in patients with spinocerebellar degeneration and slow saccades. *Ann. Neurol.* 7: 277–280.

Otis T S, Mody I (1992) Modulation of decay kinetics and frequency of GABA$_A$ receptor-mediated spontaneous inhibitory postsynaptic currents in hippocampal neurons. *Neuroscience* 49: 13–32.

Ouardouz M, Lacaille J-C (1995) Mechanisms of selective long-term potentiation of excitatory synapses in stratum oriens/alveus interneurons of rat hippocampal slices. *J. Neurophysiol.* 73: 810–819.

Ouardouz M, Lacaille J-C (1997) Properties of unitary IPSCs in hippocampal pyramidal cells originating from different types of interneurons in young rats. *J. Neurophysiol.* 77: 1939–1949.

Pantev C (1995) Evoked and induced gamma-band activity of the human cortex. *Brain Topog.* 7: 321–330.

Pantev C, Makeig S, Hoke M, Galambos R, Hampson S, Gallen C (1991) Human auditory evoked gamma-band magnetic fields. *Proc. Natl. Acad. Sci. USA* 88: 8996–9000.

Pape H-C, McCormick D A (1995) Electrophysiological and pharmacological properties of interneurons in the cat dorsal lateral geniculate nucleus. *Neuroscience* 68: 1105–1125.

Paré D, de Curtis M, Llinás R (1992) Role of the hippocampal-entorhinal loop in temporal lobe epilepsy: extra-and intracellular study in the isolated guinea pig brain *in vitro. J. Neurosci.* 12: 1867–1881.

Paré D, Steriade M, Deschênes M, Oakson G (1987) Physiological characteristics of anterior thalamic nuclei, a group devoid of inputs from reticular thalamic nucleus. *J. Neurophysiol.* 57: 1669–1685.

Pearce R A (1993) Physiological evidence for two distinct $GABA_A$ responses in rat hippocampus. *Neuron* 10: 189–200.

Pearce R A, Grunder S D, Faucher L D (1995) Different mechanisms for use-dependent depression of two $GABA_A$-mediated IPSCs in rat hippocampus. *J. Physiol.* 484: 425–435.

Pedroarena C, Llinás R (1997) Dendritic calcium conductances generate high-frequency oscillation in thalamocortical neurons. *Proc. Natl. Acad. Sci. USA* 94: 724–728.

Penttonen M, Kamondi A, Acsády L, Buzsáki G (1998) Gamma frequency oscillation in the hippocampus: intracellular analysis *in vivo. Eur. J. Neurosci.* 10: 718–728.

Perkins K L, Wong R K S (1996) Ionic basis of the postsynaptic depolarizing GABA response in hippocampal pyramidal cells. *J. Neurophysiol.* 76: 3886–3893.

Perouansky M, Kirson E D, Yaari Y (1996) Halothane blocks synaptic excitation of inhibitory interneurons. *Anesthesiology* 85: 1431–1438.

Perouansky M, Yaari Y (1993) Kinetic properties of NMDA receptor-mediated synaptic currents in rat hippocampal pyramidal cells *versus* interneurones. *J. Physiol.* 465: 223–244.

Perreault P, Avoli M (1991) Physiology and pharmacology of epileptiform activity induced by 4–aminopyridine in rat hippocampal slices. *J. Neurophysiol.* 65: 771–785.

Perreault P, Avoli M (1992) 4–Aminopyridine-induced epileptiform activity and a GABA-mediated long-lasting depolarization in the rat hippocampus. *J. Neurosci.* 12: 104–115.

Pfurtscheller G, Neuper C, Kalcher J (1993) 40–Hz oscillations during motor behavior in man. *Neurosci. Lett.* 164: 179–182.

Pinault D, Deschênes M (1992a) Voltage-dependent 40–Hz oscillations in rat reticular thalamic neurons *in vivo. Neuroscience* 51: 245–258.

Pinault D, Deschênes M (1992b) Control of 40–Hz firing of reticular thalamic cells by neurotransmitters. *Neuroscience* 51: 259–268.

Pinault D, Pumain R (1989) Antidromic firing occurs spontaneously on thalamic relay neurons: triggering of somatic intrinsic burst discharges by ectopic action potentials. *Neuroscience* 31: 625–637.

Pinsky P F, Rinzel J (1994) Intrinsic and network rhythmogenesis in a reduced Traub model for CA3 neurons. *J. Comput. Neurosci.* 1: 39–60.

Pitler T A, Alger B E (1992) Cholinergic excitation of GABAergic interneurons in the rat hippocampal slice. *J. Physiol.* 450: 127–142.

Politoff A L, Stadter R P, Monson N, Hass OP (1996) Cognition-related EEG abnormalities in nondemented Down Syndrome Subjects.

Pollin B, Rokyta R (1982) Somatotopic organization of nucleus reticularis thalami in chronic awake cats and monkeys. *Brain Res.* 250: 211–221.

Poncer J C, McKinney R A Gähwiler B H, Thompson S M (1997) Either N-or P-type calcium channels mediate GABA release at distinct hippocampal inhibitory synapses. *Neuron* 18: 463–472.

Poncer J-C, Miles R (1995) Fast and slow excitation of inhibitory cells in the CA3 region of the hippocampus. *J. Neurobiol.* 26: 386–395.

Poncer J-C, Shinozaki H, Miles R (1995) Dual modulation of synaptic inhibition by distinct metabotropic glutamate receptors in the rat hippocampus. *J. Physiol.* 485: 121–134.

Pozzo Miller L D, Petrozzino J J, Connor J A (1995) G protein-coupled receptors mediate a fast excitatory postsynaptic current in CA3 pyramidal neurons in hippocampal slices. *J. Neurosci.* 15: 8320–8330.

Preuss T M, Goldman Rakic P S (1987) Crossed corticothalamic and thalamocortical connections of macaque prefrontal cortex. *J. Comp. Neurol.* 257: 269–281.

Prezeau L, Manzoni O, Homburger V, Sladeczek F, Curry K, Bockaert J (1992) Characterization of a metabotropic glutamate receptor: direct negative coupling to adenyl cyclase and involvement of a pertussis toxin-sensitive G protein. *Proc. Natl. Acad. Sci. USA* 89: 8040–8044.

Prince D A (1968) The depolarization shift in "epileptic" neurons. *Exper. Neurol.* 21: 467–485.

Prince D A, Wilder B J (1967) Control mechanisms in cortical epileptogenic foci. *Arch. Neurol.* 16: 194–202.

Pulvermüller F, Eulitz C, Pantev C, Mohr B, Feige B, Lutzenberger W, Elbert T, Birbaumer N (1996) High-frequency cortical responses reflect lexical processing: an MEG study. *Electroenceph. Clin. Neurophysiol.* 98: 76–85.

Racca C, Catania M V, Monyer H, Sakmann B (1996) Expression of AMPA-glutamate receptor B subunit in rat hippocampal GABAergic neurons. *Eur. J. Neurosci.* 8: 1580–1590.

Rall W (1962) Theory of physiological properties of dendrites. *Ann. N.Y. Acad. Sci.* 96: 1071–1092.

Rall W (1989) Cable theory for dendritic neurons. In: Koch C, Segev I (eds.) *Methods in Neuronal Modeling.* MIT Press, Cambridge, MA, pp. 9–62.

Rall W, Rinzel J (1973) Branch input resistance and steady attenuation for input to one branch of a dendritic neuron model. *Biophys. J.* 13: 648–688.

Rall W, Shepherd G M (1968) Theoretical reconstruction of field potentials and dendrodendritic synaptic interactions in olfactory bulb. *J. Neurophysiol.* 31: 884–915.

Reece L J, Schwartzkroin P A (1991) Effects of cholinergic agonists on two non-pyramidal cell types in rat hippocampal slices. *Brain Res.* 566: 115–126.

Reid R C, Alonso J (1995) Specificity of monosynaptic connections from thalamus to visual cortex. *Nature* 378: 281–284.

Reitz J R, Milford F J (1960) *Foundations of Electromagnetic Theory.* Addison-Wesley, Reading, MA.

Reuveni I, Friedman A, Amitai Y, Gutnick M J (1993) Stepwise repolarization from Ca^{2+} plateaus in neocortical pyramidal cells: evidence for nonhomogeneous distribution of HVA Ca^{2+} channels in dendrites. *J. Neurosci.* 13: 4609–4621.

Rho J M, Donevan S D, Rogawski M A (1996) Direct activation of $GABA_A$ receptors by barbiturates in cultured rat hippocampal neurons. *J. Physiol.* 497: 509–522.

Rhodes P A, Gray C M (1994) Simulations of intrinsically bursting neocortical pyramidal neurons. *Neural Comput.* 6: 1086–1110.

Ribary U, Ioannides A A, Singh K D, Hasson R, Bolton J P, Lado F, Mogilner A, Llinás R (1991) Magnetic field tomography of coherent thalamocortical 40 Hz oscillations in humans. *Proc. Natl. Acad. Sci. USA* 88: 11,037–11,041.

Rinzel J, Rall W (1974) Transient response in a dendritic neuron model for current injected at one branch. *Biophys. J.* 14: 759–790.

Robertson R T, Kaitz S S (1981) Thalamic connections with limbic cortex. I. Thalamocortical projections. *J. Compar. Neurol.* 195: 501–525.

Roelfsema P R, Engel A K, König P, Singer W (1997) Visuomotor integration is associated with zero time-lag synchronization among cortical areas. *Nature* 385: 157–161.

Roelfsema P R, König P, Engel A K, Sireteanu R, Singer W (1994) Reduced synchronization in the visual cortex of cats with strabismic amblyopia. *Eur. J. Neurosci.* 6: 1645–1655.

Rosene D L, Van Hoesen G W (1977) Hippocampal efferents reach widespread areas of cerebral cortex and amygdala in the rhesus monkey. *Science* 198: 315–317.

Rutecki P A, Lebeda F J, Johnston D (1985) Epileptiform activity induced by changes in extracellular potassium in hippocampus. *J Neurophysiol.* 54: 1363–1374.

Rutecki P A, Lebeda F J, Johnston D (1987) 4-Aminopyridine produces epileptiform activity in hippocampus and enhances synaptic excitation and inhibition. *J. Neurophysiol.* 57: 1911–1924.

Sah P, Bekkers J M (1996) Apical dendritic location of slow afterhyperpolarization current in hippocampal pyramidal neurons: implications for the integration of long-term potentiation. *J. Neurosci.* 16: 4537–4542.

Sah P, Gibb A J, Gage P W (1988a) The sodium current underlying action potentials in guinea pig hippocampal CA1 neurons. *J. Gen. Physiol.* 91: 373–398.

Sah P, Gibb A J, Gage P W (1988b) Potassium current activated by depolarization of dissociated neurons from adult guinea pig hippocampus. *J. Gen. Physiol.* 92: 263–278.

Sah P, Hestrin S, Nicoll R A (1990) Properties of excitatory postsynaptic current recorded *in vitro* from rat hippocampal interneurones. *J. Physiol.* 430: 605–616.

Sakai K, Miyashita Y (1991) Neural organization for the long-term memory of paired associates. *Nature* 354: 152–155.

Sakatani K, Chesler M, Hassan A Z (1991) GABA$_A$ receptors modulate axonal conduction in dorsal columns of neonatal rat spinal cord. *Brain Res.* 542: 273–279.

Salin P A, Prince D A (1996) Electrophysiological mapping of GABA$_A$ receptor-mediated inhibition in adult rat somatosensory cortex. *J. Neurophysiol.* 75: 1589–1600.

Samulack D D, Lacaille J-C (1993) Hyperpolarizing synaptic potentials evoked in CA1 pyramidal cells by glutamate stimulation of interneurons from oriens/alveus border of rat hippocampal slices. II. Sensitivity to GABA antagonists. *Hippocampus* 3: 345–358.

Samulack D D, Williams S, Lacaille J-C (1993) Hyperpolarizing synaptic potentials evoked in CA1 pyramidal cells by glutamate stimulation of interneurons from oriens/alveus border of rat hippocampal slices. I. Electrophysiological response properties. *Hippocampus* 3: 331–344.

Sanchez-Vives M, Bal T, Kim U, von Krosigk M, McCormick D A (1996) Are the interlaminar zones of the ferret dorsal lateral geniculate nucleus actually part of the perigeniculate nucleus? *J. Neurosci.* 16: 5923–5941.

Sanchez-Vives M, Bal T, McCormick D A (1997) Inhibitory interactions between perigeniculate GABAergic neurons. *J. Neurosci.* 22: 8894–8908.

Sanchez-Vives M, McCormick D A (1997) Functional properties of perigeniculate inhibition of dorsal lateral geniculate nucleus thalamocortical neurons *in vitro*. *J. Neurosci.* 22: 8880–8893.

Sawyer S F, Young S J, Groves P M, Tepper J M (1994) Cerebellar-responsive neurons in the thalamic ventroanterior-ventrolateral complex of rats: in vivo electrophysiology. *Neuroscience* 63: 711–724.

Sayer R J, Friedlander M J, Redman S J (1990) The time course and amplitude of EPSPs evoked at synapses between pairs of CA3/CA1 neurons in the hippocampal slice. *J. Neurosci.* 10: 826–836.

Sayer R J, Schwindt P C, Crill W E (1992) Metabotropic glutamate receptor-mediated suppression of L-type calcium current in acutely isolated neocortical neurons. *J. Neurophysiol.* 68: 833–842.

Scanziani M, Capogna M, Gähwiler B H, Thompson S M (1992) Presynaptic inhibition of miniature excitatory synaptic currents by baclofen and adenosine in the hippocampus. *Neuron* 9: 919–927.

Scanziani M, Gähwiler B H, Thompson S M (1995) Presynaptic inhibition of excitatory synaptic transmission by muscarinic and metabotropic glutamate receptor activation in the hippocampus: are Ca^{2+} channels involved? *Neuropharmacology* 34: 1549–1557.

Scanziani M, Salin P A, Vogt K E, Malenka R C, Nicoll R A (1997) Use-dependent increases in glutamate concentration activate presynaptic metabotropic glutamate receptors. *Nature* 385: 630–634.

Scheibel M E, Scheibel A B (1966) The organization of the ventral anterior nucleus of the thalamus. A Golgi study. *Brain Res.* 1: 250–268.

Schillen T B, König P (1991) Stimulus-dependent assembly formation of oscillatory responses: II. Desynchronization. *Neural Comput.* 3: 167–178.

Schneiderman J H (1986) Low concentrations of penicillin reveal rhythmic, synchronous synaptic potentials in hippocampal slice. *Brain Res.* 398: 231–241.

Schwartzkroin P A (1978) Secondary range rhythmic spiking in hippocampal neurons. *Brain Res.* 149: 247–250.

Schwartzkroin P A, Haglund M M (1986) Spontaneous rhythmic synchronous activity in epileptic human and normal monkey temporal lobe. *Epilepsia* 27: 523–533.

Schwartzkroin P A, Slawsky M (1977) Probable calcium spikes in hippocampal neurons. *Brain Res.* 135: 157–161.

Sciancalepore M, Stratta F, Fisher N D, Cherubini E (1995) Activation of metabotropic glutamate receptors increase the frequency of spontaneous GABAergic currents through protein kinase A in neonatal rat hippocampal neurons. *J. Neurophysiol.* 74: 1118–1122.

Scoville W B, Milner B (1957) Loss of recent memory after bilateral hippocampal lesions. *J. Neurol. Neurosurg. Psychiat.* 20: 11–21.

Segal M, Barker J L (1984) Rat hippocampal neurons in culture: voltage-clamp analysis of inhibitory synaptic connections. *J. Neurophysiol.* 52: 469–487.

Sharon D, Vorobiov D, Dascal N (1997) Positive and negative coupling of the metabotropic glutamate receptors to a G protein-activated K$^+$ channel, GIKR, in *Xenopus* oocytes. *J. Gen. Physiol.* 109: 447–490.

Sheer D E (1989) Focused arousal and the cognitive 40 Hz event-related potentials: differential diagnosis of Alzheimer's disease. *Prog. Clin. Biol. Res.* 317: 79–94.

Sheridan R D, Sutor B (1990) Presynaptic M1 muscarinic cholinoceptors mediate inhibition of excitatory synaptic transmission in the hippocampus in vitro. *Neurosci. Lett.* 108: 273–278.

Shigemoto R, Kulik A, Roberts J D B, Ohishi H, Nusser Z, Kaneko T, Somogyi P (1996) Target-cell-specific concentration of a metabotropic glutamate receptor in the presynaptic active zone. *Nature* 381: 523–525.

Shirasaki T, Harata N, Akaike N (1994) Metabotropic glutamate response in acutely dissociated hippocampal CA1 pyramidal neurones of the rat. *J. Physiol.* 475: 439–453.

Siggins G R, Zieglgänsberger W (1981) Morphine and opioid peptides reduce inhibitory synaptic potentials in hippocampal pyramidal cells in vitro without alteration of membrane potential. *Proc. Natl. Acad. Sci. USA* 78: 5235–5239.

Sigvardt K A, Grillner S, Wallén P, Van Dongen P A M (1985) Activation of NMDA receptors elicits fictive locomotion and bistable membrane properties in the lamprey spinal cord. *Brain Res.* 336: 390–395.

Sik A, Penttonen M, Ylinen A, Buzsáki G (1995) Hippocampal CA1 interneurons: an *in vivo* intracellular labeling study. *J. Neurosci.* 15: 6651–6665.

Sik A, Tamamaki N, Freund T F (1993) Complete axon arborization of a single CA3 pyramidal cell in the rat hippocampus, and its relationship with postsynaptic parvalbumin-containing interneurons. *Eur. J. Neurosci.* 5: 1719–1728.

Sillito A M, Jones H E, Gerstein G L, West D C (1994) Feature-linked synchronization of thalamic relay cell firing induced by feedback from the visual cortex. *Nature* 369: 479–482.

Singer W, Gray C M (1995) Visual feature integration and the temporal correlation hypothesis. *Annual Rev. Neurosci.* 18: 555–586.

Sloviter R S. (1991) Permanently altered hippocampal structure, excitability, and inhibition after experimental status epilepticus in the rat: the "dormant basket cell" hypothesis and its possible relevance to temporal lobe epilepsy. *Hippocampus* 1: 41–66.

Smith J C, Ellenberger H H, Ballanyi K, Richter D W, Feldman J L (1991) Pre-Bötzinger complex: a brainstem region that may generate respiratory rhythm in mammals. *Science* 254: 726–729.

Snow R W, Dudek F E (1984) Electrical fields directly contribute to action potential synchronization during convulsant-induced epileptiform bursts. *Brain Res.* 323: 114–118.

Soltesz I, Deschênes M (1993) Low-and high-frequency membrane potential oscillations during theta activity in CA1 and CA3 pyramidal neurons of the rat hippocampus under ketamine-xylazine anesthesia. *J. Neurophysiol.* 70: 97–116.

Soltesz I, Mody I (1995) Ca^{2+}-dependent plasticity of miniature inhibitory postsynaptic currents after amputation of dendrites in central neurons. *J. Neurophysiol.* 73: 1763–1773.

Somogyi P, Nunzi M G, Gorio A, Smith A D (1983) A new type of specific interneuron in the monkey hippocampus forming synapses exclusively with the axon initial segments of pyramidal cells. *Brain Res.* 259: 137–142.

Spain W J, Schwindt P C, Crill W E (1991) Two transient potassium currents in layer V pyramidal neurones from cat sensorimotor cortex. *J. Physiol.* 434: 591–607.

Spencer W A, Kandel E R (1961) Electrophysiology of hippocampal neurons IV. Fast prepotentials. *J. Neurophysiol.* 24: 272–285.

Spruston N, Jonas P, Sakmann B (1995) Dendritic glutamate receptor channels in rat hippocampal CA3 and CA1 pyramidal neurons. *J. Physiol.* 482: 325–352.

Spruston N, Schiller Y, Stuart G, Sakmann B (1995) Activity-dependent action potential invasion and calcium influx into hippocampal CA1 dendrites. *Science* 268: 297–300.

Staley K J, Soldo B L, Proctor W R (1995) Ionic mechanisms of neuronal excitation by inhibitory $GABA_A$ receptors. *Science* 269: 977–981.

Stanford I M, Traub R D, Jefferys J G R (1998.) Limbic gamma rhythms. II. Synaptic and intrinsic mechanisms underlying spike doublets in oscillating subicular neurons. *J. Neurophysiol.* 80: 162–171.

Stasheff S F, Anderson W W, Clark S, Wilson W A (1989) NMDA antagonists differentiate epileptogenesis from seizure expression in an in vitro model. *Science* 245: 648–651.

Stasheff S F, Hines M, Wilson W A (1993) Axon terminal hyperexcitability associated with epileptogenesis in vitro. I. Origin of ectopic spikes. *J. Neurophysiol.* 70: 960–975.

Stasheff S F, Mott D D, Wilson W A (1993) Axon terminal hyperexcitability associated with epileptogenesis in vitro. II. Pharmacological regulation by NMDA and $GABA_A$ receptors. *J. Neurophysiol.* 70: 976–984.

Stelzer A (1992) $GABA_A$ receptors control the excitability of neuronal populations. *Intern. Rev. Neurobiol.* 33: 195–287.

Stelzer A, Kay A R, Wong R K S (1988) $GABA_A$-receptor function in hippocampal cells is maintained by phosphorylation factors. *Science* 241: 339–341.

Steriade M, Amzica F (1996) Intracortical and corticothalamic coherency of fast spontaneous oscillations. *Proc. Natl. Acad. Sci. USA* 93: 2533–2538.

Steriade M, Amzica F, Contreras D (1995) Synchronization of fast (30–40 Hz) spontaneous cortical rhythms during brain activation. *J. Neurosci.* 16: 392–417.

Steriade M, Contreras D, Amzica F, Timofeev I (1996) Synchronization of fast (30–40 Hz) spontaneous oscillations in intrathalamic and thalamocortical networks. *J. Neurosci.* 16: 2788–2808.

Steriade M, Curró Dossi R, Contreras D (1993) Electrophysiological properties of intralaminar thalamocortical cells discharging rhythmic (~40 Hz) spike-bursts at ~1000 Hz during waking and rapid eye movement sleep. *Neuroscience* 56: 1–9.

Steriade M, Curró Dossi R, Paré D, Oakson G (1991) Fast oscillations (20–40 Hz) in thalamocortical systems and their potentiation by mesopontine cholinergic nuclei in the cat. *Proc. Natl. Acad. Sci. USA* 88: 4396–4400.

Steriade M, Deschênes M (1984) The thalamus as a neuronal oscillator. *Brain Res.* 320: 1–63.

Steriade M, Domich L, Oakson G, Deschênes M (1987) The deafferented reticular thalamic nucleus generates spindle rhythmicity. *J. Neurophysiol.* 57: 260–273.

Steriade M, McCormick D A, Sejnowski T J (1993) Thalamocortical oscillations in the sleeping and aroused brain. *Science* 262: 679–685.

Steriade M, Nuñez A, Amzica F (1993) A novel slow (< 1 Hz) oscillation of neocortical neurons *in vivo*: depolarizing and hyerpolarizing components. *J. Neurosci.* 13: 3252–3265.

Steriade M, Timofeev I, Dürmüller N, Grenier F (1998) Dynamic properties of corticothalamic neurons and local cortical interneurons generating fast rhythmic (30–40 Hz) spike bursts. *J. Neurophysiol.* 79: 483–490.

Stewart M, Wong R K S (1993) Intrinsic properties and evoked responses of guinea pig subicular neurons in vitro. *J. Neurophysiol.* 70: 232–245.

Stopfer M, Bhagavan, S, Smith B H, Laurent G (1997) Impaired odour discrimination on desynchronization of odour-encoding neural assemblies. *Nature* 390: 70–74.

Storm, J. (1987) Action potential repolarization and a fast after-hyperpolarization in rat hippocampal pyramidal cells. *J. Physiol.* 385: 733–759.

Storm J (1988) Temporal integration by a slowly inactivating K^+ current in hippocampal neurons. *Nature* 336: 379–381.

Strata F, Atzori M, Molnar M, Ugolini G, Tempia F, Cherubini E (1997) A pacemaker current in dye-coupled hilar interneurons contributes to the generation of giant GABAergic potentials in developing hippocampus. *J. Neurosci.* 17: 1435–1446.

Strata F, Sciancalepore M, Cherubini E (1995) Cyclic AMP-dependent modulation of giant depolarizing potentials by metabotropic glutamate receptors in the rat hippocampus. *J. Physiol.* 489: 115–125.

Stuart G J, Sakmann B (1994) Active propagation of somatic action potentials into neocortical pyramidal cell dendrites. *Nature* 367: 69–72.

Suzuki S S, Smith G K (1988) Spontaneous EEG spikes in the normal hippocampus. II. Relations to synchronous burst discharges. *Electroenceph. Clin. Neurophysiol.* 69: 532–540.

Swann J W, Smith K L, Brady R J (1993) Localized excitatory synaptic interactions mediate the sustained depolarization of electrographic seizures in developing hippocampus. *J. Neurosci.* 13: 4680–4689.

Swartz K J, Bean B P (1992) Inhibition of calcium channels in rat CA3 pyramidal neurons by a metabotropic glutamate receptor. *J. Neurosci.* 12: 4358–4371.

Takahashi T, Forsyte I D, Tsujimoto T, Barnes-Davies M, Onodera K (1996) Presynaptic calcium current modulation by a metabotropic glutamate receptor. *Science* 274: 594–597.

Tallon-Baudry C, Bertrand O, Delpuech C, Pernier J (1997) Oscillatory γ-band (30–70 Hz) activity induced by a visual search task in humans. *J. Neurosci.* 17: 722–734.

Tamamaki N, Nojyo Y (1990) Disposition of the slab-like modules formed by axon branches originating from single CA1 pyramidal neurons in the rat hippocampus. *J. Comp. Neurol.* 291: 509–519.

Tamamaki N, Nojyo Y (1995) Preservation of topography in the connections between the subiculum, field CA1, and the entorhinal cortex in rats. *J. Compar. Neurol.* 353: 379–390.

Tamamaki N, Watanabe K, Nojyo Y (1984) A whole image of the hippocampal pyramidal neuron revealed by intracellular pressure-injection of horseradish peroxidase. *Brain Res.* 307: 336–340.

Tamás G, Buhl E H, Somogyi P (1997) Massive autaptic self-innervation of GABAergic neurons in cat visual cortex. *J. Neurosci.* 17: 6352–6364.

Tancredi V, Hwa G G C, Zona C, Brancati A, Avoli M (1990) Low magnesium epileptogenesis in the rat hippocampal slice: electrophysiological and pharmacological features. *Brain Res.* 511: 280–290.

Taube J S (1993) Electrophysiological properties of neurons in the rat subiculum in vitro. *Exp. Brain Res.* 96: 304–318.

Taube J S, Muller R U, Ranck J B Jr (1990a) Head-direction cells recorded from the postsubiculum in freely moving rats. I. Description and quantitative analysis. *J. Neurosci.* 10: 420–435.

Taube J S, Muller R U, Ranck J B Jr (1990b) Head-direction cells recorded from the postsubiculum in freely moving rats. II. Effects of environmental manipulations. *J. Neurosci.* 10: 436–447.

Taylor C P, Dudek F E (1984) Synchronization without active chemical synapses during hippocampal afterdischarges. *J. Neurophysiol.* 52: 143–155.

Taylor G W, Merlin L R, Wong R K S (1995) Synchronized oscillations in hippocampal CA3 neurons induced by metabotropic glutamate receptor activation. *J. Neurosci.* 15: 8039–8052.

Thompson S M, Gähwiler B H (1989) Activity-dependent disinhibition. I. Repetitive stimulation reduces both IPSP driving force and conductance in the hippocampus in vitro. *J. Neurophysiol.* 61: 501–511.

Thompson S M, Wong R K S (1991) Development of calcium current subtypes in isolated rat hippocampal pyramidal cells. *J. Physiol.* 439: 671–689.

Thomson A M, Deuchars J, West D C (1993) Single axon excitatory postsynaptic potentials in neocortical interneurons exhibit pronounced paired pulse facilitation. *Neuroscience* 54: 347–360.

Thomson A M, West D C, Deuchars J (1995) Properties of single axon excitatory postsynaptic potentials elicited in spiny interneurons by action potentials in pyramidal neurons in slices of rat neocortex. *Neuroscience* 69: 727–738.

Thurbon D, Field A, Redman S (1994) Electrotonic profiles of interneurons in stratum pyramidale of the CA1 region of rat hippocampus. *J. Neurophysiol.* 71: 1948–1958.

Timofeev I, Steriade M (1997) Fast (mainly 30–100 Hz) oscillations in the cat cerebellothalamic pathway and their synchronization with cortical potentials. *J. Physiol.* 504: 153–168.

Tóth K, Freund T F, Miles R (1997) Disinhibition of rat hippocampal cells by GABAergic afferents from the septum. *J. Physiol.* 500: 463–474.

Tóth K, McBain C J (1998) Afferent-specific innervation of two distinct AMPA receptor subtypes on single hippocampol interneurons. *Nature Neurosci.* 1: 572–578.

Traub R (1977) Motorneurons of different geometry and the size principle. *Biol. Cybernetics* 25: 163–176.

Traub R D (1995) Model of synchronized population bursts in electrically coupled interneurons containing active dendritic conductances. *J. Comput. Neurosci.* 2: 283–289.

Traub R D, Borck C, Colling S B, Jefferys J G R (1996) On the structure of ictal events in vitro. *Epilepsia* 37: 879–891.

Traub R D, Colling S B, Jefferys J G R J (1995) Cellular mechanisms of 4-aminopyridine-induced synchronized after-discharges in the rat hippocampal slice. *J. Physiol.* 489: 127–140.

Traub R D, Dingledine R (1990) Model of synchronized epileptiform bursts induced by high potassium in CA3 region of rat hippocampal slice. Role of spontaneous EPSPs in initiation. *J. Neurophysiol.* 64: 1009–1018.

Traub R D, Dudek F E, Snow R W, Knowles W D (1985) Computer simulations indicate that electrical field effects contribute to the shape of the epileptiform field potential. *Neuroscience* 15: 947–958.

Traub R D, Jefferys J G R, (1997) Epilepsy in vitro: electrophysiology and computer modeling. In: Engel J Jr, Pedley T A (eds.) *Epilepsy: a Comprehensive Textbook*. Lippincott-Raven, Philadelphia, pp. 405–418.

Traub R D, Jefferys J G R. Miles R (1993) Analysis of the propagation of disinhibition-induced after-discharges along the guinea-pig hippocampal slice *in vitro*. *J. Physiol*. 472: 267–287.

Traub R D, Jefferys J G R, Miles R, Whittington MA, Tóth, K. (1994) A branching dendritic model of a rodent CA3 pyramidal neurone. *J. Physiol*. 481: 79–95.

Traub R D, Jefferys J G R, Whittington M A (1994) Enhanced NMDA conductances can account for epileptiform activities induced by low Mg^{2+} in the rat hippocampal slice. *J. Physiol*. 478: 379–393.

Traub R D, Jefferys J G R, Whittington M A (1997) Simulation of gamma rhythms in networks of interneurons and pyramidal cells. *J. Comput. Neurosci*. 4: 141–150.

Traub R D, Knowles W D, Miles R, Wong R K S (1984) Synchronized afterdischarges in the hippocampus: simulation studies of the cellular mechanism. *Neuroscience* 12: 1191–1200.

Traub R D, Llinás R (1977) The spatial distribution of ionic conductances in normal and axotomized motorneurons. *Neuroscience* 2: 829–849.

Traub R D, Miles R (1991) *Neuronal Networks of the Hippocampus*. Cambridge University Press, New York.

Traub R D, Miles R (1995) Pyramidal cell-to-inhibitory cell spike transduction explicable by active dendritic conductances in inhibitory cell. *J. Comput. Neurosci*. 2: 291–298.

Traub R D, Miles R, Wong R K S (1987a) Models of synchronized hippocampal bursts in the presence of inhibition. 1. Single population events. *J. Neurophysiol*. 58: 739–751.

Traub R D, Miles R, Wong R K S (1989) Model of the origin of rhythmic population oscillations in the hippocampal slice. *Science* 243: 1319–1325.

Traub R D, Miles R, Wong R K S, Schulman L S, Schneiderman J H (1987b) Models of synchronized hippocampal bursts in the presence of inhibition. 2. Ongoing spontaneous population events. *J. Neurophysiol*. 58: 752–764.

Traub R D, Miles R, Buzsáki G (1992) Computer simulation of carbachol-driven rhythmic population oscillations in the CA3 region of the in vitro rat hippocampus. *J. Physiol*. 451: 653–672.

Traub R D, Miles R, Jefferys J G R (1993) Synaptic and intrinsic conductances shape picrotoxin-induced synchronized after-discharges in the guinea-pig hippocampal slice. *J. Physiol*. 461: 525–547.

Traub R D, Spruston N, Soltesz I, Konnerth A, Whittington MA, Jefferys J G R (1998) Gamma-frequency oscillations: a neuronal population phenomenon regulated by synaptic and intrinsic cellular processes. *Prog. Neurobiol.* 55: 1–13.

Traub R D, Whittington M A, Buhl E H, Jefferys J G R, Faulkner H J (1999) On the mechanism of the γ-β frequency shift in neuronal oscillations induced in rat hippocampal slices by tetanic stimulation. *J. Neurosci* 19: 1088–1105.

Traub R D, Whittington M A, Colling S B, Buzsáki G, Jefferys J G R (1996) Analysis of gamma rhythms in the rat hippocampus *in vitro* and *in vivo*. *J. Physiol.* 493: 471–484.

Traub R D, Whittington M A, Jefferys J G R (1997) Gamma oscillation model predicts intensity coding by phase rather than frequency. *Neural Computation* 9: 1251–1264.

Traub R D, Whittington M A, Stanford I M, Jefferys J G R (1996) A mechanism for generation of long-range synchronous fast oscillations in the cortex. *Nature* 383: 621–624.

Traub R D, Wong R K S (1982) Cellular mechanism of neuronal synchronization in epilepsy. *Science* 216: 745–747.

Traub R D, Wong R K S, Jefferys J G R Whittington M A, Michelson H (1997) Generation of temporal correlations in firing of pyramidal cells by networks of inhibitory neurons. In: Baudry M, Davis J (eds.) *Long-Term Potentiation.* Vol. 3 MIT Press, Cambridge, MA, pp. 183–197.

Traub R D, Wong R K S, Miles R, Michelson H (1991) A model of a CA3 hippocampal pyramidal neuron incorporating voltage-clamp data on intrinsic conductances. *J. Neurophysiol.* 66: 635–650.

Traynelis S F, Dingledine R (1988) Potassium-induced spontaneous electrographic seizures in the rat hippocampal slice. *J. Neurophysiol.* 59: 259–276.

Tsubokawa H, Ross W N (1996) IPSPs modulate spike backpropagation and associated Ca^{2+}_i changes in the dendrites of hippocampal CA1 pyramidal neurons. *J. Neurophysiol.* 76: 2896–2906.

Turner R W, Maler L, Deerinck T, Levinson S R, Ellisman M H (1994) TTX-sensitive dendritic sodium channels underlie oscillatory discharge in a vertebrate sensory neuron. *J. Neurosci.* 14: 6453–6471.

Valentino R J, Dingledine R (1981) Presynaptic inhibitory effect of acetylcholine in the hippocampus. *J. Neurosci.* 1: 784–792.

Van der Zee E A, Luiten P G M (1993) GABAergic neurons of the rat dorsal hippocampus express muscarinic acetylcholine receptors. *Brain Res. Bull.* 32: 601–609.

van Vreeswijk C, Abbott L F, Ermentrout G B (1994) When inhibition not excitation synchronizes neural firing. *J. Comput. Neurosci.* 1: 313–321.

Vaney D I (1993) The coupling pattern of axon-bearing horizontal cells in the mammalian retina. *Proc. Royal Soc. Lond. B* 252: 93–101.

Viana di Prisco G, Freeman W J (1985) Odor-related bulbar EEG spatial pattern analysis during appetitive conditioning in rabbits. *Behav. Neurosci.* 99: 964–978.

Vignes M, Collingridge G L (1997) The synaptic activation of kainate receptors. *Nature* 388: 179–182.

Vyklicky L Jr, Benveniste M, Mayer M L (1990) Modulation of N-methyl-D-aspartic acid receptor desensitization by glycine in mouse cultured hippocampal neurones. *J. Physiol.* 428: 313–331.

Wang X-J (1993) Ionic basis for intrinsic 40 Hz neuronal oscillations. *NeuroReport* 5: 221–224.

Wang X-J (1998) Fast burst firing and short-term synaptic plasticity: a model of neocortical chattering neurons. *Neuroscience*

Wang X-J, Buzsáki G (1996) Gamma oscillation by synaptic inhibition in a hippocampal interneuronal network model. *J. Neurosci.* 16: 6402–6413.

Wang X-J, Rinzel J (1993) Spindle rhythmicity in the reticularis thalami nucleus: synchronization among mutually inhibitory neurons. *Neuroscience* 53: 899–904.

Wang X-J, Rinzel J, Rogawski M A (1991) A model of the T-type calcium current and the low-threshold spike in thalamic neurons. *J. Neurophysiol.* 66: 839–850.

Warman E N, Durand D M, Yuen G L F (1994) Reconstruction of hippocampal CA1 pyramidal cell electrophysiology by computer simulation. *J. Neurophysiol.* 71: 2033–2045.

Warren R A, Agmon A, Jones E G (1994) Oscillatory synaptic interactions between ventroposterior and reticular neurons in mouse thalamus in vitro. *J. Neurophysiol.* 72: 1993–2003.

Wehr M, Laurent G (1996) Odour encoding by temporal sequences of firing in oscillating neural assemblies. *Nature* 384: 162–166.

Westenbroek R E, Ahlijanian M K, Catterall W A (1990) Clustering of L-type Ca^{2+} channels at the base of major dendrites in hippocampal pyramidal neurons. *Nature* 347: 281–284.

Westenbroek R E, Merrick D K, Catterall W A (1989) Differential subcellular localization of the R_I and R_{II} Na^+ channel subtypes in central neurons. *Neuron* 3: 695–704.

White E L, Hersch S M (1982) A quantitative study of thalamocortical and other synapses involving the apical dendrites of corticothalamic projection cells in mouse SmI cortex. *J. Neurocytol.* 11: 137–157.

White J A, Chow C C, Ritt J, Soto-Treviño C, Kopell N (1998) Synchronization and oscillatory dynamics in heterogeneous, mutually inhibited neurons. *J. Comput. Neurosci.* 5: 5–16.

Whittington M A, Jefferys J G R (1995) Epileptic activity outlasts disinhibition after intrahippocampal tetanus toxin in the rat. *J. Physiol.* 481: 593–604.

Whittington M A, Jefferys J G R, Traub R D, (1996) Effects of intravenous anaesthetic agents on fast inhibitory oscillations in the rat hippocampus *in vitro*. *Br. J. Pharmacol.* 118: 1977–1986. Published erratum in *Br. J. Pharmacol.* (1996) 119: 1291.

Whittington M A, Stanford I M, Colling S B, Jefferys J G R, Traub R D, (1997) Spatiotemporal patterns of gamma-frequency oscillations tetanically induced in the rat hippocampal slice. *J. Physiol.* 502: 591–607.

Whittington M A, Traub R D, Faulkner H J, Jefferys J G R, Chettiar K (1998) Morphine disrupts long-range synchrony of gamma oscillations in hippocampal slices. *Proc. Natl. Acad. Sci. USA* 94: 5807–5811.

Whittington M A, Traub R D, Faulkner H J, Stanford I M Jefferys J G R (1997) Recurrent excitatory postsynaptic potentials induced by synchronized fast cortical oscillations. *Proc. Natl. Acad. Sci. USA* 94: 12198–12203.

Whittington M A, Traub R D, Jefferys J G R (1995a) Erosion of inhibition contributes to the progression of low magnesium bursts in rat hippocampal slices. *J. Physiol.* 486: 723–734.

Whittington M A, Traub R D, Jefferys J G R (1995b) Synchronized oscillations in interneuron networks driven by metabotropic glutamate receptor activation. *Nature* 373: 612–615.

Williams J H, Kauer J A (1997) Properties of carbachol-induced oscillatory activity in rat hippocampus. *J. Neurphysiol.* 78: 2631–2640.

Williams S R, Turner J P, Anderson C M, Crunelli V (1996) Electrophysiological and morphological properties of interneurones in the rat dorsal lateral geniculate nucleus *in vitro*. *J. Physiol.* 490: 129–147.

Wilson M, Bower, J M (1992) Cortical oscillations and temporal interactions in a computer simulation of piriform cortex. *J. Neurophysiol.* 67: 981–995.

Wong R K S, Prince D A (1978) Participation of calcium spikes during intrinsic burst firing in hippocampal neurons. *Brain Res.* 159: 385–390.

Wong R K S, Prince D A (1981) Afterpotential generation in hippocampal pyramidal cells. *J. Neurophysiol.* 45: 86–97.

Wong R K S, Prince D A, Basbaum A I (1979) Intradendritic recordings from hippocampal neurons. *Proc. Nat. Acad. Sci. USA* 76: 986–990.

Wong R K S, Traub R D, (1983) Synchronized burst discharge in disinhibited hippocampal slice. I. Initiation in CA2-CA3 region. *J. Neurophysiol.* 49: 442–458.

Wong R K S, Stewart M (1992) Different firing patterns generated in dendrites and somata of CA1 pyramidal neurones in guinea-pig hippocampus. *J. Physiol.* 457: 675–687.

Wong R K S, Watkins D J (1982) Cellular factors influencing GABA response in hippocampal pyramidal cells. *J. Neurophysiol.* 48: 938–951.

Wyler A R, Ojemann G A, Ward A A Jr (1982) Neurons in human epileptic cortex: correlation between unit and EEG activity. *Ann. Neurol.* 11: 301–308.

Ylinen A, Bragin A, Nádasdy Z, Jandó G, Szabó I, Sik A, Buzsáki G (1995a) Sharp wave-associated high frequency oscillation (200 Hz) in the intact hippocampus: network and intracellular mechanisms. *J. Neurosci.* 15: 30–46.

Ylinen A, Soltész I, Bragin A, Penttonen M, Sik A, Buzsáki G (1995b) Intracellular correlates of hippocampal theta rhythm in identified pyramidal cells, granule cells and basket cells. *Hippocampus* 5: 78–90.

Young M P, Tanaka K, Yamane S (1992) On oscillating neuronal responses in the visual cortex of the monkey. *J. Neurophysiol.* 67: 1464–1474.

Zola-Morgan S, Squire L R, Amaral D G (1989) Lesions of the hippocampal formation but not lesions of the fornix or the mammillary nuclei produce long-lasting memory impairment in monkeys. *J. Neurosci.* 9: 898–913.

Index